Arthritis Sourcebook

Basic Information about Specific Forms of Arthritis and Related Rheumatic Disorders, Including Rheumatoid Arthritis, Osteoarthritis, Gout, Polymyalgia Rheumatica, Psoriatic Arthritis, Spondyloarthropathies, Juvenile Rheumatoid Arthritis, and Juvenile Ankylosing Spondylitis; Along with Information about Medical, Surgical, and Alternative Treatment Options and Including Strategies for Coping with Pain, Fatigue, and Stress

Edited by Allan R. Cook. 600 pages. 1998. 0-7808-0201-2. $78.

Back & Neck Disorders Sourcebook

Basic Information about Disorders and Injuries of the Spinal Cord and Vertebrae, Including Facts on Chiropractic Treatment, Surgical Interventions, Paralysis, and Rehabilitation, Along with Advice for Preventing Back Trouble

Edited by Karen Bellenir. 548 pages. 1997. 0-7808-0202-0. $78.

"The strength of this work is its basic, easy-to-read format. Recommended."
— *Reference and User Services Quarterly, Winter '97*

Blood & Circulatory Disorders Sourcebook

Basic Information about Blood and Its Components, Anemias, Leukemias, Bleeding Disorders, and Circulatory Disorders, Including Aplastic Anemia, Thalassemia, Sickle-Cell Disease, Hemochromatosis, Hemophilia, Von Willebrand Disease, and Vascular Diseases; Along with a Special Section on Blood Transfusions and Blood Supply Safety, a Glossary, and Source Listings for Further Help and Information

Edited by Karen Bellenir and Linda M. Shin. 575 pages. 1998. 0-7808-0203-9. $78.

Burns Sourcebook

Basic Information about Various Types of Burns and Scalds, Including Flame, Heat, Electrical, Chemical, and Sun; Along with Short- and Long-Term Treatments, Tissue Reconstruction, Plastic Surgery, Prevention Suggestions, and First Aid

Edited by Allan R. Cook. 600 pages. 1998. 0-7808-0204-7. $78.

Cancer Sourcebook, 1st Edition

Basic Information on Cancer Types, Symptoms, Diagnostic Methods, and Treatments, Including Statistics on Cancer Occurrences Worldwide and the Risks Associated with Known Carcinogens and Activities

Edited by Frank E. Bair. 932 pages. 1990. 1-55888-888-8. $78.

"Written in nontechnical language. Useful for patients, their families, medical professionals, and librarians."
— *Guide to Reference Books, '96*

"Designed with the non-medical professional in mind. Libraries and medical facilities interested in patient education should certainly consider adding the *Cancer Sourcebook* to their holdings. This compact collection of reliable information . . . is an invaluable tool for helping patients and patients' families and friends to take the first steps in coping with the many difficulties of cancer."
— *Medical Reference Services Quarterly, Winter '91*

"Specifically created for the nontechnical reader . . . an important resource for the general reader trying to understand the complexities of cancer."
— *American Reference Books Annual, '91*

"This publication's nontechnical nature and very comprehensive format make it useful for both the general public and undergraduate students." — *Choice, Oct '90*

New Cancer Sourcebook, 2nd Edition

Basic Information about Major Forms and Stages of Cancer, Featuring Facts about Primary and Secondary Tumors of the Respiratory, Nervous, Lymphatic, Circulatory, Skeletal, and Gastrointestinal Systems, and Specific Organs; Statistical and Demographic Data; Treatment Options; and Strategies for Coping

Edited by Allan R. Cook. 1,313 pages. 1996. 0-7808-0041-9. $78.

"This book is an excellent resource for patients with newly diagnosed cancer and their families. The dialogue is simple, direct, and comprehensive. Highly recommended for patients and families to aid in their understanding of cancer and its treatment"
— *Booklist Health Sciences Supplement, Oct '97*

"The amount of factual and useful information is extensive. The writing is very clear, geared to general readers. Recommended for all levels." — *Choice, Jan '97*

Cancer Sourcebook for Women

Basic Information about Specific Forms of Cancer That Affect Women, Featuring Facts about Breast Cancer, Cervical Cancer, Ovarian Cancer, Cancer of the Uterus and Uterine Sarcoma, Cancer of the Vagina, and Cancer of the Vulva; Statistical and Demographic Data; Treatments, Self-Help Management Suggestions, and Current Research Initiatives

Edited by Allan R. Cook and Peter D. Dresser. 524 pages. 1996. 0-7808-0076-1. $78.

". . . written in easily understandable, non-technical language. Recommended for public libraries or hospital and academic libraries that collect patient education or consumer health materials."
— *Medical Reference Services Quarterly, Spring '97*

Cancer Sourcebook for Women *(Continued)*

"Would be of value in a consumer health library. . . . written with the health care consumer in mind. Medical jargon is at a minimum, and medical terms are explained in clear, understandable sentences."
— *Bulletin of the MLA, Oct '96*

"The availability under one cover of all these pertinent publications, grouped under cohesive headings, makes this certainly a most useful sourcebook."
— *Choice, Jun '96*

"Presents a comprehensive knowledge base for general readers. Men and women both benefit from the gold mine of information nestled between the two covers of this book. Recommended."
— *Academic Library Book Review, Summer '96*

"This timely book is highly recommended for consumer health and patient education collections in all libraries."
— *Library Journal, Apr '96*

Cardiovascular Diseases & Disorders Sourcebook

Basic Information about Cardiovascular Diseases and Disorders, Featuring Facts about the Cardiovascular System, Demographic and Statistical Data, Descriptions of Pharmacological and Surgical Interventions, Lifestyle Modifications, and a Special Section Focusing on Heart Disorders in Children

Edited by Karen Bellenir and Peter D. Dresser. 683 pages. 1995. 0-7808-0032-X. $78.

". . . comprehensive format provides an extensive overview on this subject."
— *Choice, Jun '96*

". . . an easily understood, complete, up-to-date resource. This well executed public health tool will make valuable information available to those that need it most, patients and their families. The typeface, sturdy non-reflective paper, and library binding add a feel of quality found wanting in other publications. Highly recommended for academic and general libraries. "
— *Academic Library Book Review, Summer '96*

Communication Disorders Sourcebook

Basic Information about Deafness and Hearing Loss, Speech and Language Disorders, Voice Disorders, Balance and Vestibular Disorders, and Disorders of Smell, Taste, and Touch

Edited by Linda M. Ross. 533 pages. 1996. 0-7808-0077-X. $78.

"This is skillfully edited and is a welcome resource for the layperson. It should be found in every public and medical library."
— *Booklist Health Sciences Supplement, Oct '97*

Congenital Disorders Sourcebook

Basic Information about Disorders Acquired during Gestation, Including Spina Bifida, Hydrocephalus, Cerebral Palsy, Heart Defects, Craniofacial Abnormalities, Fetal Alcohol Syndrome, and More, Along with Current Treatment Options and Statistical Data

Edited by Karen Bellenir. 607 pages. 1997. 0-7808-0205-5. $78.

"Recommended reference source." — *Booklist, Oct '97*

Consumer Issues in Health Care Sourcebook

Basic Information about Health Care Fundamentals and Related Consumer Issues, Including Exams and Screening Tests, Physician Specialties, Choosing a Doctor, Using Prescription and Over-the-Counter Medications Safely, Avoiding Health Scams, Managing Common Health Risks in the Home, Care Options for Chronically or Terminally Ill Patients, and a List of Resources for Obtaining Help and Further Information

Edited by Karen Bellenir. 592 pages. 1998. 0-7808-0221-7. $78.

Contagious & Non-Contagious Infectious Diseases Sourcebook

Basic Information about Contagious Diseases like Measles, Polio, Hepatitis B, and Infectious Mononucleosis, and Non-Contagious Infectious Diseases like Tetanus and Toxic Shock Syndrome, and Diseases Occurring as Secondary Infections Such as Shingles and Reye Syndrome, Along with Vaccination, Prevention, and Treatment Information, and a Section Describing Emerging Infectious Disease Threats

Edited by Karen Bellenir and Peter D. Dresser. 566 pages. 1996. 0-7808-0075-3. $78.

Diabetes Sourcebook, 1st Edition

Basic Information about Insulin-Dependent and Noninsulin-Dependent Diabetes Mellitus, Gestational Diabetes, and Diabetic Complications, Symptoms, Treatment, and Research Results, Including Statistics on Prevalence, Morbidity, and Mortality, Along with Source Listings for Further Help and Information

Edited by Karen Bellenir and Peter D. Dresser. 827 pages. 1994. 1-55888-751-2. $78.

. . . very informative and understandable for the layperson without being simplistic. It provides a comprehensive overview for laypersons who want a general understanding of the disease or who want to focus on various aspects of the disease." — *Bulletin of the MLA, Jan '96*

DATE DUE

MAY 3 1 2001 JUL 2 6 2001	DEC 0 2 2006	
AUG 1 2 2001	DEC 0 6 2007 DEC 0 7 2007	
APR 0 5 2002		
MAY 0 2 2002	DEC 0 3 2012	
JUL 0 5 2002		
0 2 1 3 0 3		
DEC 0 3 2003		
1 1 2 7 0 4		
JUL 2 2 2005		
0 2 2 6 0 6		
1 0 1 7 0 7		

Health Reference Series

Health Reference Series

First Edition

SLEEP
DISORDERS
SOURCEBOOK

Basic Consumer Health Information about Sleep and Its Disorders, Including Insomnia, Sleepwalking, Sleep Apnea, Restless Leg Syndrome, and Narcolepsy; Along with Data about Shiftwork and Its Effects, Information on the Societal Costs of Sleep Deprivation, Descriptions of Treatment Options, a Glossary of Terms, and Resource Listings for Additional Help

Edited by
Jenifer Swanson

Omnigraphics, Inc.

Penobscot Building / Detroit, MI 48226

BIBLIOGRAPHIC NOTE

Because this page cannot legibly accommodate all the copyright notices, the Bibliographic Note portion of the Preface constitutes an extension of the copyright notice.

Beginning with books published in 1999, each new volume of the *Health Reference Series* will be individually titled and called a "First Edition." Subsequent updates will carry sequential edition numbers. To help avoid confusion and to provide maximum flexibility in our ability to respond to informational needs, the practice of consecutively numbering each volume will be discontinued.

Edited by Jenifer Swanson

Peter D. Dresser, Managing Editor, *Health Reference Series*
Karen Bellenir, Series Editor, *Health Reference Series*

Omnigraphics, Inc.

Tamekia N. Ashford, *Production Associate*
Matthew P. Barbour, *Manager, Production and Fulfillment*
Laurie Lanzen Harris, *Vice President, Editorial Director*
Peter E. Ruffner, *Vice President, Administration*
James A. Sellgren, *Vice President, Operations and Finance*
Jane J. Steele, *Marketing Consultant*

Robert R. Tyler, Executive Vice President and Associate Publisher
Frederick G. Ruffner, Jr., Publisher

©1999, Omnigraphics, Inc.

Library of Congress Cataloging-in-Publication Data

Sleep disorders sourcebook : basic consumer health information about sleep and its disorders including insomnia, sleepwalking, sleep apnea, restless leg syndrome, and narcolepsy; along with data about shiftwork and its effects. Information on the societal costs of sleep deprivation, descriptions of treatment options, a glossary of terms, and resource listings for additional help / edited by Jenifer Swanson. — 1st ed.
   p. cm.
  Includes bibliographical references and index.
  ISBN 0-7808-0234-9 (lib. bdg. : alk. paper)
  1. Sleep disorders. 2. Consumer education. I. Swanson, Jenifer.
RC547.S536 1998   98-37257
616.7'498—dc21   CIP

∞

This book is printed on acid-free paper meeting the ANSI Z39.48 Standard. The infinity symbol that appears above indicates that the paper in this book meets that standard.

Printed in the United States

Table of Contents

Part III: The Major Sleep Disorders

Part IV: Sleep Medications

Preface

About This Book

Sleep is a basic physiological need. Its primary function appears to be rest and restoring the body's energy levels. Its main biological function is still a great mystery. Researchers in the field do not yet agree on why we sleep, but they note that most people spend a third or more of their lives asleep. They also know that sleep disorders and disturbances cause major physical and mental problems across all ages of the lifespan. Approximately 40 million Americans are chronically ill with various sleep disorders; an additional 20 to 30 million experience intermittent sleep-related problems. Consequences of sleep disorders include reduced productivity, serious morbidity, increased mortality and decreased quality of life.

Insomnia and sleep apnea are the most prevalent sleep disorders. They occur for many differing reasons. Insomnia can be caused by environmental changes, menopause, depression, and medications. Other underlying causes include arthritis, kidney disease, heart failure, and asthma. Sleep apnea, or the repeated interruption of sleep by breathing abnormalities, is particularly prevalent in males over 50 and begins to appear in equal numbers in post-menopausal women. Physiological changes accompanying the process of aging, such as weight gain and hormonal changes, may lead to sleep apnea as well as other sleep disorders. Other sleep disorders include narcolepsy, restless leg syndrome, and sudden infant death syndrome. Treatment for many sleep disorders may include lifestyle changes, devices to aid with nighttime breathing, and medications.

This Sourcebook provides information to help the layperson identify symptoms of insomnia, sleep apnea, restless leg syndrome, narcolepsy, and the some of the other 70 disorders identified by the American Sleep Disorders Association. In addition, it provides answers to difficult problems such as adjusting to shiftwork, dealing with sleep-wake problems during cancer treatment, and how people with other disorders can adapt, in the area of sleep. A glossary, suggestions for finding sleep information on the Internet, and lists of additional reading material and resources are included to provide further help and direction.

How to Use This Book

This book is divided into parts and chapters. Parts focus on broad areas of interest. Chapters are devoted to single topics within a part.

Part I: Understanding Sleep Requirements and the Costs of Sleep Deprivation provides basic information on healthy sleep, including good sleep hygiene. It describes the important role that proper sleep plays for safety in our society, explains what problem sleepiness is, and offers an idea of what to expect when being examined for a sleep disorder.

Part II: Sleep through the Lifespan describes the differing conditions that sleep and its disorders have as we grow, change, and age. This includes topics ranging from apnea in the premature baby, sudden infant death syndrome, common bedtime disturbances in children, the sleep requirements of teenagers, the unique sleep needs of women, and sleep changes in the elderly.

Part III: The Major Sleep Disorders gives a more detailed view of the most common sleep disorders throughout all parts of our lives. It offers specific information on sleep apnea and its treatment, insomnia and the various medical approaches toward its abatement, narcolepsy, restless leg syndrome, and sleepwalking. A large chapter is devoted to shiftwork, a cause of sleep disorder that is becoming prevalent in today's society.

Part IV: Sleep Medications provides information on both the positive and negative roles various medications can play in a move towards better sleep control. This section also includes a chapter on Melatonin, a still somewhat controversial treatment.

Part V: Sleep and Other Disorders describes the effects other medical conditions can have upon one's sleep. These include mental disorders such as panic disorder and schizophrenia, substance abuse disorders like alcoholism, and major life threatening diseases such as multiple sclerosis and cancer.

Part VI: Additional Help and Information provides a glossary of sleep-related terms, a chapter on how to find information on the Internet, suggestions for further reading, and a resource list for patients with the various sleep disorders.

Bibliographic Note

This volume contains documents and excerpts from publications issued by the following government U.S. agencies: Food and Drug Administration (FDA), National Cancer Institute (NCI), National Commission on Sleep Disorders Research, National Heart, Lung, and Blood Institute (NHLBI), National Institute for Occupational Safety and Health (NIOSH), National Institute of Child Health and Human Development (NICHD), National Institute of Nursing Research (NINR), National Institutes of Health (NIH), National Institute on Alcohol Abuse and Alcoholism (NIAAA), and the U.S. Public Health Service.

In addition, this volume contains copyrighted documents from the following organizations: American Academy of Otolaryngology–Head and Neck Surgery, Inc., American Association for Respiratory Care, American Sleep Apnea Association (ASAA), American Sleep Disorders Association (ASDA), and the National Sudden Infant Death Syndrome Resource Center. Copyrighted articles from *Behavioral Health Treatment, American Family Physician, Archives of Internal Medicine, BioScience,* Jane E. Brazy, M.D., *Brown University Child and Adolescent Behavior Letter, The Brown University Long-Term Care Quality Letter, Dr. Greene's Housecalls, Drug Topics, Journal of the American Medical Association, Nation's Business, Patient Care, The Physician and Sportsmedicine, Real Living with Multiple Sclerosis,* Barton Schmitt, *Tufts Health & Nutrition Letter* are also included.

Acknowledgements

In addition to the many organizations and agencies who freely donated the material that is included in this book, thanks go to Margaret Mary Missar, Maria Franklin, Bruce Bellenir and Dawn Matthews for their assistance, deep and lasting gratitude to my mentor, Karen Bellenir, who makes this work fun, and heartfelt appreciation and love to my husband, Matt, and my daughter, Devon.

Note from the Editor

This book is part of Omnigraphics' *Health Reference Series*. The series provides basic information about a broad range of medical concerns. It is not intended to serve as a tool for diagnosing illness, in prescribing treatments, or as a substitute for the physician/patient relationship. All persons concerned about medical symptoms or the possibility of disease are encouraged to seek professional care from an appropriate health care provider.

Health Reference Series *Update Policy*

The inaugural book in the *Health Reference Series* was the first edition of *Cancer Sourcebook* published in 1992. Since then, the *Series* has been enthusiastically received by libraries and in the medical community. In order to maintain the standard of providing high-quality health information for the lay person, the editorial staff at Omnigraphics felt it was necessary to implement a policy of updating volumes when warranted.

Medical researchers have been making tremendous strides, and the challenge to stay current with the most recent advances is one our editors take seriously. Each decision to update a volume will be made on an individual basis. Some of the considerations will include how much new information is available and the feedback we receive from people who use the books. If there's a topic you would like to see added to the update list, or an area of medical concern you feel has not been adequately addressed, please write to:

Editor
Health Reference Series
Omnigraphics, Inc.
2500 Penobscot Bldg.
Detroit, MI 48226

The commitment to providing on-going coverage of important medical developments has also led to some technical changes in the *Health Reference Series*. Beginning with books published in 1999, each new volume will be individually titled and called a "First Edition." Subsequent updates will carry sequential edition numbers. To help avoid confusion and to provide maximum flexibility in our ability to respond to informational needs, the practice of consecutively numbering each volume will be discontinued.

Part One

Understanding Sleep Requirements and the Costs of Sleep Deprivation

Chapter 1

Healthy Sleep:
Our Current Understanding

The most widely accepted definition of healthy sleep is that quantity and quality of sleep required to maintain optimal alertness during desired waking hours. While health researchers in other fields of scientific inquiry have made the accumulation of normative data bases their highest priority, this has not occurred in terms of human sleep. As a result, we have only the smallest idea of the range and distribution of human sleep requirements across the population. We do know that of participants in a nine-year longitudinal study by the California State Department of Health, who stated that they slept six hours or less a night, 70 percent had a higher mortality rate than those who reported sleeping seven to eight hours. This association remains significant even after controlling for age, sex, race, physical health status, physical activity, and several other potentially confounding influences.

Normal sleep constitutes a portion of a cyclic circadian ("about a day") alternation of sleep and wakefulness. The circadian sleep-wake rhythm is regulated by a neural pacemaker located in a region of the brain called the supra-chiasmatic nucleus (SCN). The timing of the SCN is influenced by time cues, such as light and darkness, and controls many other (if not all) physiologic circadian rhythms, such as body temperature and various hormone secretion patterns.

From *Wake Up America: A National Sleep Alert*, Volume 1, Executive Summary and Executive Report, Report of the National Commission on Sleep Disorders Research, Submitted to the United States Congress and to the Secretary U.S. Department of Health and Human Services, January 1993.

Sleep actually includes two distinct states: non-rapid eye movement (non-REM) sleep, and rapid eye movement (REM) sleep. These states exist in virtually all mammals and birds. Scientific study has found that the sleep states are as different from one another as each is from the waking state. In adult humans, non-REM sleep alternates cyclically with REM sleep approximately every 90-100 minutes throughout the night; non-REM sleep normally occurs first in the transition from wakefulness to sleep and occupies 75-80 percent of sleep. Non-REM sleep is subdivided into four stages that roughly parallel sleep depth; the lightest is called stage 1 and the deepest, stage 4. The deepest stages of non-REM sleep are concentrated in the 90-minute sleep cycles of the early night. Brain function in non-REM sleep, markedly different from waking brain activity, continues to regulate and maintain vital bodily functions, often at a slowed rate (e.g., heart rate, respiration rate). REM sleep, which occupies 20-25 percent of sleep in adult humans, is characterized by a high level of brain activity, bursts of rapid eye movement, increased heart and respiration rates, and paralysis of many muscles. REM sleep takes up an increasing proportion of the 90-minute sleep cycle in the later portion of the night; 80 percent of arousals from REM sleep elicit vivid dream recall. The brain's regulation of bodily functions in REM sleep changes markedly as compared to waking or non-REM. Certain functions, for example, temperature regulation, are inactivated or greatly suppressed in REM sleep.

Chapter 2

Why Do We Sleep?

A New Hypothesis Suggests That We Sleep to Refuel Energy Stores in the Brain

We humans have been known to do strange things when our sleep gets disordered. A Canadian man murdered his mother-in-law while sleepwalking. Another man, while dreaming that he was fleeing from an intruder, drove his car to his parents' house without mishap. Then there is the woman who drew a map of the United States on her bedroom wall and filled in all 50 state capitals while asleep. The American Sleep Disorders Association in an advertisement last year noted that one woman had gained 40 pounds because she ate chocolates while deep in slumber, and another had awakened at the grocery store while pushing along a cart that contained 56 boxes of corn flakes.

Disrupted nights hit more than 30 million Americans who suffer from serious sleep problems such as chronic insomnia, apnea, and narcolepsy. Most of us, though, only occasionally have restless nights, waking the next morning bleary-eyed and sleep deprived. If sleep problems large and small are to be managed, it would be helpful to know which molecules floating through our bodies ultimately trigger sleep and the chain of events that lead to activation of those molecules. Could the most important instigators of sleep be molecules already

Reprinted with permission from *BioScience*, June 1996, Volume 46, Number 6, pp. 391-393. ©1996 by American Institute of Biological Sciences, 1444 Eye Street, N.W., Suite 200, Washington, D.C., USA, 20005.

known to induce sleep, or might an as-yet-undiscovered class of compounds be responsible?

The root causes of sleep gone haywire may not be discovered until sleep researchers determine why our ancestors first developed the highly risky habit of snoozing. The main biological function of so-called normal sleep is still a great mystery, say researchers in the field, who are nowhere close to agreement on a reason for an activity that takes up a third or more of human life.

Researchers, however, have clarified that, contrary to general belief, sleep is not about resting the body. After all, several sets of tennis or a hard run in the morning do not drive us into nap mode at noon just because our muscles are tired. There is consensus that sleeping mostly does something good for the brain.

Puzzle Pieces

Decades of research have given scientists a plethora of details about the events that occur during sleep. Use of electroencephalograms (EEG) made it possible to study the variations in brain waves that characterize the two broad stages of sleep. REM (rapid-eye-movement) is the more active phase, during which we dream. Non-REM sleep is of longer duration, and high-amplitude, low-frequency EEG waves are produced.

Scientists know, for instance, that echidnas, which are primitive, egg-laying mammals, only experience non-REM sleep. Many other mammals, including us, spend 80% of sleep time in non-REM.

Scientists have measured the physiological changes that hearts, lungs, and other organs undergo during sleep, and psychiatrists have picked apart dreams. Much of the genetic basis for circadian rhythms has been worked out, and recent studies indicate that melatonin can set the biological clock right and compensate for the jet lag that accompanies travel across time zones. Scientists can even measure the activity of individual neurons in sleeping animals.

Researchers know that mental acuity declines with sleep deprivation. There is also evidence that a little sleep deprivation can relieve the symptoms of severe depression.

Clearly, sleep serves a survival function when one considers that extreme sleep deprivation is fatal—at least in rats. A pivotal study carried out more than a decade ago by Allan Rechtschaffen and colleagues of the University of Chicago showed that rats deprived of sleep experienced a doubling of their metabolic rates. Despite eating considerably more than rats allowed to sleep normally, the sleep-deprived animals lost weight. They also could not maintain their body temperatures, and they developed unusual skin disorders. The animals died after two-and-a-half weeks, says Rechtschaffen. "The specific cause of death has never been determined."

But despite having tantalizing clues about what occurs during sleep, and about the need for shuteye, modern researchers are, at the most fundamental level, as confounded by the purpose and ultimate control of sleep as were Hippocrates and Aristotle more than 2500 years ago. Hippocrates thought that because sleeping bodies feel cool to the touch, sleep was caused by blood retreating to the inner regions of the body, says sleep researcher James M. Krueger, a physiologist at the University of Tennessee Medical School in Memphis.

In Aristotle's view, the instigator of sleep was digestion. He hypothesized that food digesting in the stomach emitted vapors that were carried by the humors—blood, phlegm, black bile, yellow bile—to various parts of the body. The moving of the vapors induced sleep. Aristotle's idea held sway for more than two millennia in the scientific community, and, in today's popular culture, a residue of that notion remains. Who does not know that a postprandial snooze is inevitable following a rich meal?

During the nineteenth century there was a hypothesis that flooding the brain with blood drives one to sleep. A competing theory suggested just the opposite.

Hypotheses today run a gamut of possibilities. Perhaps our brains use sleep as cleanup time, reordering our jumbled thoughts and memories, tossing out those that just create mental clutter. Could one of sleep's jobs be to keep the immune system in good fettle, ready to do battle with undesirable invaders? Might it have a thermoregulatory function and keep the brain from overheating? Does sleep give our neurons time to mature or our bodies time to manufacture proteins?

There are more theories about the purpose of sleep than can possibly be correct, says Rechtschaffen, who points out that there is evidence for and against all of the major theories. "None has commanded the universal enthusiasm of sleep researchers," he says.

A New Restorative Hypothesis

Intuitively we know that sleeping, like drinking and eating, returns us to a physiological even keel when we feel out of sorts. The drives to sate these basic desires that ensure survival are managed constantly by homeostatic mechanisms that were finely tuned deep in our evolutionary past to respond to changes in particular substances. "Thirst and hunger are reasonably well understood. With sleep, there is a long way to go," says Joel Benington, a researcher at Stanford University.

Benington and Craig Heller, also of Stanford, hypothesize that sleep's homeostatic purpose is to replenish glycogen stores in the brain. In papers published late last year in *Brain Research* and *Progress in Neurobiology*, Benington and Heller described experiments that support their belief, and they fingered adenosine as a likely instigator of sleep.

The brain chugs along using glucose to fuel its workings. But glycogen, which is stored throughout the brain, is also mobilized and broken down steadily throughout waking in anticipation of extra energy needs, says Benington.

After an extended period of wakefulness, Benington and Heller suggest that those depleted reserves must somehow be refilled during non-REM sleep. "Sleep takes the brain off-line to do the job," says Heller.

It would be maladaptive to replenish glycogen while an animal is awake because the process would compete with its ability to sort through the information needed to survive. "Sleep has therefore evolved as a state in which animals retreat to a safe environment, behavior is suppressed, and glycogen stores are replenished," Benington and Heller say in *Progress in Neurobiology* (45:347-360).

When the brain has run out of its back-up fuel after hours of mental alertness, Benington and Heller think that changes in adenosine levels influence the drive to sleep. They speculate that as the need for sleep increases adenosine production rises; the amount of adenosine produced in turn may determine how big the EEG waves in non-REM sleep get. (Size of the waves on an EEG during non-REM sleep is important because scientists consider it the best physiological measurement of how deeply we are sleeping. Also, it is a measure of how sleep deprived we were to begin with—a person who has gone an extended period without sleep will generate larger-than-normal slow waves on their EEGs.)

Benington and Heller decided to test how various levels of N6-cyclopentyladenosine (CPA), an analog of adenosine might influence the slow wave patterns of rats that were sleep sated. (Studies in another lab had already shown that treated rats fell into a deep sleep.) The researchers found that rats that had already had plenty of sleep would go back to sleep and generate EEG slow-waves characteristic of the deep sleep that follows a period of extended wakefulness. The bigger the dose of CPA, the larger the waves generated. "A key symptom of sleep need is increase in slow waves," says Benington. "We showed adenosine analogs produced this fingerprint of sleep need and did it in animals that didn't theoretically need to sleep."

There have been previous indirect and direct hints that adenosine has a role in sleep. Several years ago is was shown that nerve-jangling eye-openers such as caffeine and theophylline, an active ingredient in tea, block adenosine receptors and disrupt non-REM sleep.

Misha Radulovacki at the University of Illinois in Chicago says he first became curious about adenosine's importance in the 1980s. He asked, "Would stimulation of adenosine receptors produce sleep?" He found that certain adenosine analogs increased sleep, whereas antagonists decreased it. "We know that in the brain, adenosine calms the firing of neurons. Once we block the receptors, the neurons fire wildly," says Radulovacki.

There has been a resurgence of interest in adenosine and sleep. According to Harvard University's Peter Shiromani, editor of the *Sleep Research Society's Bulletin*, an upcoming issue will deal with just this topic.

If adenosine is the messenger in the homeostatic feedback mechanism that controls sleep, how might it work? Heller suggests that when enough adenosine molecules bind to their receptors in the brain, ion channels in nearby neurons open and positive potassium ions seep out of the cells. The movement of the ions causes the neurons to be less excitable and to fire in synchrony, producing the big, slow waves of non-REM sleep. The analogy Heller uses is that, in sleep, the neurons are like singers in an auditorium who all sing the same song. But when we are awake, neuromodulators like serotonin and norepinephrine keep the neurons constantly firing, creating an auditorium filled with static sounds and discordant voices.

Benington and Heller are now conducting studies in which they will deprive animals of sleep and determine how much glycogen is depleted and how much adenosine is released. In the process, if they find that glycogen stores are not decreased during the experiment "we'll have to reject the glycogen hypothesis," says Benington.

A collaboration also is underway with Raymond Swanson at the Veterans Affairs Medical Center in San Francisco to clarify how glycogen is used in the brain. Glycogen is stored in glial cells called astrocytes, which exist only in the brain. The function of astrocytes is unclear, Swanson says. Historically, they have been thought of as a brain filler of sorts. Now, they are perceived as being important for maintaining homeostasis in the brain.

Using cell cultures, Swanson wants to determine whether energy demand causes glycogen breakdown in the astrocytes. He says it is not clear whether glycogen is broken down in the astrocytes to produce glucose for neurons or whether the astrocytes use the glycogen themselves for some unknown purpose.

But if the purpose of sleep is to restore glycogen and if that occurs only during non-REM sleep, why waste time in the REM world? Because REM sleep may be needed to push us back into non-REM sleep to ensure that we get enough restorative sleep, say Benington and Heller. The brain activity of REM sleep may be needed to pump positive ions into brain cells so that another cycle of non-REM sleep can begin.

The Stanford team's suggestion challenges the standard interpretation of REM sleep. Scientists have tended to associate the need for REM sleep with waking. This viewpoint is a result of an early emphasis on the dreaming that occurs during REM, say the researchers.

Not Accepted Yet

If Heller's and Benington's hypothesis is substantiated, the result would be a theory general enough to explain a purpose of sleep across species, says Alexander A. Borbely at the University of Zurich in Switzerland, who points out that a sleeplike state exists even in invertebrates. He calls the Heller-Benington hypothesis "provocative" and "novel in that it proposes specific biochemical processes in the brain occurring during sleep and waking. It is testable, and one of its aspects is that it accounts for effects of sleep deprivation."

Other researchers are undecided about the merit of the hypothesis. "A major problem of the Heller-Benington theory is that the one study that directly assessed brain glycogen levels during wake and sleep did not find much of a difference," says Rechtschaffen. "Perhaps future studies might reverse that result. It is too early to reach a final decision on the matter."

Whether adenosine is most critical in sleep regulation remains to be seen. "There is a consensus within the field of the biochemical regulation of sleep that no behavior as complex as sleep is regulated by a single substance. This consensus is based on a very large literature," says Krueger.

Many other substances in the body induce sleep. For instance, interleukin-1, tumor necrosis factor, and growth-hormone releasing hormone have all been implicated in non-REM sleep regulation, says Krueger, who specializes in the biochemical regulation of sleep and immune responses.

"What's important about the Heller-Benington hypothesis is not the mechanism. There are other ideas we have better data on," says Krueger. "What is important is their emphasis that sleep is driven by local metabolism. It is thus dependent on neuronal use not prior wakefulness per se. In the past, the emphasis was on regulatory centers or sleep neural networks imposing the state."

Krueger himself proposed several years ago that sleep starts at the local level in the brain. The collective output of small groups of localized neurons triggers sleep for the purpose of preserving synapses, he says. "Our theory is built on the idea that there are critical synaptic populations that are important for survival, but that are not maintained enough during waking. So sleep's job is to 'use them or lose them.'"

Benington expects skepticism. In fact, he will remain somewhat skeptical himself until they have more data. The proof will be in the studies now underway, he says.

If further investigations show that adenosine levels in the brain are critical to the non-REM stage, it potentially means that adenosine-like compounds could be used to treat sleep problems.

Such substances might be particularly useful for elderly people, who tend to spend less time in the deepest stages of non-REM sleep, and for whom insomnia is common, says Heller.

Now when people have a tough time getting to sleep, their physicians often prescribe benzodiazepines, which work by reducing the excitability of neurons just as adenosine does. But, after extended use, people get used to benzodiazepines, and they lose their effectiveness. Coming off benzodiazepines can also make insomnia worse.

What makes adenosine different from some substances currently used to treat sleep problems is that it is a natural substance and it modulates the depth of sleep, says Heller. "If you're sleep deprived, you can make it up by having a deeper, more intense sleep."

Benington says, even if adenosine is shown to be critical for sleep, it will not be a cure for all the troubles we experience trying to get to sleep. It seems such a simple explanation would be too much to hope for, given how mysterious sleep is.

—*by Anna Maria Gillis*

Chapter 3

Test Your Sleep I.Q.

The following true or false statements test what you know about sleep. Be sure to read the correct answers and explanations at the bottom of this test.

True or False?

1. Sleep is a time when your body and brain shut down for rest and relaxation.

2. If you regularly doze off unintentionally during the day, you may need more than just a good night's sleep.

3. If you snore loudly and persistently at night and are sleepy during the day, you may have a sleep disorder

4. Opening the car window or turning the radio up will keep the drowsy driver awake

5. Narcolepsy is a sleep disorder marked by "sleep attacks."

6. The primary cause of insomnia is worry.

7. One cause of not getting enough sleep is restless legs syndrome.

NIH Pub. No. 96-3797, October 1996.

13

8. The body has a natural ability to adjust to different sleep schedules such as working different shifts or traveling through multiple time zones quickly.

9. People need less sleep as they grow older.

10. More people doze off at the wheel of a car in the early morning or midafternoon than in the evening.

Answers to the Sleep I.Q. Quiz

1. *False*. Although it is a time when your body rests and restores its energy levels, sleep is an active state that affects both your physical and mental well-being. Adequate restful sleep, like diet and exercise, is critical to good health. Insufficient restful sleep can result in mental and physical health problems and possibly premature death.

2. *True*. Many people doze off unintentionally during the day despite getting their usual night of sleep. This could be a sign of a sleep disorder. Approximately 40 million Americans suffer from sleep disorders, including sleep apnea, insomnia, narcolepsy, and restless legs syndrome. An untreated sleep disorder can reduce your daytime productivity, increase your risk of accidents, and put you at risk for illness and even early death.

3. *True*. Persistent loud snoring at night and daytime sleepiness are the main symptoms of a common and serious sleep disorder, sleep apnea. Another symptom is frequent long pauses in breathing during sleep, followed by choking and gasping for breath. People with sleep apnea don't get enough restful sleep, and their daytime performance is often seriously affected. Sleep apnea may also lead to hypertension, heart disease, heart attack, and stroke. However, it can be treated, and the sleep apnea patient can live a normal life.

4. *False*. Opening the car window or turning the radio up may arouse a drowsy driver briefly, but this won't keep that person alert behind the wheel. Even mild drowsiness is enough to reduce concentration and reaction time. The sleep-deprived driver may nod off for a couple of seconds at a time without even knowing it—enough time to kill himself or someone else.

It has been estimated that drowsy driving may account for an average of 56,000 reported accidents each year—claiming over 1,500 lives.

5. *True*. People with narcolepsy fall asleep uncontrollably —at any time of the day, in all types of situations— regardless of the amount or quality of sleep they've had the night before. Narcolepsy is characterized by these "sleep attacks," as well as by daytime sleepiness episodes of muscle weakness or paralysis, and disrupted nighttime sleep. Although there is no known cure, medications and behavioral treatments can control symptoms, and people with narcolepsy can live normal lives.

6. *False*. Insomnia has many different causes, including physical and mental conditions and stress. Insomnia is the perception that you don't get enough sleep because you can't fall asleep or stay asleep or get back to sleep once you've awakened during the night. It affects people of all ages, usually for just an occasional night or two, but sometimes for weeks, months, or even years. Because insomnia can become a chronic problem, it is important to get it diagnosed and treated if it persists for more than a month.

7. *True*. Restless legs syndrome (RLS) is a medical condition distinguished by tingling sensations in the legs—and sometimes the arms—while sitting or lying still, especially at bedtime. The person with RLS needs to constantly stretch or move the legs to try to relieve these uncomfortable or painful symptoms. As a result, he or she has difficulty falling asleep or staying asleep and usually feels extremely sleepy and unable to function fully during the day. Good sleep habits and medication can help the person with RLS.

8. *False*. The human body's biological clock programs each person to feel sleepy during the nighttime hours and to be active during the daylight hours. So people who work the night shift and try to sleep during the day are constantly fighting their biological clocks. This puts them at risk of error and accident at work and of disturbed sleep. The same is true for people who travel through multiple time zones quickly; they get "jet lag" because they cannot maintain a regular sleep-wake schedule. Sleeping during the day in a dark, quiet bedroom

and getting exposure to sufficient bright light at the right time can help improve daytime alertness.

9. *False.* As we get older, we don't need less sleep, but we often get less sleep. That's because our ability to sleep for long periods of time and to get into the deep restful stages of sleep decreases with age. Older people have more fragile sleep and are more easily disturbed by light, noise, and pain. They also may have medical conditions that contribute to sleep problems. Going to bed at the same time every night and getting up at the same time every morning, getting exposure to natural outdoor light during the day, and sleeping in a cool, dark, quiet place at night may help.

10. *True.* Our bodies are programmed by our biological clock to experience two natural periods of sleepiness during the 24-hour day, regardless of the amount of sleep we've had in the previous 24 hours. The primary period is between about midnight and 7:00 a.m. A second period of less intense sleepiness is in the midafternoon, between about 1:00 and 3:00. This means that we are more at risk of falling asleep at the wheel at these times than in the evening—especially if we haven't been getting enough sleep.

How Many Answers Did You Get Correct?

9-10 Correct
Congratulations! You know a lot about sleep. Share this information with your family and friends.

7-8 Correct
Very Good.

Fewer Than 7 Correct
Go over the answers and try to learn more about sleep.

For More Information

NHLBI Information Center
P.O. Box 30105
Bethesda, MD 20824-0105
(301) 251-1222
(301) 251-1223 (Fax)

Chapter 4

The National Cost of Sleep Deprivation

As a Nation, we have been transformed over the course of this century. Our knowledge and technology have expanded exponentially, altering irrevocably the fabric of society. As we have changed our society, we, too, have been changed. Competitiveness and drive have been heightened, perhaps excessively. We think nothing of ignoring the clock, often pushing our bodies and minds to work or play far beyond the sunrise to sunset cycle. Our lives appear to demand something close to perpetual motion, or at least motion minimally tempered by rest. The student studies all night for an examination and hopes to remain awake to take the test; the mother works out of the home by day and attempts to maintain the home and care for her family by night; the shiftworker takes a part-time day job to supplement income from the full-time swing or night shift job. Pilots, truckers, line-workers, soldiers, physicians, business executives, housewives and children, to a greater or lesser extent, all make similar trade-offs. Ironically, these efforts, apparently in pursuit of the "American Dream," have left little time for the true dream state—sleep.

The failure to acknowledge the importance of sleep and its effect on the full 24 hours of existence has given rise to a constellation of problems, both actual and potential. Sleep deprivation has become one of the most significant causes of error and accident throughout our

Excerpted from *Wake Up America: A National Sleep Alert*, Volume 1, Executive Summary and Executive Report, Report of the National Commission on Sleep Disorders Research, Submitted to the United States Congress and to the Secretary U.S. Department of Health and Human Services, January 1993.

society. Annual sleep-related accidents in transportation alone claim over 5,000 lives, cause hundreds of thousands of injuries, and assess a cost in the billions in health care costs, death, lost productivity, and damage to property.

In addition to the millions of Americans who suffer from pathologies of sleep and wakefulness, millions more—either chronically or intermittently—obtain insufficient sleep due to a variety of workplace and lifestyle determinants. On any given day, a substantial number of Americans, perhaps the majority, are functionally handicapped on the job, in the class room, or behind the wheel. The effects of sleepiness on healthy citizens permeate all aspects of our lives: our health, our education, our careers, and our overall quality of life. Despite these significant consequences, the burden on society remains largely unrecognized. Public education, leading to behavior change, can correct much of this problem.

The Commission has concluded that a major factor in the pervasive sleepiness found in American society is the failure to educate Americans about the facts related to sleep and sleep deprivation. Many aspects of our modern technological society are involved in causing sleep deprivation—the need to work long hours, competitiveness, and the need to work and sleep at the wrong times. The failure to educate does not even provide individuals at risk with the understanding that could enable them to counter and mitigate the effects of sleep deprivation and to organize their lives in a more rational manner.

Causes of Sleepiness

Each human being requires a specific amount of sleep in each 24-hour period to maintain optimal waking function. If an individual obtains less than this optimal dose, he will be less alert the following day. Moreover, sleep loss accumulates from one night to the next as a "sleep debt." Therefore, sleep of durations that represent only a modest loss of sleep on a single night may produce a serious sleep debt when sustained over several nights. The more sleep lost each day, the greater the sleep debt and the larger the impairment.

In the laboratory, sleep debt can be measured by assessing increased sleep tendency, negative mood, and performance decrements. In the real world, the consequences include learning impairments, discord in interpersonal relationships, errors, and accidents. Because individuals often do not recognize that they are sleepy, they seldom guard against inappropriate sleep episodes. Much like the intoxicated driver, sleepy drivers do not realize they are incapable of adequate performance and may deny drowsiness and impairment. When the individual does acknowledge sleepiness, it is often attributed mistakenly to boredom, to an overly warm environment, or to a heavy meal; rarely is drowsiness linked to the true cause—the quality and quantity of prior sleep. Sleepiness also may result from medication, alcohol consumption, or age-related deterioration of sleep found in the elderly.

America's massive sleep debt results from a complex interplay of technological advances, needs that compete with sleep, widespread ignorance, and to the ubiquitous disorders of sleep.

Voluntary Chronic Sleep Deprivation

Over the past 100-125 years, we have reduced our average nightly total sleep time by over 20 percent. Yet, no available scientific evidence suggests that we have developed a reduced need for sleep or that our ancestors slept too much. The change in our sleep behavior has paralleled technological change in our society. While our ancestors had few choices of activity for the evening hours, we can now choose from a wide variety of activities. The invention of electricity has enabled much activity to continue past sunset; now, 24-hour operations are commonplace.

A convincing body of scientific evidence leads the Commission to the conclusion that many Americans are sleep-deprived and, therefore, are sleepy during the day. Surveys of children's and adolescents' sleep habits conducted in 1910-1911 found that 8 to 12-year-old children averaged about 10.5 hours of sleep per night; 13 to 17-year-old adolescents averaged 9.5 hours. A 1968 survey found that the average number of hours of sleep experienced by each group had declined by 1.5 hours. It is assumed that the appropriate amount of sleep is the amount that will allow the individual to awaken voluntarily, without the use of an alarm or other environmental influences. When allowed to sleep without environmental influences for 14 consecutive days, young adults, who report typical nightly sleep durations of 7.5 hours, have been shown to average 8.6 hours per day. In a second study, when time in bed was limited to eight hours for ten consecutive days, time asleep averaged 7.4 hours. For the next 10 nights, when allowed to sleep *ad libitum*, the same individuals averaged 8.9 hours—nearly 1.5 hours *more* each night.

Younger Americans are not the only ones who short-change their sleep needs. Similarly, adults of all ages report average nightly sleep durations that are insufficient to avoid daytime sleepiness. In a 1960 study of over 800,000 Americans between the ages of 30 and 65, 13 percent of males and 15 percent of females reported obtaining less than seven hours of sleep each night. Nearly 48 percent of men and of women reported obtaining less than eight hours of sleep nightly. Moreover, every indication provided to the Commission suggests that these percentages are likely to be higher in 1992 than they were in 1960. Although definitive research on sleep need has not yet been performed, evidence to date suggests that the vast majority of adults requires an average of at least seven hours each night to avoid the serious consequences of sleep deprivation. Many individuals require more than eight hours of sleep each night.

Moreover, a 1992 study reports that Americans have added approximately 158 hours—nearly one full month of working hours—to their annual working/commuting time since 1969. It is logical to suggest that the increased time expended working and commuting forces many Americans to reduce sleep time. Young parents (ages 18-39) are affected the most; working, commuting young mothers add 241 more hours per year, fathers add 189 hours. Thus, survey, laboratory, and other types of studies indicate that many Americans are chronically sleep deprived.

Neither survey studies of large populations nor investigations of individual incidents address what appears to be the most serious issue: jobs that actually cause sleep deprivation. In our society, specific groups of workers are employed in jobs that tend to produce inordinate, prolonged sleep deprivation. Furthermore, these jobs tend to be hazardous; interstate commercial trucking is an excellent example. In a recent study, all but a handful of interstate truck drivers were found habitually to obtain fewer than five hours of sleep per day. Bus drivers, locomotive engineers, medical house staff, fire prevention workers, and police officers have similarly demanding work schedules that entail severe levels of sleep deprivation. All of these workers continually find themselves in situations in which impaired performance and unintended sleep can be catastrophic. The Commission believes that these special components require immediate attention.

The Role of the Biological Clock in Sleep Deprivation

Recent research has identified a circadian rhythm of sleepiness that is partially independent of the duration and quality of recent sleep. Most people experience two natural dips in alertness during the twenty-four hour day, regardless of the amount of sleep in the previous 24 hours. Both periods of sleepiness are more dramatic if an individual has not met his or her sleep needs in recent days. The primary period of sleepiness occurs between 2 a.m. and 8 a.m. The other daily period of sleepiness—commonly called the post-lunch dip—occurs in the mid-afternoon. One common practice to counteract this normal physiological dip in daytime alertness is to consume caffeine. In other cultures, a siesta is a popular response to mid-day sleepiness.

Circadian rhythm-related sleepiness pervades American society. Between the hours of 2 a.m. and 8 a.m., the physiological alertness of a night worker (even one who has slept reasonably well the prior day) is comparable to that of a dayshift worker who has obtained only four hours of sleep for two consecutive nights. Because most nightshift workers do not sleep well during the day, on-the-job sleepiness is even more severe. In some cases, night work, sleep loss, and circadian sleep tendency prove to be a particularly dangerous combination.

The same circadian increase in sleepiness affects people who must work after traversing multiple time zones. After transmeridian travel, flight crews, business executives, government officials, and others often find that they must go to work in what is the trough of the circadian alertness rhythm. Physiological adaptation to a new time zone generally takes three to 10 days; however, work/travel schedules rarely allow adequate time for adaptation.

Consequences of Sleepiness and Short Sleep

The consequences of reduced sleep time—whether caused by sleep disorders, voluntary sleep deprivation, or circadian factors—include diminished mental and physical health, increased mortality, lowered productivity, and increased incidence of errors and accidents.

Increased Morbidity and Mortality

The Commission found that habitual short sleepers are at risk of increased morbidity and mortality. According to several studies, individuals who report sleeping six hours or less a night experienced poorer health than those sleeping seven to eight hours a night. Moreover, a nine-year follow-up study found that individuals sleeping fewer than six hours each night had a 70 percent higher mortality rate in comparison to those who slept seven or eight hours a night. This association remains significant even after controlling for age, gender, race, physical health, smoking history, physical inactivity, alcohol consumption, and social support.

The Commission found abundant information suggesting that the relatively short habitual sleep duration associated with shiftwork significantly increases the risk of morbidity and mortality. Shift-workers suffer a higher incidence of illness than non-shiftworkers, including gastrointestinal and cardiovascular disorders. Although the psychosocial consequences of sleep loss and shiftwork have received little scientific attention, the toll is likely to be great. Sleep deprivation is known to result in more negative mood. For example, a recent study reduced the nightly sleep of adolescents by two hours for five consecutive nights, from the usual 8 to 9.5 hours to 7 to 8.5 hours. At the end of just five nights of restricted sleep, the study group showed significant increases in dysphoria, feelings of poor health, and unhappiness. Prior research involving longer periods of sleep restriction indicates that the negative mood swings may persist for weeks or months.

Night workers and rotating shiftworkers have a three to five-fold increase in psychosocial problems, such as an inability to find time for family obligations, community service, or other routine activities. Shiftwork has enormous social consequences that are exacerbated by the emotional vulnerability associated with reduced sleep time. The congressional Office of Technology Assessment has documented marital problems and community alienation as just two of the results of the strain imposed by work schedules.

> I have been a police officer for 12 years. The graveyard shift has always been difficult for me—hour on hour of futilely counting cracks in ceilings. I would sleep only 2-3 hours a day. I made adjustments. I cancelled many of my outside activities. I did not socialize with friends. Family relationships suffered dearly.
>
> —Witness, Commission Hearing, Portland, OR

Diminished Productivity and Impaired Performance

Over 30 years of laboratory research document the influence of sleep loss on human functioning. Sleepy individuals are less ambitious and less productive. Sleep loss impairs performance on cognitive tasks involving memory, learning, logical reasoning, arithmetic calculations, pattern recognition, complex verbal processing, and decision making. For example, reduction of sleep time to five hours a night for only two nights significantly reduces physiological levels of alertness, impairs vigilance, and worsens arithmetic ability and creative thinking. Loss of as little as three hours of sleep in a single night can slow human reaction time significantly, a change which can be dangerous in situations such as driving. Sleepiness due to normal circadian variation also clearly influences performance. A recent survey of 784 individuals who often experience jet lag found that 90 percent reported daytime sleepiness or fatigue; 78 percent noted difficulty sleeping at night; 69 percent reported impaired concentration; 66 percent experienced slowed physical reflexes; 50 percent noted irritability; 47 percent reported abnormal digestion, and 31 percent experienced depression. These findings are not new. As early as 1949, a study demonstrated that switchboard operators worked more slowly between midnight and 7:30 a.m.

Reports of low productivity or occasional errors during laboratory studies cannot convey the significance and impact of sleepiness in the real world. Sleepiness affects our safety each day, whether on the road, at home, or at work, where we may be vulnerable to the effects of our own sleepiness or the mistakes of other sleepy persons. Sleepiness on the job is widespread. In one study, 52 to 63 percent of night workers (in the utility, manufacturing, petroleum, and chemical industries) admitted to falling asleep on the job at least once a week. A study of train drivers found that 11 percent fell asleep on most or all night shifts; five percent of drivers reported falling asleep on most or all early morning shifts.

Increased Numbers of Accidents

Performance decrements due to sleepiness have been cited in reports about countless accidents. James Danaher, Chief of the Human Performance Division of the National Transportation Safety Board (NTSB), offered the following statement in testimony to the Commission:

> In recent years the [Safety] Board has investigated a number of major transportation accidents in which the effects of fatigue, sleepiness, sleep disorders and circadian factors contributed to the accidents. These and other experiences indicate that poor scheduling of work and rest time continue to adversely affect the performance of operating personnel in virtually all modes of transportation .... (and that) most employees and supervisors in the transportation industry do not receive training on the problems associated with work and rest schedules and the effects such schedules have on performance and safety.
>
> —Witness, Commission Hearing, Washington, DC

In the transportation field, the consequences of drowsiness can be especially serious because of the dangerous or valuable cargo carried and the traveling speeds of trains, airplanes, trucks, and buses. The consequences may be all the more serious when an accident occurs near a heavily populated site or a fragile ecosystem.

Accidents on the Road

Examination of single-vehicle, fatal-to-the-driver truck accidents (not due to alcohol consumption, drug use, or road conditions) showed that accidents are most common during the sleepy phase of the circadian alertness rhythm, despite the fact that fewer trucks are on the road at these times of day. Other similar data show fatigue-related accidents for all motor vehicles peak at times of day that correspond to the nighttime and mid-day troughs in alertness. Night and rotating shiftworkers are almost always out of synchrony with their biological clocks and are at higher risk for motor vehicle accidents.

Truck drivers, as others in the transportation industry, work long and irregular hours; sleepiness is pervasive, often with disastrous results. A study by the NTSB found that fatigue was the most common cause of fatal-to-the-driver truck accidents, involving 31 percent of such accidents. One example illustrates the potential consequences of a tanker truck crash. On the morning of May 20, 1991, at 7: 00 a.m., a tanker carrying 8,800 gallons of gasoline went off the road and exploded, and, according to a local newspaper, sparked "a fast-moving fire and halting northbound traffic for more than six hours." The 31-year-old driver admitted that he had fallen asleep at the wheel. He explained to authorities that "he was driving at about 67mph when he was jolted awake by the trailer hitting the guard rail. He swerved and lost control before the truck and its volatile cargo overturned and skidded down the pavement, (California Highway Patrol) Sgt. Doug Howell said."

There is reason to be concerned about other modes of transportation, such as taxis and school buses. It is not uncommon for these drivers to work around the clock. Intercity buses, in particular, are on the roads 24 hours a day, forcing some personnel, including drivers and mechanics, to work during the hours of high risk of falling asleep. Greyhound (which provides the country's only nationwide intercity bus service) transports 18 million passengers each year. A number of accidents involving Greyhound buses have been investigated by the NTSB; sleepiness was found to be a factor in several. En route to Buffalo, New York, on June 27, 1990, a driver fell asleep at the wheel (having attempted unsuccessfully to stay awake by smoking a cigarette, drinking coffee, and listening to loud music). The driver and 13 of the 21 passengers were injured. In late June 1991, another Greyhound driver dozed off at the wheel. According to newspaper reports, the driver "punched in at the Cleveland station at 3 a.m. Wednesday, and took over driving the bus at 7:20 a.m." After a stop in Pittsburgh, the bus left at 12:20 p.m. for Washington, D.C., traveling about 60 miles before the driver lost control of the bus and drove off a 20-foot embankment on the Pennsylvania Turnpike. One woman was killed and 15 others injured. On August 3, 1991, passengers on another Greyhound bus fell victim to a sleepy driver when the bus went off a New York highway and overturned at 6:15 a.m. A sheriff's deputy told the Associated Press, "It appears that from speaking to the individuals on the bus that the driver fell asleep several times on the way up (to Buffalo) and then he finally just fell asleep and lost control of the bus." More than 30 passengers suffered broken bones, cuts, and internal injuries; none was critically injured.

Sleep-related accidents on the highway are not limited to commercial vehicles; each day drivers have accidents while commuting to and from work, travelling for pleasure, or running personal errands. A causal relation between motor vehicle accidents and sleepiness is certain; the exact percentage of motor vehicle accidents directly caused by sleepy drivers is difficult to establish. According to the National Highway Transportation Safety Administration's Office of Crash Avoidance Research, of accidents reported to the police each year, driver fatigue/ drowsiness is cited as a factor in 72,000 of them, or in 1. 1 percent of all such crashes. Of all such accidents resulting in a serious injury, 14,000 or 3 percent are caused at least in part by driver fatigue; of those that result in fatalities, 1,550, or 3 percent, are caused by a fatigued driver.

The NHTSA believes that the number of accidents caused by driver fatigue is *actually much higher*. Many people simply are unwilling to blame sleepiness for the accident; police officers tend to cite factors other than fatigue (such as alcohol consumption or bad weather). A 1973 survey supports this belief. It reported that 69 percent of 1,500 drivers questioned had been drowsy at times while driving. Of that 69 percent, a full 10 percent admitted to having been involved in a fatigue-related accident and another 10 percent, to having come close to being involved in an accident. Statistics from Australia show driver fatigue and sleepiness to be major contributing factors in approximately 15 percent of fatal motor vehicle accidents and in 25 percent of all accidents on main highways.

In 1988, an 18-year-old high school senior from Oregon died in a car accident on his way home from his part-time job at a fast food restaurant. On the Sunday before the accident, he had worked from

6:00 p.m. until 11:30 p.m., and then drove 45 minutes to reach his home. He woke up on Monday morning at 6:30 a.m., as usual, in time to attend school. After school that afternoon, he reported to work for the 3:30 p.m. to 7:30 p.m. shift; he returned at midnight to clean, until he clocked out at 8:21 a.m. At 8:40 a.m.—having obtained only seven hours of sleep in the previous 48 hours—he apparently fell asleep at the wheel and was killed in a head-on collision with another vehicle. The driver of the other car still suffers the effects of a serious injury to his left leg and cannot return to his previous occupation.

On February 23, 1990, at around 5:00 p.m., while driving home on a New Hampshire highway, a young man, who had been designated as America's Safest Teen Driver, fell asleep at the wheel, killing himself and the 19-year-old female driver of another car. The police determined that alcohol was not involved in the accident; a witness stated that the young man's car slowed down without braking, and then drifted over the yellow line into oncoming traffic. The police believe that the teenager, who had won the use of the car in which he died at the National Driver's Excellence contest in July of 1989, had simply fallen asleep a short distance from his home. One newspaper quoted his father as saying, "Safe driving was an obsession with him. The question of why he didn't recognize the fatigue and respond to it is something we will never know."

One mother told the Commission at its Houston, Texas, hearing that her son "was killed, two years ago, in a car accident because he fell asleep at the wheel while coming home from working the night shift as a prison guard." Her son, who had worked nights in order to see his young daughter during the day, drove an hour to and from work. Although he wanted to transfer to a prison closer to home, he was required to work there for a few months before he could apply for another position. Tragically, "on October 29, 1989, he fell asleep at the wheel, drove off the road and struck a tree. The police say he was killed instantly." His mother went on to testify that since that day, "there have been two other accidents... involving prison guards driving home from the night shift at the Angleton Unit."

Rail Accidents

On Friday, November 22, 1991, just before 7:30 a.m., two trains collided and derailed on tracks outside Eugene, Oregon, causing serious damage to both trains. More than 8,000 gallons of diesel fuel were spilled and, subsequently, were ignited, creating significant traffic problems. The engineer of the train at fault admitted that he had fallen asleep while on duty. According to newspaper reports, the engineer, Barber, "awoke just in time to see a yellow warning signal through the fog as the train passed the north end of the siding. The caution signal indicated that the next signal ... would be red and that the engineer should be prepared to stop the train." He "activated the train's emergency braking system shortly before it struck the northbound train" but did not activate it soon enough, given the train's speed. Barber was certain that the cause of the accident was "fatigue stress" as he "was dead tired even before (his) shift began." Alcohol and drug testing revealed that drugs were not a factor in the accident. Considering his accumulated sleep debt and the time of the morning, it is not surprising that he fell asleep.

The following are additional examples:

- In 1984, Burlington Northern trains collided: five crew killed, two injured; $3.9 million in damages; probable cause, engineer of one train fell asleep.

- In 1988, Conrail trains collide: four crew killed; $6 million in damages; probable cause, sleep deprived condition of engineer and crew.

- In 1990, Santa Fe railway crash: four crew killed, two injured; $4.4 million in damages; probable cause, all of three-person crew on one train were sleeping.

Maritime Accidents

Shipboard personnel, also subject to excessive hours and shifting work schedules, have been implicated in sleepiness-related accidents as well. The *Exxon Valdez* disaster is the most well known sleep-related maritime accident, indeed, perhaps the most serious sleep-related accident in recent history. Although many believe the captain's alcohol impairment to have been the cause of the accident, in fact, he had left the ship's bridge almost 20 minutes before the grounding occurred. It was the third mate—who had slept only six hours the night prior to the grounding in addition to a brief afternoon nap after two tiring days of loading cargo—who was in charge of the ship at the time of the accident. Responsible for both navigating the ship and plotting its course, the third mate made errors guiding the vessel through the islands and ice of Prince William Sound. Despite two warning reports from the lookout, shortly after midnight on the night of March 24,

1989, the ship hit Bligh Reef. The NTSB named as the immediate cause of the disaster "the failure of the third mate to properly maneuver the vessel because of fatigue and excessive workload..."

The accident of the Greek tanker, *World Prodigy*, off the coast of Rhode Island on June 23, 1989, also was found to be related to sleepiness. The NTSB determined that the probable cause of the accident was "the master's impaired judgment from acute fatigue, which led to his decisions to decrease the bridge watch and to attend to nonessential tasks during a crucial period in the ship's navigation." While under the master's control, the Prodigy was grounded on a reef in Rhode Island Sound, causing 7,000 barrels of diesel oil to spill into the sound and causing damage in excess of a million dollars to the ship itself. The ship's master had been on duty for more than 33 hours when the accident occurred.

In one case, a passenger-car ferry ran aground near a small island off the coast of Puerto Rico; the NTSB ruled that the master's "assuming a watch while on medication and in a fatigued physical condition and his failure to maintain an adequate lookout" contributed to the accident. The master was fatigued as "insomnia and operational responsibilities had deprived (him) of sleep for a period of about 42 hours at the time of the grounding." The ship, worth $5 million, was considered a complete loss.

Airway Accidents

In the words of one airline pilot: "There have been times I've been so sleepy [that] I was nodding off as we were taxiing to get into takeoff position." Air traffic controllers and mechanics can be affected by both sleep deprivation and sleep disturbances. One tragic example of an accident, possibly related to performance on the night shift, is the 1988 Aloha Airlines flight in which a flight attendant was sucked out of the plane and killed after part of the airplane's fuselage broke off. The NTSB determined that a number of cracks in the rivet holes of the fuselage should have been noticed in a routine examination of the plane. To ensure that planes are available for daytime schedules, most maintenance examinations are conducted at night. This means that the maintenance of passenger airplanes is vulnerable to all the negative consequences of night work; the NTSB acknowledged this factor in its report.

Accidents in the Nuclear Industry

On March 28, 1979, around 4 a.m., a mechanical failure, unrecognized by tired shiftworkers, almost led to a meltdown in the unit two reactor of the Three Mile Island nuclear power plant. The U.S. Nuclear Regulatory Commission found that the human error of failing to recognize the loss of core coolant water (caused by a stuck valve), coupled with subsequent flawed corrective action, caused the reactor's near meltdown.

Accidents in Hospitals

By its very nature, the health care field is active 24 hours a day. In fact, a disproportionate number of emergency cases occur during the night shift. Thus, by necessity, many health workers are engaged in shiftwork. The sleep-related problems caused by shiftwork are complicated further by staff who work excessive hours each day. Medical residents notoriously have difficult schedules; when on call, they may work as many as 36 hours in a single shift. Estimates indicate that house staff rarely get more than three hours of sleep a night. Nurses and emergency personnel often are subjected to excessive hours, particularly in times of nursing shortages, when double shifts may be necessary.

Studies have demonstrated that sleep-deprived physicians commit a greater number of errors than do rested physicians. The consequences of this sleep deprivation can be extremely serious. Studies have shown that a disproportionate number of emergency cases occur during the night shift, the time at which the greatest number of shiftwork-related errors take place. A news magazine cover-story, appearing in November 1991, told of a medical resident who "fell asleep while sewing up a woman's uterus—and toppled onto the patient." In another incident, a fatigued "resident forgot to order a diabetic patient's nightly insulin shot and, instead, prescribed another medication. The man went into a coma." Not only are the physicians' mental skills impaired, their bedside manner may be improper as they lack the patience to deal with their patients calmly: "One young doctor admitted to abruptly cutting off the questions of a man who had just been told he had AIDS: 'All I could think of was going home to bed.'"

In 1984, in a widely publicized incident, an 18-year-old woman died in a New York hospital after receiving improper treatment for her condition, bilateral bronchopneumonia. An investigation into the patient's death, in part, implicated the fatigue experienced by the residents who treated her between the hours of 11:30 p.m. and 6:30 a.m. when she died. By 2:00 a.m., when the woman was admitted officially as an inpatient, the intern and junior resident caring for her had each been at work for 18 hours. Her condition was misdiagnosed; moreover, one resident prescribed an injection for one drug that was contraindicated. It seems likely that his sleepiness—compounded by the time of day—may have contributed to these errors.

Accidents in Military Operations

The consequences of sleep deprivation are of both human and economic concern to the military due to the high cost of the equipment and the nature of military activities, many of which occur at night. The impact of circadian factors on performance must be considered when decisions about nighttime activities are made; currently such consideration is rare.

Sleepiness in the military has had significant consequences. On April 21, 1987, a few minutes after midnight, a guided-missile frigate, the USS *Richard L Page*, hit a fishing ship which sank and was judged a total loss. At the time of the accident, despite limited visibility, the captain of the Page was testing his vessel's maximum speed. The Officer of the Deck (OOD) noted intermittent contacts on the radarscope, but since he could not identify the contact, decided that it was not an actual vessel, and thus did not report the contact to the captain. The NTSB found fault with the officer's actions and "attributed the OOD's behavior on the day of the accident partly to his long working hours and disrupted sleep pattern during the several days before the accident."

This sleep-related accident, unfortunately, is not an isolated incident. Around 4:45 on the morning of June 14, 1989, a U.S. Navy nuclear-powered attack submarine made contact with a civilian tug towing two barges in the San Pedro Channel off the coast of California. The antenna of the black, 360-foot-long submarine snagged the steel cable that linked the *Barcona* and the two barges. The 6,000 ton submarine easily dragged the 97-ton *Barcona* backwards. The tug sank; one tug crew member drowned. An investigation of the accident by the NTSB revealed that the crew of the Navy vessel had not ascertained adequately that the area was free of other ships; moreover, the watch duty engineer's sleep-deprived condition may have played a part in the accident. At 4:34 a.m., the submarine began its ascent; then, as the periscope surfaced, the engineer on watch duty "made three quick sweeps and reported 'no close contacts,' although the lights on the tiny Barcona and its two barges were just 300 yards away.

Because much military activity takes place at night, military personnel often need to sleep during the day, despite the influences of their circadian rhythm. To override the circadian rhythm, military forces in some countries have used medications to promote sleep. For example, during the Falkland Islands conflict, a benzodiazepine (temazepam) was administered to aviation crews during off-duty hours to induce sleep before they returned to flying duties. Israeli forces administered sleep-promoting hypnotics to troops during the deployment phase of the Entebbe raid. Yet, researchers are concerned about this practice. Specifically, a number of issues about their use remain unanswered, such as the amount and quality of sleep/rest obtained with particular drug doses, the capacity to awaken easily during drug-induced sleep, and the potential for lingering effects on performance after awakening.

Alcohol and Sleep Deprivation Are a Deadly Combination

Alcohol, rightfully, is regarded as a leading cause of motor vehicle accidents; it is not widely known that the combination of alcohol and sleepiness may be more deadly than alcohol alone. The finding that mild alcohol consumption exacerbates sleepiness markedly has led investigators to hypothesize that the addition of the sedative effects of alcohol to an already sleepy individual may cause accidents, due not to motor or visual impairment from drunkenness, but to falling asleep at the wheel. While studies have shown that ethanol consumption increases one's sleep latency, a Danish study examined the visual-motor reaction time of intoxicated drivers to determine whether feelings of fatigue increased the effects of alcohol. The study found that those who stated they were very tired reacted significantly slower than the other two groups who considered themselves to be either tired or rested. The difference between the reaction time of those who were rested and those who were very tired was large—approximately 30 percent. The study concluded that fatigue is more important as a factor in road safety that it is currently considered.

A recent study of the sedative effects of alcohol showed that the same low dose of alcohol produced no sedation in individuals given the dose immediately after 10 hours of nighttime sleep. Moderate sedation was experienced by individuals who had been spending eight hours in bed at night. Those who had slept for only five hours in nighttime sleep felt marked sedation. When one considers that, in general, we are likely to feel more sleepy on a Friday evening than on a Monday evening, the potential consequences of the common "Friday evening happy hour after work are frightening.

Despite these findings, many drivers continue to operate motor vehicles while under the influence of medications and/or alcohol, endangering themselves and others. In fact, according to a Gallup poll, 61 percent of those who take allergy medications that warn against driving say they ignore the warning and drive anyway.

Cost of Sleep Deprivation

The dearth of available data precludes a precise assessment of the direct costs of sleep-related errors and accidents. However, extrapolations from existing information suggest that these costs may be in the tens of billions of dollars. For example, a recent report estimated the cost of diminished productivity due to shiftwork at $70 billion per year. A health care economist working with the Commission developed an estimate of the cost of sleep-related accidents, using both data on accidents and injuries in America and best estimates from the scientific literature on sleep deprivation. He arrived at an estimate of $46 billion a year for these sleep-related accidents. In comparison, the effect of stress on workplace productivity has been estimated at $150 billion a year.

The precise cost of accidents related to sleepiness is difficult to calculate because investigators tend to ignore the role of sleepiness in determining the cause of accidents. Sleepiness is not a standard consideration in assessing the causes of accidents, as is alcohol or drug consumption, or faulty equipment. This is true, in part, because sleepiness is not a concrete factor but more often a contributing factor (not to mention that the feeling of tiredness is subjective) and not usually determined to be the cause of the accident; thus, many minor accidents associated with sleepiness remain unidentified. Yet, the Commission's review of a number of accidents shows that all too often, sleepiness is a factor in tragedies; a portion of the cost of accidents of all types is attributable to sleepiness.

The cost of accidents in certain industries, such as transportation and manufacturing, can be extreme. For example, the property damage-related costs of the 1991 Oregon train accident are estimated at no less than $3.3 million. Additional costs include those associated with the government investigation into the accident, with the need to extinguish the fire caused by the spilled diesel fuel and to clean the accident's residue, and with the lost commerce caused by the closing of the track and a nearby highway. An example of even greater magnitude is the *Exxon Valdez*. Property damage and clean-up expenses were in excess of $2.5 billion; the environmental damage is incalculable.

The National Safety Council estimated that workplace accidents in 1990 cost our Nation $63.8 billion. (This figure includes medical expenses, lost wages as a result of increased morbidity and mortality rates, property damage, insurance administration, and uninsured work loss—defined as the value of time lost by uninjured workers affected by the accident, perhaps by investigating and reporting injuries, giving first aid, and losing production time.)

Further, the cost of lawsuits is not included in the estimate of sleep-related accidents. This cost is not insignificant. For example, a serious trucking accident in Texas generated three lawsuits. Two were settled out of court: the first with the trucking company's insurance carrier paying the survivors of the deceased $5 million; and the second with the automobile manufacturer paying $325,000 to the same. While the third suit, brought against the manufacturers of the tractor and trailer, was decided in favor of the manufacturers, the cost of defending the suit was approximately $3 million. These costs, considered related costs, must be considered as part of the cost of accidents related to sleepiness.

Despite the association between mortality and habitual short sleep duration, the absence of data precludes us from calculating the cost of this presumably higher mortality rate to society. Equally, we cannot calculate the cost associated with increased morbidity. However, a simple extrapolation provides some insight. If one considers that there are a minimum of seven million full-time night and rotating shiftworkers, and that the 1990 mean fee for an office visit to a physician for an established patient was $39.87 and for a new patient was $74.84, the resulting estimated cost is not trivial. The evidence that this sleepiness imposes a substantial toll on our Nation is clear; now, steps to reduce this cost must be taken.

Conclusions

Few Americans appear to know the facts that are most important. One, sleep loss is cumulative. Two, the sleep debt and chronic sleep deprivation are camouflaged by endogenous and exogenous stimulation and circadian rhythm effects. Thus, an individual may not feel sleepy at one time of the day, but may experience the sudden onset of completely disabling drowsiness when all stimulating influences are withdrawn. This is what happened to the third mate on the bridge of the *Exxon Valdez* a few minutes after midnight on the night of the grounding, as well as to countless drivers at about the same time of the day. Three, adolescents appear to need as much sleep as older children and perhaps more and, thus, the marked reduction of time in bed that occurs during adolescence has profound and far reaching consequences. Four, napping can immediately relieve dangerous drowsiness. In their uneducated state, most Americans attribute causality to situations or activities that actually only reduce stimulation and unmask the sleep debt or sleep drive. These include monotony, a heavy meal which reduces the stimulation of hunger, a warm room, and relaxation (muscle activity is the best way to postpone falling asleep). None of these activities or situations causes sleepiness if an individual has had all the sleep that he or she needs.

The Commission has found that the mission of society is seriously undermined by chronic sleep deprivation and fatigue. Knowing the facts of sleep and sleep deprivation can only help our citizens foster the growth of a safe and productive society. Such education will also provide the knowledge to create a mandate for the research that will lead to more effective countermeasures to sleepiness, whatever the cause.

The purpose of calculating the costs of sleep deprivation to American society is to guide priorities in dealing with the various causes and consequences of sleep deprivation. The Commission has found that very little effort has been made to develop either methodology or databases that would make such an effort feasible. In addition, sleep deprivation as a cause of sleepiness is often intertwined with sleep disorders and circadian factors. However, the initial focus of estimating costs of workplace errors, accidents, and diminished productivity should be on the consequences of severe, dangerous sleepiness and impaired performance, regardless of cause.

The Commission believes that sleep deprivation and its consequences could be largely reversed if society had the motivation to do so. Such motivation, particularly in the workplace and transportation industry, is more likely to be enhanced by accurate cost estimates than by appeals to humanitarian concerns. The Commission believes that an accountable entity is essential to provide leadership in such an effort.

Chapter 5

Problem Sleepiness

What Is Problem Sleepiness?

Everyone feels sleepy at times. However, when sleepiness interferes with daily routines and activities, or reduces the ability to function, it is called "problem sleepiness." A person can be sleepy without realizing it. For example, a person may not feel sleepy during activities such as talking and listening to music at a party, but the same person can fall asleep while driving home afterward.

You may have problem sleepiness if you:

- consistently do not get enough sleep, or get poor quality sleep;
- fall asleep while driving;
- struggle to stay awake when inactive, such as when watching television or reading;
- have difficulty paying attention or concentrating at work, school, or home;
- have performance problems at work or school;
- are often told by others that you are sleepy;
- have difficulty remembering;
- have slowed responses;
- difficulty controlling your emotions; or
- take naps on most days.

NIH Pub. No. 97-407, September 1997

What Causes Problem Sleepiness?

Sleepiness can be due to the body's natural daily sleep-wake cycles, inadequate sleep, sleep disorders, or certain drugs.

Sleep-Wake Cycle

Each day there are two periods when the body experiences a natural tendency toward sleepiness: during the late night hours (generally between midnight and 7 a.m.) and again during the midafternoon (generally between 1 p.m. and 4 p.m.). If people are awake during these times, they have a higher risk of falling asleep unintentionally, especially if they haven't been getting enough sleep.

Inadequate Sleep

The amount of sleep needed each night varies among people. Each person needs a particular amount of sleep in order to be fully alert throughout the day. Research has shown that when healthy adults are allowed to sleep unrestricted, the average time slept is 8 to 8.5 hours. Some people need more than that to avoid problem sleepiness; others need less.

If a person does not get enough sleep, even on one night, a "sleep debt" begins to build and increases until enough sleep is obtained. Problem sleepiness occurs as the debt accumulates. Many people do not get enough sleep during the work week and then sleep longer on the weekends or days off to reduce their sleep debt. If too much sleep has been lost, sleeping in on the weekend may not completely reverse the effects of not getting enough sleep during the week.

Sleep Disorders

Sleep disorders such as sleep apnea, narcolepsy, restless legs syndrome, and insomnia can cause problem sleepiness. *Sleep apnea* is a serious disorder in which a person's breathing is interrupted during sleep, causing the individual to awaken many times during the night and experience problem sleepiness during the day. People with *narcolepsy* have excessive sleepiness during the day, even after sleeping enough at night. They may fall asleep at inappropriate times and places. *Restless legs syndrome* (RLS) causes a person to experience unpleasant sensations in the legs, often described as creeping, crawling, pulling, or painful. These sensations frequently occur in the evening, making it difficult for people with RLS to fall asleep, leading to problem sleepiness during the day.

Insomnia is the perception of poor-quality sleep due to difficulty falling asleep, waking up during the night with difficulty returning to sleep, waking up too early in the morning, or unrefreshing sleep. Any of these sleep disorders can cause problem sleepiness.

Medical Conditions/Drugs

Certain medical conditions and drugs, including prescription medications, can also disrupt sleep and cause problem sleepiness. Examples include:

- Chronic illnesses such as asthma, congestive heart failure, rheumatoid arthritis, or any other chronically painful disorder;

- Some medications to treat high blood pressure, some heart medications, and asthma medications such as theophylline;

- Alcohol—Although some people use alcohol to help themselves fall asleep, it causes sleep disruption during the night, which can lead to problem sleepiness during the day. Alcohol is also a sedating drug that can, even in small amounts, make a sleepy person much more sleepy and at greater risk for car crashes and performance problems;

- Caffeine—Whether consumed in coffee, tea, soft drinks, or medications, caffeine makes it harder for many people to fall asleep and stay asleep. Caffeine stays in the body for about 3 to 7 hours, so even when taken earlier in the day it can cause problems with sleep at night; and

- Nicotine from cigarettes or a skin patch is a stimulant and makes it harder to fall asleep and stay asleep.

Problem Sleepiness and Adolescents

Many U.S. high school and college students have signs of problem sleepiness, such as:

- difficulty getting up for school;
- failing asleep at school; and/or
- struggling to stay awake while doing homework.

The need for sleep may be 9 hours or more per night as a person goes through adolescence. At the same time, many teens begin to show a preference for a later bed time, which may be due to a biological change. Teens tend to stay up later but have to get up early for school, resulting in their getting much less sleep than they need.

Many factors contribute to problem sleepiness in teens and young adults, but the main causes are not getting enough sleep and irregular sleep schedules. Some of the factors that influence adolescent sleep include:

- social activities with peers that lead to later bedtimes;
- homework to be done in the evenings;
- early wake-up times due to early school start times;
- parents being less involved in setting and enforcing bedtimes; and
- employment, sports, or other extracurricular activities that decrease the time available for sleep.

Teens and young adults who do not get enough sleep are at risk for problems such as:

- automobile crashes;
- poor performance in school and poor grades;
- depressed moods; and
- problems with peer and adult relationships.

Many adolescents have part-time jobs in addition to their classes and other activities. High school students who work more than 20 hours per week have more problem sleepiness and may use more caffeine, nicotine, and alcohol than those who work less than 20 hours per week or not at all.

Shift Work and Problem Sleepiness

About 20 million Americans (20 to 25 percent of workers) perform shift work. Most shift workers get less sleep over 24 hours than day workers. Sleep loss is greatest for night shift workers, those who work early morning shifts, and female shift workers with children at home. About 60 to 70 percent of shift workers have difficulty sleeping and/or problem sleepiness.

The human sleep-wake system is designed to prepare the body and mind for sleep at night and wakefulness during the day. These natural rhythms make it difficult to sleep during daylight hours and to stay awake during the night hours, even in people who are well rested.

It is possible that the human body never completely adjusts to night-time activity and daytime sleep, even in those who work permanent night shifts.

In addition to the sleep-wake system, environmental factors can influence sleepiness in shift workers. Because our society is strongly day-oriented, shift workers who try to sleep during the day are often interrupted by noise, light, telephones, family members, and other distractions. In contrast, the nighttime sleep of day workers is largely protected by social customs that keep noises and interruptions to a minimum.

Problem sleepiness in shift workers may result in:

- increased risk for automobile crashes, especially while driving home after the night shift;

- decreased quality of life;

- decreased productivity (night work performance may be slower and less accurate than day performance); and/or

- increased risk of accidents and injuries at work.

What Can Help?

Sleep—There Is No Substitute!

Many people simply do not allow enough time for sleep on a regular basis. A first step may be to evaluate daily activities and sleep-wake patterns to determine how much sleep is obtained. If you are consistently getting less than 8 hours of sleep per night, more sleep may be needed. A good approach is to gradually move to an earlier bedtime. For example, if an extra hour of sleep is needed, try going to bed 15 minutes earlier each night for four nights and then keep the last bedtime. This method will increase the amount of time in bed without causing a sudden change in schedule. However, if work or family schedules do not permit the earlier bedtime, a 30- to 60-minute daily nap may help.

Medications/Drugs

In general, medications do not help problem sleepiness, and some make it worse. Caffeine can reduce sleepiness and increase alertness, but only temporarily. It can also cause problem sleepiness to become worse by interrupting sleep.

While alcohol may shorten the time it takes to fall asleep, it can disrupt sleep later in the night, and therefore add to the problem sleepiness.

Medications may be prescribed for patients in certain situations. For example, the short-term use of sleeping pills has been shown to be helpful in patients diagnosed with acute insomnia. Long-term use of sleep medication is recommended only for the treatment of specific sleep disorders.

If You're Sleepy—Don't Drive!

A person who is sleepy and drives is at high risk for an automobile crash. Planning ahead may help reduce that risk. For example, the following tips may help when planning a long distance car trip:

- Get a good night's sleep before leaving.

- Avoid driving between midnight and 7 a.m.

- Change drivers often to allow for rest periods.

- Schedule frequent breaks.

If you are a shift worker, the following may help:

- decreasing the amount of night work;

- increasing the total amount of sleep by adding naps and lengthening the amount of time allotted for sleep;

- increasing the intensity of light at work;

- having a predictable schedule of night shifts;

- eliminating sound and light in the bedroom during daytime sleep;

- using caffeine (only during the first part of the shift) to promote alertness at night; or

- possibly using prescription sleeping pills to help daytime sleep on an occasional basis (check with your doctor).

If you think you are getting enough sleep, but still feel sleepy during the day, check with your doctor to be sure your sleepiness is not due to a sleep disorder.

Where to Get More Information

For additional information on sleep and sleep disorders, contact the following offices of the National Heart, Lung, and Blood Institute of the National Institutes of Health:

National Center on Sleep Disorders Research (NCSDR)

The NCSDR supports research, scientist training, dissemination of health information, and other activities on sleep and sleep disorders. The NCSDR also coordinates sleep research activities with other Federal agencies and with public and nonprofit organizations.

National Center on Sleep Disorders Research
National Institutes of Health
Two Rockledge Centre Suite 7024 6701
Rockledge Drive, MSC 7920
Bethesda, MD 20892-7920
(301) 435-0199
(301) 480-3451 (fax)

National Heart, Lung, and Blood Institute Information Center

The Information Center acquires, analyzes, promotes, maintains, and disseminates programmatic and educational information related to sleep and sleep disorders. Write for a list of available publications or to order additional copies of this fact sheet.

NHLBI Information Center
P.O. Box 30105
Bethesda, MD 20824-0105
(301) 251-1222
(301) 251-1223 (fax)
http://www.nhlbi.nih.gov/nhlbi/nhlbi.htm

Chapter 6

Does Exercise Truly Enhance Sleep?

In Brief: Two recent studies support the common sense view that exercise improves sleep in individuals with insomnia, but questions still abound. Do patients have to be fit to reap the benefits of exercise? Does exposure to bright light during exercise enhance sleep? Is shorter, more intense exercise more helpful than longer, more moderate activities? Does exercising too close to bedtime inhibit sleep? In considering recent research on sleep and exercise, this article addresses such questions and also looks at the relationship of exercise and sleep to anxiety, depression, circadian rhythms, and age-associated problems, such as sleep apnea.

Insomnia afflicts about a third of the adult population and is associated with increased mortality, psychiatric disturbances, and decreased work productivity (1,2). Because sleeping pills—the most common treatment for insomnia—are associated with increased mortality (2), medication tolerance and dependence, and a host of negative side effects (3), they are seldom recommended for long-term use. Hence, clinicians and patients have shown increased interest in cognitive and behavioral strategies for improving sleep.

One behavioral strategy is exercise. Epidemiologic survey studies (4,5) indicate that daytime exercise is the behavior most closely associated with improved sleep in the general populace. Since exercise

Reprinted with permission from *The Physician and Sportsmedicine*, Volume 25, Number 10, October 1997. © 1997 The McGraw-Hill Companies.

elicits physical fatigue and because its physiologic and psychological calming effects are well established, the notion that exercise promotes sleep may seem like common sense. This common sense view has been reinforced for years in the lay and scientific literature, but the experimental evidence that exercise promotes sleep is not compelling. In addition, the changes in sleep that follow exercise have not been shown to influence daytime cognitive functioning or alertness, and little is known about the effects of exercise on people who have sleep disturbances.

Exercise and Insomnia

Two recent studies (6,7), however, suggest that exercise training may improve sleep among insomniacs. Guilleminault et al. (6) randomly assigned 30 individuals (average age 44) who had psychophysiologic insomnia to three different 4-week treatments. One treatment consisted of sleep hygiene education, such as encouraging the subjects to maintain a fixed sleep-wake schedule and to avoid daytime napping. Another treatment included sleep hygiene education and light therapy that involved patients sitting in front of a bright light (3,000 lux) for 45 minutes beginning 5 minutes after awakening. (Bright light exposure can improve sleep, particularly for people with abnormally phased circadian rhythms (8)). A third treatment involved sleep hygiene education and 45 minutes of brisk daily walking in the early evening.

Wrist actigraphy measurements taken the week before and after each 4-week protocol indicated that the regimens that included exercise and light elicited greater improvements in sleep (an increase of 17 and 54 min/night respectively) compared with sleep hygiene education alone (a decrease of 3 min/night). Similar findings were observed from self-reported sleep assessments via sleep diaries.

Though the data suggest that exercise can relieve insomnia, other issues may confound the study's findings. The exercise-related improvements in sleep could have been linked to the subjects' exposure to outdoor light during exercise and at other times of the day. Unfortunately, the study did not provide information regarding such exposure, nor about patient adherence to the treatments. Another confounder may have been the subjects' different expectations for improved sleep associated with each protocol.

In another study, King et al. (7) randomly assigned 43 older individuals (ages 50 to 76) with moderate sleep complaints to a 16-week exercise program or to a waiting list control condition. The exercise group performed 30 to 40 minutes of moderate aerobic exercise four times per week during the day or early evening. Based on sleep diaries and the Pittsburgh Sleep Quality Index (9)—a standardized, subjective measure of sleep quality—the exercise group showed significantly greater improvements in sleep.

Self-reported measures of sleep, however, do not always correspond with objective measures of sleep, especially in insomniacs. Self-reported measures can be skewed because individuals commonly expect exercise to promote sleep. The data may also have been confounded by environmental influences, such as exposure to bright light, or by the adoption of sleep-promoting habits that were not assessed, such as reduced caffeine consumption. Moreover, the data failed to delineate whether the reported sleep improvements were the result of chronic or repeated acute exercise.

Despite the limitations of these pioneering studies, they provide tantalizing evidence that exercise may promote sleep in individuals with insomnia. Whether exercise promotes sleep among all individuals or whether improvements in sleep can be attributed to exercise per se will require further research.

Acute Exercise and Sleep

Most studies on the relationship between exercise and sleep have focused on the influence of acute exercise. A recent meta-analysis by Youngstedt et al. (10) of 38 studies examined the average effect of acute exercise on sleep and the variables that may moderate this effect. In all studies, sleep was assessed by polysomnography, and the stages of sleep were determined by standard criteria.

The analysis concluded that a single bout of exercise:

- had no effect on the time it took to fall asleep;

- elicited statistically significant but small increases in total sleep time (average, 10 minutes) and in the amount of slow-wave sleep (average, 4 minutes); and

- elicited statistically significant but small decreases in rapid eye movement (REM) sleep (average, 7 minutes) and increases in the time for REM sleep to occur following sleep onset (average, 13 minutes).

These studies focused exclusively on subjects who are good sleepers. Although these findings indicate that the effects of acute exercise are small, these effects may still be noteworthy. Since even sleeping pills can have little influence on good sleepers (11,12), the small size of the exercise-related effects doesn't necessarily undermine their importance. On the other hand, because the studies focus on good sleepers, the findings indicate nothing about the effects of acute exercise on individuals suffering from sleep disturbances. In fact, I am unaware of any studies that have examined the effects of acute exercise in these individuals.

Factors Affecting Exercise and Sleep

Several factors may potentially moderate the effects of sleep on exercise, including the subjects' level of fitness, the heat load and duration of exercise, when exercise is performed, and the subjects' exposure to bright light. Analyzing these factors may help us understand the mechanisms by which exercise influences sleep and the parameters that most influence sleep.

Fitness. Some researchers (13) have speculated that only fit subjects are capable of performing the intense, exhaustive exercise assumed necessary for sleep enhancement. Since unfit subjects cannot achieve the level of exercise that may be required for improved sleep, the argument goes, exercise may benefit them less than it benefits fit individuals. An alternative explanation might be that exercise benefits the unfit less because it elicits more prolonged physiologic arousal in the unfit, thus inhibiting their sleep. However, experimental evidence (10) indicates that fitness does not influence the effects of acute exercise on sleep, and these data are consistent with surveys that show that exercise promotes sleep in the general population.

Body temperature. A popular explanation for the effects of exercise on sleep has been the thermogenic hypothesis, which posits that exercise promotes sleep by heating the body or brain. This hypothesis is consistent with evidence that passive body heating—via hot tub or sauna—increases slow-wave sleep (14). Neurophysiologic evidence (15) also suggests an interaction between heat loss and sleep mechanisms in the anterior hypothalamus that are activated when temperature is elevated. Hence, exercise may act as a thermogenic stimulus to enhance sleep.

The primary impetus behind the thermogenic hypothesis has been a study by Horne and Moore (16) showing that increases in slow-wave sleep following exercise were reversed by cooling the body during exercise. The results of this study, though, are questionable because body temperature during sleep was not assessed, and exercise was performed approximately 6 hours before bedtime, apparently enough time for the body to return to a normal temperature before sleep. Furthermore, our meta-analysis (10) revealed no modulating thermogenic effect of exercise on sleep. These inconsistencies suggest the need for further testing of the thermogenic hypothesis.

Another issue for such research is the level of exercise that would benefit the most people. Since body temperature increases during exercise as a function of exercise intensity, the thermogenic hypothesis would suggest that the more intense the exercise, the greater the sleep enhancement. Since the general public tends to exercise at lower intensities, the thermogenic hypothesis would also suggest that exercise would not enhance most people's sleep. However, if less intense exercise is just as efficacious for sleep, as evidence suggests (10), then more people may be able to improve their sleep with exercise.

Exercise duration. Our recent meta-analysis indicated that exercise duration was one of the most important factors modulating the influence of exercise on sleep. For example, as exercise duration increased beyond 1 hour per day, total sleep time became progressively greater. Further research is needed to confirm whether very prolonged exercise may increase total sleep time. Even if research does so, the practical usefulness of such evidence is questionable since most people are unlikely to exercise for the 1 hour per day that the studies found necessary to reliably improve sleep.

Exercise timing. A common assumption is that vigorous exercise right before bedtime disrupts sleep. However, this issue has not been adequately addressed in the literature because most studies' exercise protocols were completed at least 4 hours before sleep.

Recent evidence (17) challenges the assumption that late-night exercise disturbs sleep. In aerobically fit subjects, sleep was not adversely affected by a 1-hour bout of exercise at 60% VO2 max or by 3 hours of exercise at 70% VO2 max completed 30 minutes before bedtime. These results could be explained by quicker postexercise physiologic recovery among physically fit individuals. On the other hand, a population survey (5) indicated that exercise within 2 hours of bedtime improved or had no effect on sleep for most individuals. Since the evening is often convenient for exercise, individuals should include evening as they experiment to find the most suitable exercise time.

Exposure to bright light. Inadequate exposure to bright light has been associated with disturbed sleep. Conversely, bright light exposure can elicit quick and dramatic improvements in sleep. While the average adult receives only about 20 minutes of daily exposure to bright light—more than 2,500 lux (18)—it is reasonable to suppose that individuals who exercise regularly outdoors receive at least three times this much.

Though our meta-analysis (10) generally failed to reveal whether exercise performed indoors or outdoors affected subjects' sleep differently, our analysis was limited by the studies' lack of information about their subjects' illumination during exercise and throughout the day. In light of the recent study (6) suggesting that bright light exposure may enhance sleep more than exercise, this issue needs to be examined more carefully. There may be interesting synergistic effects of exercise and bright light on sleep.

Anxiety and Depression

Anxiety is perhaps the primary cause of insomnia, particularly transitory, situational insomnia. Since exercise has been shown to reduce psychophysiologic and subjective indices of anxiety, and anxiolytic behavioral treatments have been effective for insomnia, it is plausible that exercise may promote sleep by reducing anxiety. The one study (19) that explored this mechanism was inconclusive: Although subjects who exercised had significantly reduced anxiety 20 minutes after exercise when compared with sedentary controls, there was no difference between the two groups' anxiety levels at bedtime (4 to 6 hours after exercise) and no association between anxiety level at bedtime and sleep.

Chronic exercise may also promote sleep by its antidepressant effects. Depression is associated with disturbed sleep and REM sleep abnormalities, which are frequently reversed with remission of depression. Acute exercise delays REM onset and reduces the total amount of REM sleep (10). Vogel et al (20) have argued that these REM effects are the mechanism by which all antidepressant treatments work.

The Biological Clock

Poor sleep is one of the primary symptoms resulting from working different shifts (shift work) or jetting across multiple time zones. It can largely be attributed to a person's circadian pacemaker—which controls sleep and wakefulness—being out of synchrony with his or her changed sleep-wake schedule. (Poor sleep is also associated with aging [see "Exercise and Sleep Problems of Older Patients," below]). Because about 48 million passengers return from international flights annually and 50 million people in the United States are engaged in some form of shift work (21), the potential health consequences of air travel and shift work are significant.

Evidence now suggests that exercise can elicit substantial shifts in circadian rhythm phase in humans (22) and rodents (23), comparable to shifts that occur in response to bright light. Moreover, research on rodents suggests that appropriately timed exercise and exposure to light can have synergistic phase-shifting effects (24). Therefore, it is plausible that appropriately timed exercise can improve sleep for shift workers and air travelers.

Circadian phase delays have been consistently observed following late-night or early-morning exercise (10 pm to 4 am). Recently, Eastman et al. (25) found that exercise during a simulated graveyard shift (midnight to 8 am) allowed subjects to adjust more quickly to a daytime-sleep and nighttime-work schedule.

Exercise before bedtime (10 pm to midnight local time) following westward travel across two to five time zones might similarly enhance circadian adjustment and, therefore, improve sleep. It is unknown whether exercise in humans might have analogous circadian phase-advancing effects appropriate for eastward travel across multiple time zones.

The Exercise-Sleep Riddle

While most people have assumed that exercise promotes sleep, the potential adverse effects of exercise on sleep have received little attention. Anecdotal evidence suggests that overtraining can disturb sleep. Overtraining occurs in competitive athletes and fitness enthusiasts and is associated with other physiologic and psychological markers of distress such as elevated cortisol and depression. Experimental (26) and anecdotal (4) evidence demonstrates that discontinuing regular exercise will cause disrupted sleep, a sign of possible dependency. Such evidence may mean that exercise, like other sleep medicine, could have limitations and potential dangers.

Clearly, further research is needed to explore the effects of exercise on sleep and to establish whether they can be attributed to exercise or associated factors. A formal exercise prescription for sleep problems is not justified until such research results are available.

Nonetheless, clinicians and scientists still can suggest exercise as a means of improving sleep (see "Steps to Promote Sleep," below). Based on epidemiologic evidence and recent experimental evidence with insomniacs, the suggestions seem reasonable, especially if exercise is part of an overall treatment program and suggested with the patient's understanding that it may produce little or no improvement in sleep. Even if exercise does not improve sleep, it should still be recommended because exercise can reduce overall mortality and morbidity.

References

1. National Commission on Sleep Disorders Research: *Wake Up America: A National Sleep Alert, Executive Summary and Executive Report*. 1993;1:1-76

2. Kripke DF, Simons RN, Garfinkel L, et al: Short and long sleep and sleeping pills: is increased mortality associated? *Arch Gen Psychiatry* 1979;36(1):103-116

3. American Psychiatric Association. *Benzodiazepine Dependence, Toxicity, and Abuse: A Task Force Report of the American Psychiatric Association*. Washington DC, American Psychiatric Association, 1990

4. Vuori I, Urponen H, Hasan J, et al: Epidemiology of exercise effects on sleep. *Acta Physiol Scand* 1988;574:3-7

5. Hasan J, Urponen H, Vuori I, et al: Exercise habits and sleep in a middle-aged Finnish population. *Acta Physiol Scand* 1988;574:33-35

6. Guilleminault C, Clerk A, Black J, et al: Nondrug treatment trials in psychophysiologic insomnia. *Ann Intern Med* 1995;155(8):838-844

7. King AC, Oman RF, Brassington GS, et al: Moderate-intensity exercise and self-rated quality of sleep in older adults: a randomized controlled trial. *JAMA* 1997;277(1):32-37

8. Campbell SS, Dawson D, Anderson MW: Alleviation of sleep maintenance insomnia with timed exposure to bright light. *J Am Geriatr Soc* 1993;41:829-836

9. Buysse DJ, Reynolds CF III, Monk TH, et al: The Pittsburgh Sleep Quality Index: a new instrument for psychiatric practice and research. *Psychiatry Res* 1989;28(2):193-213

10. Youngstedt SD, O'Connor PJ, Dishman RK: The effects of acute exercise on sleep: a quantitative synthesis. *Sleep* 1997;20(3):203-214

11. Mendelson WB: Effects of flurazepam and zolpidem on the perception of sleep in normal volunteers. *Sleep* 1995;18(2):88-91

12. Terzano MG, Parrino L: Evaluation of EEG cyclic alternating pattern during sleep in insomniacs and controls under placebo and acute treatment with zolpidem. *Sleep* 1992;15(1):64-70

13. Horne JA: The effects of exercise upon sleep: a critical review. *Biol Psychol* 1981;12(4):241-290

14. Bunnell DE, Agnew JA, Horvath SM, et al: Passive body heating and sleep: influence of proximity to sleep. *Sleep* 1988; 11(2):210-219

15. McGinty D, Szymusiak R: Keeping cool: a hypothesis about the mechanisms and functions of slow wave sleep. *Trends Neurosci* 1990;13(12):480-487

16. Horne JA, Moore VJ: Sleep EEG effects of exercise with and without additional body cooling. *Electroencephal Clin Neurophysiol* 1985;60(1):33-38

17. Youngstedt SD, Kripke DF: Late night exercise does not disrupt sleep in physically active individuals. *Sleep Res* 1997;26:222

18. Espiritu RC, Kripke DF, Ancoli-Israel S, et al: Low illumination by San Diego adults: association with atypical depressive symptoms. *Biol Psychiatry* 1994;35(16):403-407

19. Youngstedt SD, O'Connor PJ, Dishman RK, et al: Influence of exercise on caffeine-induced insomnia. *Sleep Res* 1995;24:144

20. Vogel GW, Buffenstein A, Minter K, et al: Drug effects on REM sleep and on endogenous depression. *Neurosci Biobehav Rev* 1990;14(1):49-63

21. Monk TH: Shift work, in Kryger MH, Roth T, Dement WC (eds): *Principles and Practices of Sleep Medicine*, Philadelphia, WB Saunders, 1994, pp 471-476

22. Van Reeth O, Sturis J, Byrne MM, et al: Nocturnal exercise phase delays circadian rhythms of melatonin and thyrotropin secretion in normal men. *Am J Physiol* 1994;266(6 pt 1):E964-E974

23. Reebs SG, Mrosovsky N: Large phase-shifts of circadian rhythms caused by induced running in a re-entrainment paradigm: the role of pulse duration and light. *J Comp Physiol (A)* 1989;165(6):819-825

24. Mrosovsky N: Double-pulse experiments with nonphotic and photic phase-shifting stimuli. *J Biol Rhythms* 1991;6(2):167-179

25. Eastman CI, Hoese EK, Youngstedt SD, et al: Phase-shifting human circadian rhythms with exercise during the night shift. *Physiol Behav* 1995;58(6):1287-1291

26. Baekeland F: Exercise deprivation: sleep and psychological reactions. *Arch Gen Psychiatry* 1970;22(4):365-369

Exercise and Sleep Problems of Older Patients

Many of the sleep problems associated with aging, including sleep fragmentation, early-morning awakening, daytime sleepiness, and frequent napping, may be attributed to abnormal circadian phase or a dampened circadian rhythm amplitude, thought to indicate reduced strength of the circadian oscillator. In addition to shifting circadian phase, regular exercise may also strengthen the circadian oscillator, thus helping the older person to sleep at night and remain awake in the day.

Support for this hypothesis is provided by studies that show that complete activity restriction results in dramatic fragmentation of sleep throughout the day, even in young, healthy individuals (1) Further, a recent study by Van Someren et al. (2) found that 3 months of exercise training significantly reduced fragmentation of the rest-activity rhythm in older men (average age 73), a change that may enhance daytime wakefulness and nighttime sleep.

Sleep apnea. Sleep apnea and periodic leg movements during sleep (PLMS) increase with age and have been associated with disturbed sleep. Obstructive sleep apnea can often be attributed to excessive fat deposits in the upper airway. This condition is treated by surgery or with the use of a nasal mask that provides continuous positive pressure to the upper airway.

Many patients, however, cannot tolerate the masks, and surgery is not always effective. Exercise may be an effective alternative or adjuvant treatment because it may reduce the upper-airway fat deposits.

Leg movements. Exercise may also help patients whose sleep is disturbed by leg movements. In our lab, we have observed that PLMS can occur from 100 to 1,000 times throughout the night. PLMS is related to restless legs syndrome (RLS), characterized by "creepy-crawly" sensations in the lower legs and an irresistible urge to move the legs that occur just after lying down for sleep. Both conditions may be attributed to inadequate dopamine stores or neurotransmission. Dopaminergic drugs have been used to treat PLMS and RLS but have adverse side effects.

Leg exercise such as walking is the only known behavioral method for temporary relief of RLS. This exercise-induced attenuation of symptoms suggests that these conditions are related to dopamine stores, since body movement is integrally related to dopamine systems, and chronic exercise increases dopamine synthesis and metabolism in many brain regions (3). Regular exercise may effectively treat both conditions, but, to my knowledge, this hypothesis has not been tested.

References

1. Campbell SS: Duration and placement of sleep in a 'disentrained' environment. *Psychophysiol* 1984;21(1):106-11

2. Van Someren EJ, Lijzenga C, Mirmiran G, et al: Long-term fitness training improves the circadian rest-activity rhythm in healthy elderly males. *J Biol Rhythms* 1997;12(2):146-156

3. Chaouloff F: Physical exercise and brain monoamines: a review. *Acta Physiol Scand* 1989;137(1):1-13

Steps to Promote Sleep

Though current research does not offer compelling evidence that exercise promotes sleep, several practical recommendations seem prudent in light of current knowledge on exercise and sleep:

- exercise in bright outdoor light if possible.

- experiment with exercise at different times of the day in order to find a convenient time; late-night exercise does not necessarily disrupt sleep.

- whether you are fit or unfit, try exercise to enhance sleep, since level of fitness does not determine the effects of exercise on sleep.

- exercise duration is more important than intensity. Thirty minutes of moderate exercise most days is the standard recommendation for general health, and sleep time seems to increase when exercise continues an hour or longer.

—by Shawn D. Youngerstedt, Phd.

Dr. Youngstedt is a postdoctoral fellow in the Department of Psychiatry at the Sam and Rose Stein Institute for Research on Aging at the University of California, San Diego. Address correspondence to Shawn D. Youngstedt, PhD, Dept of Psychiatry, 0667, University of California, San Diego, 9500 Gilman Dr, La Jolla, CA 92093-0667.

Chapter 7

Sleep Hygiene:
Tips to Help You Sleep Better

For most people, falling asleep and staying asleep are parts of a natural process. Good sleepers are likely to have developed certain lifestyle and dietary habits that promote sound sleep. These habits or behaviors—known as sleep hygiene—can have positive effects on sleep before, during, and after time spent in bed. For the most part, sleep hygiene is a matter of common sense, and the techniques suggested in this chapter will help people sleep better.

For Better Sleep

Stimulants

Caffeine stimulates the brain and interferes with sleep. Coffee, tea, colas, cocoa, chocolate, and prescription and nonprescription drugs that contain caffeine should not be taken within three to four hours of bedtime. Although moderate daytime use of caffeine usually does not interfere with sleep at night, heavy or regular use during the day can lead to withdrawal symptoms and to sleep problems at night.

Nicotine is another stimulating drug that interferes with sleep, and nicotine withdrawal can also disrupt sleep throughout the night. Cigarettes and some drugs contain substantial quantities of nicotine. Smokers who break the habit, once they overcome the withdrawal

Reprinted with permission. © 1991 American Sleep Disorders Association, 6301 Bandel Road, Suite 101, Rochester, MN 55901. Web site - http://www.asda.org

effects of the drug, can expect to fall asleep faster and wake up less during the night.

Alcohol

One of the effects of alcohol is a slowing of brain activity. When taken at bedtime, alcohol may help induce sleep at first, but will disrupt sleep later in the night. A "nightcap" before bed can result in awakenings during the night, nightmares, and early morning headaches. Alcoholic beverages should be avoided within four to six hours of bedtime.

Exercise

Regular exercise helps people sleep better; the benefits of exercise on sleep, however, depend on the time of day it is undertaken and on your overall fitness level. People who are physically fit should avoid exercising within six hours of bedtime. Exercise in the morning is not likely to affect sleep at night, but the same amount of exercise—if done too close to bedtime—can disrupt sleep. On the other hand, too little exercise and limited activity during the day can also lead to sleeplessness at night. Consult a healthcare provider before beginning an exercise program.

Environment

A comfortable bed in a dark, quiet room is the best setting for a good night's sleep. Some people seem to adjust easily to changes in sleep environment, but others (such as insomniacs and the elderly) can be easily disturbed by small changes in sleep surroundings. When excessive light is a problem, blackout curtains and spot lighting can be helpful. Noise problems can be alleviated with the use of background sound ("white noise") or earplugs.

Diet

Eating a full meal shortly before bedtime can interfere with the ability to fall asleep and stay asleep, as can heavy meals eaten at any time of day or foods that cause indigestion. A light snack at bedtime, however, can promote sleep. Milk and other dairy products, which contain the natural sleep-promoting substance tryptophan, are especially good as bedtime snacks.

Decreasing Time Awake in Bed

Stress contributes to many sleep problems. People who have trouble sleeping sometimes begin to rely on certain strategies—such as regular napping, excessive use of caffeine, use of alcoholic beverages at bedtime, working at night, and sleeping at irregular times—to help adapt to a disturbed sleep schedule. After the source of stress that led to the sleep problem is eliminated, these behaviors can sometimes cause sleep problems to continue. A cycle of repeated difficulty in falling asleep develops, and tension and a fear of sleeplessness can result. The bedroom itself can come to be associated with unsuccessful attempts to sleep and with tension and anxiety. Some people who have trouble sleeping will begin sleeping on a sofa or in a chair because they are no longer able to sleep in the bedroom. This phenomenon, termed conditioning, may respond to one of two treatment techniques: stimulus control and sleep restriction.

Stimulus control attempts to reestablish the connection between sleep and the bedroom. This is done by reducing the amount of time spent lying awake in bed. Table 7.1 at the end of this chapter lists instructions for stimulus control treatment. The principles of good sleep hygiene and stimulus control are often used together to relieve sleeplessness.

Sleep restriction works by reducing the amount of time spent in bed to the estimated time period spent actually sleeping. Sleep restriction techniques, which can be learned from a sleep specialist, include recording the time you spend in bed and the time you spend asleep each day for one to two weeks. The amount of time spent in bed is then restricted to the time spent actually sleeping. As sleep quality improves, the sleep schedule is adjusted as appropriate. Sleep restriction prescribes a specific amount of sleep but not a mandatory time period in bed. Stimulus control and sleep hygiene guidelines may be used in combination with sleep restriction.

Clock-watching should be avoided by people experiencing sleep problems, especially those with insomnia. It can be helpful to set the alarm for the desired morning arise time, and then hide the clock and watches in a dresser drawer across the room. Most people experiencing sleep problems sleep best when time pressures are relieved.

Managing Stress

As mentioned earlier, the stress that stems from common life situations often contributes to sleep problems. A relaxing activity around bedtime can help relieve tension and encourage sleep. Consciously attempting to clarify problems and formulate solutions can have a positive effect on sleep quality. Talking with a trusted friend or colleague to "air out" troubling issues can be helpful. Relaxation exercises, meditation, biofeedback, and hypnosis are sometimes beneficial in controlling sleep problems. These techniques should be learned from a psychologist, physician, or other healthcare professional.

Designating "Worry Time"

Another technique that can be helpful is to designate a particular time for worry. This time is dedicated to sorting out problems and coming up with possible solutions. Set aside 30 minutes in the evening to sit alone and undisturbed. On 3 x 5 cards, write down each of your worries as it comes to mind (one worry per card). These worries can range from the mundane (needing to call someone in the morning or remembering an anniversary) to the serious (financial concerns or problems with a relationship). When all worries have been written down, sort the cards into three to five piles according to the priority of the worry. Next, look at each card and formulate a possible solution to that worry. While not all worries will have easy solutions, even small progress in remedying a worry can yield helpful results. The morning after recording your worries, review the worry cards and begin to work on resolving the worries you've identified.

Summary

Good sleep hygiene will improve the sleep of many people (see Table 7.2 at the end of this article). Stimulus control and sleep restriction strategies, although they are challenging techniques to master, improve the likelihood of a successful outcome. If sleeplessness persists after four to six weeks of modifying sleep and daytime habits as described earlier, it's time to consider seeking professional help from a healthcare provider or an expert in sleep disorders.

Further Reading on Sleep Hygiene

Bodyrhythms: Chronobiology and Peak Performance by Lynne Lamberg (William Morrow and Company, Inc., 1994)

No More Sleepless Nights by Peter Hauri, PhD, and Shirley Linde, PhD (John Wiley and Sons, Inc. 1990)

Encyclopedia of Sleep and Dreaming edited by Mary A. Caskadon, PhD (New York: Macmillan, 1992)

Table 7.1. Instructions for Stimulus Control Management for Sleep Problems

1. Try to sleep only when you are drowsy.

2. If you are unable to fall asleep or stay asleep, leave your bedroom and engage in a quiet activity elsewhere. Do not permit yourself to fall asleep outside the bedroom. Return to bed when—and only when—you are sleepy. Repeat this process as often as necessary throughout the night.

3. Maintain a regular arise time, even on days off work and on weekends.

4. Use your bedroom only for sleep and sex.

5. Avoid napping during the daytime. If daytime sleepiness becomes overwhelming, limit nap time to a single nap of less than 1 hour, no later than 3 p.m.

Table 7.2. Sleep Hygiene Instructions

1. Avoid caffeine within four to six hours of bedtime.

2. Avoid the use of nicotine close to bedtime or during the night.

3. Do not drink alcoholic beverages within four to six hours of bedtime.

4. While a light snack before bedtime can help promote sound sleep, avoid large meals.

5. Avoid strenuous exercise within 6 hours of bedtime.

6. Minimize light, noise, and extremes in temperature in the bedroom.

Chapter 8

Power Napping: Benefits of Midday Sleeping

It's not even noon, but you can't keep your eyes open another second. Now the hard, polished surface of the conference table looks like the perfect resting place. In fact, you'd trade anything for a short nap.

If you feel sleepy during your busy work day, you're not alone. According to a 1992 report by the National Commission on Sleep Disorders Research, which was created by Congress in 1989, Americans in general are grossly sleep-deprived. Most of them get 20 percent less sleep than people did 100 years ago, the commission's report says.

The cost of this national need for shut-eye is staggering. The commission estimated that in 1990 the cost of accidents, lost productivity, and poor decision making related to sleepiness was $15.9 billion.

In a January 1994 survey conducted by the Better Sleep Council, a nonprofit organization supported by the bedding industry, one in five adults surveyed said they have at some time called in sick or have showed up late for work because they didn't sleep well the night before.

This national sleep deficit could be easily reduced if exhausted employees and employers alike simply napped once a day. But napping still bears a heavy social stigma in our highly productive, fast-paced society.

"It's associated with laziness because we don't put a very high value on sleep," explains Andrea Herman, director of the Better Sleep

Council, based in Alexandria, Va. The group wants to restore sleep to its rightful place in what it calls the triumvirate of health—eating properly, exercising regularly, and sleeping well.

Nightly sleep requirements vary among adults, but 7 to 10 hours is the norm. During that time, the body moves in and out of physically healing NREM (nonrapid eye movement) sleep in cycles of about 90 minutes. This is when the body's metabolism slows down enough to permit repair of the daily wear and tear on the whole system.

Roughly a fifth of slumber time is spent in REM (rapid eye movement) sleep, or dreamland, where a lot of psychological healing is accomplished. Interruption or shortening of either sleep cycle intensifies the midday sleepiness already determined by the body's circadian rhythms, which set sleep and other physiological patterns.

The midday slump, say researchers at the Institute for Circadian Physiology, in Cambridge, Mass., is totally natural and has virtually nothing to do with lunchtime dietary indiscretions. People who rise and shine around 7 o'clock usually conk out between 2 and 4 in the afternoon. Earlier risers start dragging at noon and don't perk up until 2 o'clock. But because the slump is exacerbated by sleep debt, some doctors are becoming strong advocates of napping.

Dr. Jeffrey Migdow, who practices holistic medicine and directs yoga programs at the Kripalu Center for Yoga and Health, in Lenox, Mass., says napping has a venerable tradition. Ancient yogis, having discovered how napping relieved stress on the nervous and immune systems, built 20 to 30 minutes of it into their daily practices.

"In 10 to 15 minutes, today's business person can get the same benefits," Migdow says. "The body is a very resilient system that to rejuvenate. If you take time to turn the nervous system off, the whole system recharges."

Dr. Karl Doghramji, director of the Sleep Disorders Center at Thomas Jefferson University Hospital, in Philadelphia, recommends naps only for people who suffer sleep deprivation, not for sufferers of sleep disorders such as sleep apnea, in which breathing stops temporarily, or narcolepsy, a frequent and uncontrollable desire for sleep. "I do not recommend napping, in fact I forbid it, for people who are insomniacs, or who have a weak sleep drive," he cautions. "If you're getting eight hours of sleep at night and still need a daily nap, then something else might be going on in your sleep that needs medical attention."

If you're not getting eight hours of sleep and suspect a daytime snooze might boost your creativity, productivity, and mood, here's how to make it work:

- To avoid disrupting your circadian rhythms, schedule your nap about eight hours after waking and eight hours before bedding down for the night.

- Create a routine that includes napping even on days you don't feel particularly tired.

- Lie down to nap if possible—it's the optimal position.

- Close your office door and turn off your phone so you don't subliminally worry about being disturbed.

- Take a minute for some slow, deep breaths before hunkering down. These will help your body relax into sleep.

- After you wake up, take a minute to reorient yourself by taking a few more deep breaths and stretching. Don't kick into gear too abruptly. Such a shock to the nervous system undermines the wonderful benefits of napping.

—by Meredith Gould

Chapter 9

What to Expect at an Overnight Sleep Study

A sleep study, or polysomnogram, is a recording that contains several types of measurements used to identify different sleep stages and classify various sleep problems. This study will probably be a new experience and we urge you to learn more about it before you arrive at the sleep disorders center so that it will be an easy and interesting experience for you.

Sleep is not a simple process. Many parts of the brain control it and influence its different stages. These levels or stages of sleep include drowsiness, light sleep, deep sleep, and dream sleep. We can tell which stage of sleep a person is in by measuring different activities of the brain and body. These activities include brain waves, eye movements, muscle tone, heart rate, and respiration. Your sleep also may be videotaped for later review of any abnormalities observed during the study. The sleep technician will let you know if this is done. The activities that occur during sleep (brain waves, muscle movements, and eye movements, breathing through your mouth and nose, snoring, heart rate, leg movements) are monitored by applying small metal discs called electrodes to the head and skin. These electrodes are attached with an adhesive. Flexible elastic belts are placed around your chest and abdomen to measure your breathing. The level of oxygen in your blood and your heart rate are monitored by a clip that fits on your index finger or earlobe.

None of these devices hurt and all are designed to be as comfortable as possible. If you have questions or concerns about the application of these electrodes (e.g., hair pieces, beards, prostheses, hearing aids, dentures), please contact your doctor or ask the technician before you arrive at the center.

Why Do I Need a Sleep Study?

Many different events occur in the brain and body during sleep. In order to fully understand your sleep and any potential problems, we need to look at various brain activities and body systems and their relationships throughout the night. After the study, your sleep specialist will review and interpret the record to help you and your doctor understand your specific sleep patterns. Treatment recommendations will be made if evidence of a sleep disorder is found.

The sleep study and its analysis and interpretation involve a complex process. Many hours of work are required by specially trained people, including sleep technologists who process or "score" the large amount of data from the night.

The information is then interpreted by a sleep specialist with special knowledge of and training in sleep and its disorders. A typical sleep study is more than 800 pages of different types of data (e.g., brain waves, muscle movements, eye movements). Due to this time-consuming and labor-intensive process, sleep studies are usually not evaluated immediately and it may take some time to receive the results of your study. A representative from the sleep center should be able to give you some idea of how long it will take to receive your results.

How Will I Be Able to Sleep In Such a Different Environment With All Those Wires On Me?

This is the question most frequently asked by patients prior to their sleep studies. Many people think the sleep center will be cold, bright, technical, and impersonal-looking. At most sleep centers, however, an attempt has been made to make the surroundings, particularly the bedroom, very homey and comfortable, something like a hotel room.

The technical equipment and technicians will be in a room separate from your sleeping room, and the electrode wires are gathered together in a kind of ponytail behind your head so that you will be able to roll over and change position almost as easily as you would at home.

The day of your sleep study, avoid caffeine (coffee, tea, cola, chocolate) after 2 p.m. and try not to nap. Before coming to the sleep center, wash and dry your hair and do not apply hair sprays, oils, or gels.

You may feel strange at first with the electrodes on your skin, however, most people do not find them uncomfortable or an obstacle to falling asleep. The sleep specialist recognizes that you may not sleep in the center exactly as you do at home, but in most cases this does not cause a problem in obtaining the necessary information from your study. Before coming to the center you should pack an overnight bag with anything you will need, as you would for an overnight stay at a hotel or a friend's house. If you have special needs, please advise the sleep center personnel so that they can accommodate you.

What Will Happen When I Arrive at the Sleep Center?

When you arrive at the center, anywhere from 5:30 p.m. to 9:30 p.m. (check with the center to be certain of the right time), the technician will greet you and show you to your bedroom. The technician will then show you the equipment and answer any questions you may have about it and the electrode application. You should inform the technician of any changes in your sleep or specific difficulties that you might not have already have discussed with your doctor.

You will have time to change and get ready for bed, as you do at home. There may be a waiting period before the technician applies your electrodes and you should feel free to read, watch TV, or relax. If you have a commitment in the morning (if, for example you have to be at work at a certain time), be sure to inform the sleep technician prior to your study, so that a wake-up time can be arranged. You also should confirm your desired wake-up time upon arrival at the sleep center.

While you are sleeping, various important body functions and measurements are recorded. The technician will monitor your sleep from a nearby room throughout the night. If a respiratory or breathing problem is observed during sleep, the technician may awaken you to ask you to try a device that treats breathing problems. Patients are always notified about this possibility before going to bed and the use and purpose of the device are explained in full on the night of the study.

This device, called a nasal positive airway pressure device, includes a small mask which fits around your nose or nose and mouth. If you are unsure whether you will be having a nasal positive airway pressure trial during your study, call your doctor or the sleep center to ask. If you will be trying this device during your sleep study night, the technician will adjust the mask in advance to ensure a comfortable fit and will usually give you a chance to practice with the device before going to bed. You will be able to ask questions about the device and/or your sleep study, and discuss your impressions and the study results with your doctor during your follow-up visit.

What Happens If I Am Scheduled For a Nap Study?

Your doctor may order an additional test, called a multiple sleep latency test (MSLT) as part of your overall sleep evaluation. This means that you will need to stay at the center for most of the next day for a series of brief naps that begin the morning after your sleepover in the center. The naps are scheduled at intervals throughout the day. You will wear most of the same recording equipment you wore to bed the night before.

The amount and type of sleep you get during the naps can help your doctor understand complaints of sleepiness better and make decisions about specific sleep disorders and treatments.

Be sure you know whether you will be staying at the center the next day so that you can plan ahead. Call the center in advance to find out specific breakfast and lunch arrangements and approximately when you will be able to leave.

Should I Take My Medication As I Usually Do?

It is important for your sleep professional to know if you are taking any regularly prescribed or over-the-counter medications since certain medications can affect sleep and the interpretation of your sleep study. Sometimes specific medications are gradually discontinued during the weeks prior to the sleep study in order for the results of your study to be interpreted correctly. It is important that you discuss your medication use with your doctor before your sleep study. Do not discontinue any prescription medication without first talking with your doctor. You should avoid coffee and alcohol on the day/evening of your study.

What Happens After My Sleep Study?

After you have completed your sleep study, you will probably have a follow-up visit with your doctor to discuss the results and recommendations for treatment. Be sure to inquire at your doctor's office about scheduling a follow-up visit. Some doctors' offices prefer that you wait until the sleep study results have been received by the office before scheduling the follow-up appointment. Sleep study results are not generally discussed over the telephone because of their complex nature.

To fully understand your sleep study results, their implications, and any treatment recommendations that are made, it is best to meet face-to-face with your doctor. It is possible that one of your doctor's recommendations may be that you have another test in the sleep center. If so, do not be alarmed or disappointed. Sometimes additional procedures are needed to provide more information to establish a diagnosis or evaluate a treatment.

In Summary

We hope that your experience at the sleep center will be positive and helpful. By informing you of the specifics involved in evaluating sleep and its disorders we hope that you will understand more about sleep and take an active role in your own care.

For More Information

Sleep is not merely a "time out" from daily life. It is an active state, essential for physical and mental restoration. Yet, more than 100 million Americans of all ages regularly fail to get a good night's sleep.

For more information about specific sleep disorders, contact your healthcare provider, for a list of accredited, member, sleep-disorders centers near you write to:

The American Sleep Disorders Association
1610 14th Street NW, Suite 300
Rochester, MN 55901

Further Reading on Overnight Sleep Studies

Sleep, Dreaming and Sleep Disorders by William H. Moorcroft (Lanham, MD: University Press of America, 1989)

Snoring and Sleep Apnea by Ralph A. Pascualy, MD and Sally Warren Soest (New York: Raven Press, 1994)

No More Sleepless Nights by Peter Hauri, MD and Shirley Linde, PhD (John Wiley & Sons, Inc, 1990)

Part Two

Sleep through the Lifespan

Chapter 10

Sleep Disturbances Affect the Entire Lifespan

Sleep disorders and disturbances occur at all points in the lifespan; babies, children, adolescents, adults, and the elderly all experience sleep problems. The epidemiological data available offer only the most conservative estimates on prevalence in each age group. Even so, the numbers are startling.

Sleep in Infants, Children, and Adolescents

In the United States, two of every 1,000 babies born will die from sudden infant death syndrome (SIDS). SIDS claims more lives between the ages of one month and one year than all other causes of death combined. SIDS is linked inextricably to sleep; more than 70 percent of its victims are found in the early morning hours after the nighttime sleep. While a number of theories have been proposed to explain the mechanisms of SIDS, none has received unequivocal substantiation. The medical profession, therefore, remains unable to recommend specific preventive measures, therapies, or other interventions.

With no warning my healthy baby died silently in her sleep. I cannot begin to describe for you how devastating our daughter's death has been for us....Because there is no known cause, I've

Excerpted from *Wake Up America: A National Sleep Alert*, Volume 1, Executive Summary and Executive Report, Report of the National Commission on Sleep Disorders Research, Submitted to the United States Congress and to the Secretary U.S. Department of Health and Human Services, January 1993.

73

had a tremendous burden of guilt, wondering if I did something that would have contributed to her death..

—Witness, Commission Hearing, Charleston, WV

Because sleep is especially important during periods of growth and development, children and adolescents may be particularly vulnerable to the effects of sleep loss. Approximately 25 percent of children between the ages of one and five experience some type of sleep disturbance, including sleep talking, nightmares, sleepwalking, bedwetting, and night terrors. A significant number of children experience obstruction of their upper airway during sleep, often causing a reduction in the amount of oxygen in the blood and, therefore, the brain. In about 70 percent of such cases, symptoms are relieved when the adenoids and tonsils are removed. Childhood sleep disturbances tend to persist if untreated. Furthermore, children with sleep-waking disorders during the first year of life often experience multiple sleep problems in later years

Although insomnia and sleep loss are prevalent in children and adolescents, the effects of these sleep problems on the young have not been established definitively. Sleep problems may be associated with difficult temperament in children. According to parents, children behave differently during the day after a poor night's sleep. Instead of appearing sleepy, the overtired child may appear overactive and inattentive. A label of "problem child" may be applied early on; once made, it is difficult to shed. Poor sleep—childhood insomnia—may cause a child to be more vulnerable to physical illness, may limit parent-child bonding and later interaction, and may affect a child's self-esteem. Somewhat older children with poor sleep are more likely than those who are good sleepers to report negative emotional states, such as daytime tiredness, tension, moodiness, and depressed feelings.

Sleep problems in the school-age child may move out of the bedroom and become a problem of dally life. The child may have difficulty concentrating in school and may develop secondary behavior problems in the classroom. Children with inadequate or disrupted sleep often appear irritable, have decreased attention spans, are oppositional, and can appear hyperactive. Children with primary sleep problems even may be misdiagnosed as learning disabled or hyperactive.

One hundred years ago, Dr. Hill published a paper in the British Medical Journal about children with "enlargement of the lymphoid (tonsilar) tissues...[who were] described by their parents and teachers as being backward and even stupid." He, in fact, describes obstruction in children with the resulting sleep deprivation causing the child to be labeled lazy, or even worse, retarded. He cautions that "the stupid looking lazy child who frequently suffers from headache at school, breathes through his mouth instead of his nose, snores, and is restless at night... is well worthy of the solicitous attention of the school medical officer."...The way we treat our children sets the tone for the citizens of this country for the next 60 years. The child who is considered to be a "poor student" because of a sleep disorder is being unfairly denied the opportunity to grow and develop into a productive citizen of the United States.

—Witness, Commission Hearing, Cleveland, OH

A problem concomitant with childhood sleep disorders is family stress. Research has shown that parents of infants with sleep disturbances typically report more depressive symptomatology, decreased satisfaction in their marriage, and greater anxiety than do parents of children with normal sleep patterns.

Chronic, frequent night wakenings by the child result in a severely stressed, sleep deprived, and out-of-control family. Desperate parents feel overwhelmed, inadequate as parents, and develop negative feelings toward the child. Occasionally, they turn to sedative medications, and in the worst case scenario, after months of struggle, the parents can lose control and hurt their children at the peak of the night frustration.

—Witness, Commission Hearing, Pittsburgh, PA

Sleep problems in adolescence span a number of specific disorders, including both disorders common in younger children and those more prevalent in adults. Some sleep disorders, such as narcolepsy, characteristically emerge in the adolescent years.

My symptoms of narcolepsy started during the seventh grade... Cataplexy, hypnagogic hallucinations, and sleep paralysis began to gradually appear over the next two years. I was convinced that I was a "bad" person. So I learned early...to lie in order to hide my problems. This was a critical dynamic in the development of my personality during adolescence, the consequences of which I continue to struggle with as an adult.

—Witness, Commission Hearing, Washington, DC

I hated my days because of the way the other kids teased me for falling asleep. I hated my nights because of my "dreams" when I tried to fall asleep. My talking, crying, and screams disturbed everyone in the house...I slowly became a misfit at home and at school. I remember going to my mother when I was fifteen and asking her to get me help and I was told not to ever tell anyone about my dreams and my fits (cataplexy) because they would lock me away.

—Witness, Commission Hearing, Portland, OR

A 1990 report estimated that greater than 15 percent of American youth have significant behavioral or emotional problems. Given the disturbing proportions of child and adolescent psychopathology, there is a compelling need for a better understanding of the relationship of adequate amounts of sleep for optimal emotional and behavioral states. Seventy-five percent of depressed adolescents suffer from insomnia; 20 percent suffer with hypersomnia. Among adolescents, depression, substance abuse, and sleep/schedule problems seem to overlap; depressed adolescents frequently have problems with erratic schedules, delayed sleep onset, and difficulty awakening for school.

...[I]n our studies of major depressive disorders in adolescents, we frequently see difficulty falling asleep, late night schedules, and...daytime fatigue (meeting criteria for delayed sleep phase syndrome). There are also provocative questions with respect to the relationship between alcohol and substance abuse and sleep schedule disorders in adolescents.

—Witness, Commission Hearing, Pittsburgh, PA

Sleep disturbances may disrupt sexual maturation by interfering with the normally preferential secretion of specific hormones during sleep. Physical growth, too, may be affected by disturbed sleep that impedes the normal secretion of growth hormone. Waking function—school performance, mood, socialization—may be impaired by sleep disturbances, compromising education and future opportunities.

76

Sleep in Mid-life

Numerous sleep disorders appear during the second through fifth decades of life. During this period, most adults will experience an increase in workload and family responsibilities. Insomnia associated with depression and chronic stress increases during these years. In addition, the body undergoes significant physiological changes that may be accompanied by disrupted sleep.

Sleep disturbances occur concomitant with post-partum psychosis and post-partum depression, disorders that affect 10-15 percent of women following childbirth. Little research has examined sleep of pregnant women and new mothers, notwithstanding the fact that both sleep disturbances and mood alterations are prevalent in these two groups. Equally, only a limited number of studies have investigated the effects of maternal sleep disorders on pregnancy outcome. Additional factors for both parents are the erratic sleep patterns of even the perfectly healthy newborn and the potential development of childhood sleep problems.

This age group suffers the highest incidence of insomnia related to shiftwork and other environmental stresses. The greatest number of shiftworkers are between the ages of 30 and 45. As we age, the disruption of rhythms is less well-tolerated. For example, a college student can recover from lost sleep easily, but a middle-aged executive or shiftworker, frequently, cannot. Chronic sleep debt produces a loss of alertness and mental efficiency during the day, inappropriate mood, and greater vulnerability to life events.

The prevalence of insomnia in women over 40 years of age is upwards of 40 percent; yet, research has examined neither the chronicity nor the severity of such complaints. By 1992, more than one-third of all American women will reach menopause. During menopause, 75 percent of women experience hot flashes and other physical symptoms that interrupt sleep; in some, this sleep disruption causes insomnia, leading to excessive daytime sleepiness and fatigue.

..As 21 million baby boom women approach mid-life I expect we're going to see a dramatic change in the way society views menopause and aging.. With the increasing life expectancy, 50 million North American women will live one-third of their life beyond their menopausal age...Hot flashes, which do occur at night, are often associated with arousal from sleep and, in many, the intensity is such that they are termed night sweats necessitating a change of nightclothes and bed linens...Possibly the increasing use of hypnotic sedative medication by women as they age may be related to sleep complaints beginning during the menopause.

—Witness, Commission Hearing, Chicago, IL

Sleep apnea is particularly prevalent in males over 50 and begins to appear in equal numbers in post-menopausal women. Physiological changes accompanying the process of aging, such as weight gain and hormonal changes, may potentiate sleep apnea as well as other sleep disorders.

As many as two-thirds of post-menopausal women experience episodes of sleep disordered breathing and nocturnal oxygen desaturation. More than enough evidence exists to link the hormonal changes of menopause to sleep related disorders. Yet, 85 percent of the normative database in sleep research has been conducted on men.

—Witness, Commission Hearing, Chicago, IL

Sleep in the Older American

Altered daily sleep patterns are among the most prominent behavioral and symptomatic changes that occur with advancing age. These changes are so common that, frequently, they are mistaken as part of the normal aging process. However, new information indicates that many of these disturbances are not normal; they are, in fact, serious sleep disorders. Recent estimates suggest that over half of the 19 million people now over the age of 65 experience some disruption of sleep, including chronic and recurrent insomnias, excessive daytime sleepiness, circadian rhythm disruptions, and primary sleep disorders such as apnea, REM behavior disorder, and periodic limb movements.

Disturbances of sleep found in the older population may be the result of a variety of factors: retirement and changes in social patterns, death of a spouse and close friends, and increased use of medications. An older person's risk of developing depression appears to be greater among those suffering from insomnia than among those without insomnia. Moreover, aging persons frequently suffer from physical problems—cardiovascular disease, pulmonary disease, arthritis, pain syndromes, prostatic disease, endocrine imbalances, and others—that often are associated with disturbances of sleep. Moreover, impaired sleep frequently is associated with abnormalities of brain function, such as Alzheimer's disease. Over the course of the night, orderly sleep cycles are disrupted; less deep sleep and less REM sleep (dream sleep) are experienced. Daytime napping is increased as a form of compensation. Sleep problems in the elderly may result in evening and nighttime agitation, confusion, and disruptive behavior, a disorder known as "sundowning," occurring in an estimated 12-20 percent of demented patients. These changes become increasingly severe as the dementia progresses.

The importance of identifying and treating these disorders is highlighted by research findings in which 70 percent of the caregivers of older demented elders cited the influence of the elders' nocturnal problems as a factor in a decision to institutionalize the elder, often because their own sleep was disrupted. Another study found that among families of hospitalized, aged psychiatric patients, sleep disturbance and "troublesome" behavior at night were among the most frequent problem relieved by institutionalization. The costs of this nursing home care are not inconsequential. As many as 63 percent of those over age 65 are institutionalized at some time in their lives, at an annual cost of around $25,000 per person, or $40.6 billion per year. Improved sleep for the aged could reduce these costs significantly.

Yet, for the aging person, institutionalization, frequently, is not the solution to the sleep problems. *One study found that patients in a typical nursing home were never asleep for a full hour and never awake for a full hour throughout a 24-hour day*. Well-meaning, but uninformed practices, such as heavy sedation, serve to worsen sleep problems and to compromise waking function.

The goal of therapy for sleep disorders and disturbances in the aged is to reduce morbidity, to reduce excess mortality, and to improve the quality of life. The principal sleep complaints of older persons are hypersomnia and insomnia, complaints that frequently reflect underlying psychiatric or physical disorders. Research could help disclose appropriate interventions that respond to the special needs of the elderly and that do not rely solely on pharmacologic interventions that may increase disability. Education could help improve compliance with home-based therapy for sleep disorders and disturbances, and could provide greater understanding and involvement by nursing home staff in appropriate nonpharmacologic interventive strategies.

Chapter 11

Sudden Infant Death Syndrome (SIDS)

Sudden Infant Death Syndrome (SIDS) is the diagnosis given for the sudden death of an infant under one year of age that remains unexplained after a complete investigation, which includes an autopsy, examination of the death scene, and review of the symptoms or illnesses the infant had prior to dying and any other pertinent medical history. Because most cases of SIDS occur when a baby is sleeping in a crib, SIDS is also commonly known as "crib death".

SIDS is the leading cause of death in infants between 1 month and 1 year of age. Most SIDS deaths occur when a baby is between 1 and 4 months of age. African American children are two to three times more likely than white babies to die of SIDS, and Native American babies are about three times more susceptible. Also, more boys are SIDS victims than girls.

What Are the Risk Factors for SIDS?

A number of factors seem to put a baby at higher risk of dying from SIDS. Babies who sleep on their stomachs are more likely to die of SIDS than those who sleep on their backs. Mothers who smoke during pregnancy are three times more likely to have a SIDS baby, and exposure to passive smoke from smoking by mothers, fathers, and others in the household doubles a baby's risk of SIDS. Other risk factors include mothers who are less than 20 years old at the time of their

National Institute of Child Health and Human Development (NICHD) Public Information and Communications Branch, April 1997.

first pregnancy, babies born to mothers who had no or late prenatal care, and premature or low birth weight babies.

What Causes SIDS?

Mounting evidence suggests that some SIDS babies are born with brain abnormalities that make them vulnerable to sudden death during infancy. Studies of SIDS victims reveal that many SIDS infants have abnormalities in the arcuate nucleus, a portion of the brain that is likely to be involved in controlling breathing and waking during sleep. Babies born with defects in other portions of the brain or body may also be more prone to a sudden death. These abnormalities may stem from prenatal exposure to a toxic substance, or lack of a vital compound in the prenatal environment, such as sufficient oxygen. Cigarette smoking during pregnancy, for example, can reduce the amount of oxygen the fetus receives.

Scientists believe that the abnormalities that are present at birth may not be sufficient to cause death. Other possibly important events occur after birth such as lack of oxygen, excessive carbon dioxide intake, overheating or an infection. For example, many babies experience a lack of oxygen and excessive carbon dioxide levels when they have respiratory infections that hamper breathing, or they rebreathe exhaled air trapped in underlying bedding when they sleep on their stomachs. Normally, infants sense such inadequate air intake, and the brain triggers the babies to wake from sleep and cry, and changes their heartbeat or breathing patterns to compensate for the insufficient oxygen and excess carbon dioxide. A baby with a flawed arcuate nucleus, however, might lack this protective mechanism and succumb to SIDS. Such a scenario might explain why babies who sleep on their stomachs are more susceptible to SIDS, and why a disproportionately large number of SIDS babies have been reported to have respiratory infections prior to their deaths. Infections as a trigger for sudden infant death may explain why more SIDS cases occur during the colder months of the year, when respiratory and intestinal infections are more common.

The numbers of cells and proteins generated by the immune system of some SIDS babies have been reported to be higher than normal. Some of these proteins can interact with the brain to alter heart rate and breathing during sleep, or can put the baby into a deep sleep. Such effects might be strong enough to cause the baby's death, particularly if the baby has an underlying brain defect. Some babies who die suddenly may be born with a metabolic disorder. One such disorder is medium chain acylCoA dehydrogenase deficiency, which prevents the infant from properly processing fatty acids. A build-up of these acid metabolites could eventually lead to a rapid and fatal disruption in breathing and heart functioning. If there is a family history of this disorder or childhood death of unknown cause, genetic screening of the parents by a blood test can determine if they are carriers of this disorder. If one or both parents is found to be a carrier, the baby can be tested soon after birth.

What Might Help Lower the Risk of SIDS?

There currently is no way of predicting which newborns will succumb to SIDS; however, there are a few measures parents can take to lower the risk of their child dying from SIDS.

Good prenatal care, which includes proper nutrition, no smoking or drug or alcohol use by the mother, and frequent medical check-ups beginning early in pregnancy, might help prevent a baby from developing an abnormality that could put him or her at risk for sudden death. These measures may also reduce the chance of having a premature or low birthweight baby, which also increases the risk for SIDS. Once the baby is born, parents should keep the baby in a smoke-free environment.

Parents and other caregivers should put babies to sleep on their backs as opposed to on their stomachs. Studies have shown that placing babies on their backs to sleep has reduced the number of SIDS cases by as much as a half in countries where infants had traditionally slept on their stomachs. Although babies placed on their sides to sleep have a lower risk of SIDS than those placed on their stomachs, the back sleep position is the best position for infants from 1 month to 1 year. Babies positioned on their sides to sleep should be placed with their lower arm forward to help prevent them from rolling onto their stomachs.

Many parents place babies on their stomachs to sleep because they think it prevents them from choking on spit-up or vomit during sleep. But studies in countries where there has been a switch from babies sleeping predominantly on their stomachs to sleeping mainly on their backs have not found any evidence of increased risk of choking or other problems.

In some instances, doctors may recommend that babies be placed on their stomachs to sleep if they have disorders such as gastroesophageal reflux or certain upper airway disorders which predispose them to choking or breathing problems while lying on their backs. If a parent is unsure about the best sleep position for their baby, it is always a good idea to talk to the baby's doctor or other health care provider.

A certain amount of "tummy time" while the infant is awake and being observed is recommended for motor development of the shoulder. In addition, awake time on the stomach may help prevent flat spots from developing on the back of the baby's head. Such physical signs are almost always temporary and will disappear soon after the baby begins to sit up.

Parents should make sure their baby sleeps on a firm mattress or other firm surface. They should avoid using fluffy blankets or covering as well as pillows, sheepskins, blankets, or comforters under the baby. Infants should not be placed to sleep on a waterbed or with soft stuffed toys.

Recently, scientific studies have demonstrated that bedsharing, between mother and baby, can alter sleep patterns of the mother and baby. These studies have led to speculation that bedsharing, sometimes referred to as co-sleeping, may also reduce the risk of SIDS. While bedsharing may have certain benefits (such as encouraging breast feeding), there are not scientific studies demonstrating that bedsharing reduces SIDS. Some studies actually suggest that bedsharing, under certain conditions, may increase the risk of SIDS. If mothers choose to sleep in the same beds with their babies, care should be taken to avoid using soft sleep surfaces. Quilts, blankets, pillows, comforters, or other similar soft materials should not be placed under the baby. The bedsharer should not smoke or use substances such as alcohol or drugs which may impair arousal. It is also important to be aware that unlike cribs, which are designed to meet safety standards for infants, adult beds are not so designed and may carry a risk of accidental entrapment and suffocation.

Babies should be kept warm, but they should not be allowed to get too warm because an overheated baby is more likely to go into a deep sleep from which it is difficult to arouse. The temperature in the baby's room should feel comfortable to an adult and overdressing the baby should be avoided.

There is some evidence to suggest that breast feeding might reduce the risk of SIDS. A few studies have found SIDS to be less common in infants who have been breast fed. This may be because breast milk can provide protection from some infections that can trigger sudden death in infants.

Parents should take their babies to their health care provider for regular well baby check-ups and routine immunizations. Claims that immunizations increase the risk of SIDS are not supported by data, and babies who receive their scheduled immunizations are less likely to die of SIDS. If an infant ever has an incident where he or she stops breathing and turns blue or limp, the baby should be medically evaluated for the cause of such an incident.

Although some electronic home monitors can detect and sound an alarm when a baby stops breathing, there is no evidence that such monitors can prevent SIDS. A panel of experts convened by the National Institutes of Health in 1986 recommended that home monitors not be used for babies who do not have an increased risk of sudden unexpected death. The monitors are recommended, however, for infants who have experienced one or more severe episodes during which they stopped breathing and required resuscitation or stimulation, premature infants with apnea, and siblings of two or more SIDS infants. If an incident has occurred or if an infant is on a monitor, parents need to know how to properly use and maintain the device, as well as how to resuscitate their baby if the alarm sounds.

How Does a SIDS Baby Affect the Family?

A SIDS death is a tragedy that can prompt intense emotional reactions among surviving family members. After the initial disbelief, denial, or numbness begins to wear off, parents often fall into a prolonged depression. This depression can affect their sleeping, eating, ability to concentrate, and general energy level. Crying, weeping, incessant talking, and strong feelings of guilt or anger are all normal reactions. Many parents experience unreasonable fears that they, or someone in their family, may be in danger. Over-protection of surviving children and fears for future children is a common reaction.

As the finality of the child's death becomes a reality for the parents, recovery occurs. Parents begin to take a more active part in their own lives, which begin to have meaning once again. The pain of their child's death becomes less intense but not forgotten. Birthdays, holidays, and the anniversary of the child's death can trigger periods of intense pain and suffering.

Children will also be affected by the baby's death. They may fear that other members of the family, including themselves, will also suddenly die. Children often also feel guilty about the death of a sibling and may feel that they had something to do with the death. Children may not show their feelings in obvious ways. Although they may deny being upset and seem unconcerned, signs that they are disturbed include intensified clinging to parents, misbehaving, bed wetting, difficulties in school, and nightmares. It is important to talk to children about the death and explain to them that the baby died because of a medical program that occurs only in infants in rare instances and cannot occur in them. The National Institute of Child Health and Human Development (NICHD) continues to support research aimed at uncovering what causes SIDS, who is at risk for the disorder, and ways to lower the risk of sudden infant death. Inquiries regarding research programs should be directed to Dr. Marian Willinger, 301-496-5575.

Families with a baby who has died from SIDS may be aided by counseling and support groups. Examples of these groups include the following:

Association of SIDS and Infant Mortality Programs
630 West Fayette Street
Room 5-684
Baltimore, MD 21201
1-410-706-5062

National SIDS Resource Center
2070 Chain Bridge Road
Suite 450
Vienna, VA 22181
1-703-821-8955

SIDS Alliance (a national network of SIDS support groups)
1314 Bedford Avenue
Suite 210
Baltimore, MD 21208
1-800-221-7437 or 1-410-653-8226

Chapter 12

What Is Sudden Infant Death Syndrome (SIDS)?

Sudden Infant Death Syndrome (SIDS) is the "sudden death of an infant under one year of age which remains unexplained after a thorough case investigation, including performance of a complete autopsy, examination of the death scene, and review of the clinical history" (Willinger, et al., 1991).

What Are the Most Common Characteristics of SIDS?

Most researchers now believe that babies who die of SIDS are born with one or more conditions that make them especially vulnerable to stresses that occur in the normal life of an infant, including both internal and external influences. SIDS occurs in all types of families and is largely indifferent to race or socioeconomic level. SIDS is unexpected, usually occurring in otherwise apparently healthy infants from 1 month to 1 year of age. Most deaths from SIDS occur by the end of the sixth month, with the greatest number taking place between 2 and 4 months of age. A SIDS death occurs quickly and is often associated with sleep, with no signs of suffering. More deaths are reported in the fall and winter (in both the Northern and Southern Hemispheres) and there is a 60- to 40-percent male-to-female ratio. A death is diagnosed as SIDS only after all other alternatives have been eliminated: SIDS is a diagnosis of exclusion.

This publication was produced by the National Sudden Infant Death Syndrome Resource Center, 2070 Chain Bridge Road, Suite 450, Vienna, VA 22182, (703) 821-8955, (operated by Circle Solutions, Inc.).

87

What Are Risk Factors for SIDS?

Risk factors are those environmental and behavioral influences that can provoke ill health. Any risk factor may be a clue to finding the cause of a disease, but risk factors in and of themselves are not causes.

Researchers now know that the mother's health and behavior during her pregnancy and the baby's health before birth seem to influence the occurrence of SIDS, but these variables are not reliable in predicting how, when, why, or if SIDS will occur. Maternal risk factors include cigarette smoking during pregnancy; maternal age less than 20 years; poor prenatal care; low weight gain; anemia; use of illegal drugs; and history of sexually transmitted disease or urinary tract infection. These factors, which often may be subtle and undetected, suggest that SIDS is somehow associated with a harmful prenatal environment.

How Many Babies Die From SIDS?

From year to year, the number of SIDS deaths tends to remain constant despite fluctuations in the overall number of infant deaths. The National Center for Health Statistics (NCHS) reported that, in 1988 in the United States, 5,476 infants under 1 year of age died from SIDS; in 1989, the number of SIDS deaths was 5,634 (NCHS, 1990, 1992). However, other sources estimate that the number of SIDS deaths in this country each year may actually be closer to 7,000 (Goyco and Beckerman, 1990). The larger estimate represents additional cases that are unreported or underreported (i.e., cases that should have been reported as SIDS but were not).

When considering the overall number of live births each year, SIDS remains the leading cause of death in the United States among infants between 1 month and 1 year of age and second only to congenital anomalies as the leading overall cause of death for all infants less than 1 year of age.

How Do Professionals Diagnose SIDS?

Often the cause of an infant death can be determined only through a process of collecting information, conducting sometimes complex forensic tests and procedures, and talking with parents and physicians. When a death is sudden and unexplained, investigators, including medical examiners and coroners, use the special expertise of forensic medicine (application of medical knowledge to legal issues). SIDS is no exception.

Health professionals make use of three avenues of investigation in determining a SIDS death:

(1) the autopsy,

(2) death scene investigation, and,

(3) review of victim and family case history.

The Autopsy

The autopsy provides anatomical evidence through microscopic examination of tissue samples and vital organs. An autopsy is important because SIDS is a diagnosis of exclusion. A definitive diagnosis cannot be made without a thorough postmortem examination that fails to point to any other possible cause of death. Also, if a cause of SIDS is ever to be uncovered, scientists will most likely detect that cause through evidence gathered from a thorough pathological examination.

A Thorough Death Scene Investigation

A thorough death scene investigation involves interviewing the parents, other caregivers, and family members; collecting items from the death scene; and evaluating that information. Although painful for the family, a detailed scene investigation may shed light on the cause, sometimes revealing a recognizable and possibly preventable cause of death.

Review of the Victim and Family Case History

A comprehensive history of the infant and family is especially critical to determine a SIDS death. Often, a careful review of documented and anecdotal information about the victim's or family's history of previous illnesses, accidents, or behaviors may further corroborate what is detected in the autopsy or death scene investigation.

Investigators should be sensitive and understand that the family may view this process as an intrusion, even a violation of their grief. It should be noted that, although stressful, a careful investigation that reveals no preventable cause of death may actually be a means of giving solace to a grieving family.

What SIDS Is and What SIDS Is Not

SIDS Is:

- the major cause of death in infants from 1 month to 1 year of age, with most deaths occurring between 2 and 4 months

- sudden and silent—the infant was seemingly healthy

- currently, unpredictable and unpreventable

- a death that occurs quickly, often associated with sleep and with no signs of suffering

- determined only after an autopsy, an examination of the death scene, and a review of the clinical history

- designated as a diagnosis of exclusion

- a recognized medical disorder listed in the International Classification of Diseases, 9th Revision (ICD-9)

- an infant death that leaves unanswered questions, causing intense grief for parents and families

SIDS Is Not:

- caused by vomiting and choking, or minor illnesses such as colds or infections

- caused by the diphtheria, pertussis, tetanus (DPT) vaccines, or other immunizations

- contagious

- child abuse

- the cause of every unexpected infant death

Any sudden, unexpected death threatens one's sense of safety and security. We are forced to confront our own mortality (Corr, 1991). This is particularly true in a sudden infant death. Quite simply, babies are not supposed to die. Because the death of an infant is a disruption of the natural order, it is traumatic for parents, family, and friends. The lack of a discernible cause, the suddenness of the tragedy, and the involvement of the legal system make a SIDS death especially difficult, leaving a great sense of loss and a need for understanding.

For Additional Information On SIDS, Contact

American SIDS Institute
6065 Roswell Road, Suite 876
Atlanta, GA 30328
(800) 232-7437, (800) 847-7437 (within GA)
(404) 843-1030, (404) 843-0577 (fax)

Association of SIDS Program Professionals (ASPP)
c/o Massachusetts Center for SIDS
Boston City Hospital
818 Harrison Avenue
Boston, MA 02118
(617) 534-7437, (617) 534-5555 (fax)

National Sudden Infant Death Syndrome Resource Center (NSRC)
2070 Chain Bridge Road, Suite 450
Vienna, VA 22182
(703) 821-8955, (703) 821-2098 (fax)

Southwest SIDS Research Institute, Inc.
Brazosport Memorial Hospital
100 Medical Drive
Lake Jackson, TX 77566
(409) 299-2814, (800) 245-7437, (409) 297-6905 (fax)

Sudden Infant Death Syndrome Alliance
1314 Bedford Avenue, Suite 210
Baltimore, MD 21208
(800) 221-7437,(410) 653-8226, (410) 653-8709 (fax)

References

Corr, C.A., Fuller, H., Barnickol, C.A., and Corr, D.M. (Eds). *Sudden Infant Death Syndrome: Who Can Help and How.* New York: Springer Publishing Co., 1991.

Goyco, P.G., and Beckerman, R.C. "Sudden Infant Death Syndrome." *Current Problems in Pediatrics* 20(6):299-346, June 1990.

National Center for Health Statistics. "Advanced Mortality Statistics for 1989." *Monthly Vital Statistics Report,* Vol. 40, No. 8, Supp. 2, January 7, 1992, p. 44.

National Center for Health Statistics. "Advance Report of Final Mortality Statistics, 1988." *Monthly Vital Statistics Report*, Vol. 39, No. 7, Supp. 1990, p. 33.

Willinger, M., James, L.S., and Catz, C. "Defining the Sudden Infant Death Syndrome (SIDS): Deliberations of an Expert Panel Convened by the National Institute of Child Health and Human Development." *Pediatric Pathology* 11:677-684, 1991.

Chapter 13

How to Reduce the Risk of Sudden Infant Death Syndrome (SIDS)

Sudden Infant Death Syndrome (SIDS) is the sudden and unexplained death of an infant under one year of age. SIDS, sometimes known as crib death, strikes nearly 5,000 babies in the United States every year. Doctors and nurses don't know what causes SIDS, but they have found some things you can do to make your baby safer.

Healthy Babies Should Sleep on Their Back

One of the most important things you can do to help reduce the risk of SIDS is to put your healthy baby on his or her back to sleep. Do this when your baby is being put down for a nap or to bed for the night.

This is new. Your mother was told and, if you have other children, you may have been told that babies should sleep on their tummy. Now, doctors and nurses believe that fewer babies will die of SIDS if most infants sleep on their back.

Check With Your Doctor or Nurse

Most babies should sleep on their back. But a few babies have health conditions that might require them to sleep on their tummy.

This chapter consists of an undated document from the U. S. Public Health Service, American Academy of Pediatrics, SIDS Alliance, and Association of SIDS and Infant Mortality Programs and "...bottoms up.(daycare workers still put infants to sleep on their stomachs)" from *The Brown University Child and Adolescent Behavior Letter*, Volume 13, Number 9, pp. 3, September 1997. © 1997 Manisses Communications Group, Inc.; Manisses customer service phone number 1-800-333-7771. Reprinted with permission.

If your baby was born with a birth defect, often spits up after eating, or has a breathing, lung or heart problem, be sure to talk to a doctor or nurse about which sleep position to use.

Some mothers worry that babies sleeping on their back may choke on spit-up or vomit during sleep. There is no evidence that sleeping on the back causes choking. Millions of babies around the world now sleep on their back and doctors have not found an increase in choking or other problems.

Some babies at first don't like sleeping on their back, but most get used to it and this is the best sleep position for your baby. Although back sleeping is the best sleep position, your baby can be placed on his or her side. Side position does not provide as much protection against SIDS as back sleeping, but it is much better than placing your baby on his or her tummy.

Your baby can be placed on his or her stomach when awake. Some "tummy time" during awake hours is good for your baby. Talk to your doctor or nurse if you have questions about your baby's sleep position.

Other Things You Can Do to Help Reduce the Risk of SIDS

Bedding. Make sure that your baby sleeps on a firm mattress or other firm surface. Don't use fluffy blankets or comforters under the baby. Don't let the baby sleep on a waterbed, sheepskin, a pillow, or other soft materials. When your baby is very young, don't place soft stuffed toys or pillows in the crib with him or her. Some babies have smothered with these soft materials in the crib.

Temperature. Babies should be kept warm, but they should not be allowed to get too warm. Keep the temperature in your baby's room so that it feels comfortable to you.

Smoke-free. Create a smoke-free zone around your baby. No one should smoke around your baby. Babies and young children exposed to smoke have more colds and other diseases, as well as an increased risk of SIDS.

Doctor or clinic visits. If your baby seems sick, call your doctor or clinic right away. Make sure your baby receives his or her shots on schedule.

Prenatal care. Early and regular prenatal care can also help reduce the risk of SIDS. The risk of SIDS is higher for babies whose mothers smoked during pregnancy. For your baby's well being, you should not use alcohol or drugs during pregnancy unless prescribed by a doctor.

Breastfeeding. If possible, you should consider breastfeeding your baby. Breast milk helps to keep your baby healthy.

Enjoy your baby! Remember, most babies are born healthy and most stay that way. Don't let the fear of SIDS spoil your joy and enjoyment of having a new baby.

Best Sleep Position

Make sure your baby goes to sleep on his or her back. This provides the best protection against SIDS.

Alternative Sleep Position

If you choose to use the side sleep position, make sure your baby's lower arm is forward to stop him or her from rolling over onto the stomach.

If you have any questions about your baby's sleep position or health, first talk to your doctor or nurse.

For More Information

Back to Sleep
P.O. Box 29111
Washington, D.C. 20040
1-800-505-2742

What Is SIDS?

Sudden Infant Death Syndrome (SIDS) is the sudden and unexplained death of an infant under one year of age.

SIDS, sometimes known as crib death, is the major cause of death in babies from 1 month to 1 year of age. Most SIDS deaths occur when a baby is between 1 and 4 months old. More boys than girls are victims, and most deaths occur during the fall, winter and early spring months.

The death is sudden and unpredictable; in most cases, the baby seems healthy. Death occurs quickly, usually during a sleep time.

After 30 years of research, scientists still cannot find one definite cause or causes for SIDS. There is no way to predict or prevent SIDS. But, as this article describes, research has found some things that can help reduce the risk of SIDS.

... Bottoms Up: Day Care Workers Still Put Infants to Sleep on Their Stomachs

Despite evidence that infants' sleep positions are closely related to the incidence of sudden infant death syndrome (SIDS), many child-care workers still put babies to sleep on their stomachs, according to a recent article in *Pediatrics*, the journal of the American Academy of Pediatrics (AAP).

The article reported on a study of 131 child-care facilities caring for infants younger than 6 months old in Washington, DC, and Montgomery and Prince Georges counties in Maryland. Researchers found that 49 percent of the workers placed babies on their stomachs to sleep at least some of the time and 20 percent did so exclusively. Researchers from the Children's National Medical Center in Washington also found that even when child-care staff were aware of the SIDS risk, they followed parental requests for positioning infants for naps in the manner to which they are accustomed.

The authors concluded that parents and child-care workers need more education about the importance of proper infant sleep positioning. In 1992, the AAP recommended that infants be placed on their backs or sides to reduce the risk of SIDS.

Chapter 14

Confirmed Deficits in the Brainstems of Sudden Infant Death Syndrome (SIDS) Victims

Researchers have discovered that some infants who have died of sudden infant death syndrome (SIDS) show abnormalities in not just one—but two—receptors located in an area of the brainstem thought to be involved in the control of breathing, carbon dioxide sensitivity, and blood pressure responses. This discovery confirms earlier evidence of a similar brain abnormality in another receptor and provides additional support for the theory that malfunctions in the brain region known as the arcuate nucleus may be a strong factor in SIDS.

SIDS, the sudden, unexplained death of an infant under one year of age, strikes nearly 3,000 infants each year and is the leading cause of death among infants one month to one year of age.

The study, partially funded by the National Institute of Child Health and Human Development (NICHD), appears in the November issue of the *Journal of Neuropathology and Experimental Neurology*.

Specifically, researchers found a significant decrease in kainate binding to kainate neurotransmitter receptors in the arcuate nucleus of the brainstem in a group of SIDS infants. "Brain and nerve cells communicate by means of molecules called neurotransmitters," explained Dr. Hannah Kinney, study author, NICHD grantee, and researcher at Children's Hospital and Harvard Medical School in Boston.

Neurotransmitters produced in one brain cell bind to special receptor molecules on neighboring brain cells, in much the same way

NIH News Alert, NICHD, November 24, 1997.

the key fits into a lock. In the case of SIDS victims, it appears that the decreased binding to the kainate receptor results in faulty communication among nerve cells and may prevent infants from responding to life-threatening cardiorespiratory events during sleep.

Earlier reported findings suggested that a significant decrease in binding of another receptor, the muscarinic cholinergic receptor (mAChR) in the arcuate nucleus, could prevent SIDS victims from responding to potentially life-threatening, but frequent events, that occur during sleep. These events include responding to the rising levels of carbon dioxide or decreasing levels of oxygen that might occur when infants, lying face down in heavy bedding or blankets, rebreathe trapped air.

"This finding is exciting in that it confirms our earlier discovery of the mAChR receptor, and strengthens the argument that a deficit in the arcuate nucleus—specifically in two receptors involved in signaling neurons—may be partially responsible for some SIDS deaths," explained Dr. Kinney.

The kainate and muscarinic cholinergic receptors, located in the arcuate nucleus on the ventral or front surface of the brainstem, are thought to be directly involved in the body's ability to respond to rising levels of carbon dioxide, according to experimental animal studies.

Dr. Kinney and a scientific team studied the brainstems of 79 infants who had succumbed to SIDS and other causes. The scientific team included Dr. J. Filiano of Children's Hospital at Dartmouth; Dr. L. Sleeper of the New England Research Institutes; Dr. M. Valdes-Dapena of the University of Miami; Dr. W. White of Pfizer Central Research; Dr. H. Krous of San Diego Children's Hospital; and Dr. F. Mandell, L. Rava, and A. Panigraphy of Children's Hospital and Harvard Medical School.

In this study, the average receptor binding in the arcuate nucleus was significantly different between SIDS and the control groups. In addition, the average decrease in receptor binding for SIDS, relative to the control group of infants who had died suddenly from other causes, is greater for the kainate receptor (52%) than the mAChR receptor (27%).

"We now have a clue about the region of the brain that is involved—and that there may be a more global, neural cell defect in the arcuate nucleus. We know two of the neurotransmitters involved. Our next step is to find out how and why this occurs," said Kinney.

One of the goals of this research is to eventually develop a screening test to identify infants at risk or a standard of measurement of kainate receptor binding that could be used for diagnosis at autopsy.

"This finding is also extremely important for the back sleeping recommendation," said Kinney. "We think this new finding fits in with the rebreathing theory—that infants sleeping in the prone (stomach) position are rebreathing trapped air and, unable to sense and respond to the excess carbon dioxide, die suddenly."

In 1992, the American Academy of Pediatrics (AAP), after reviewing studies that had linked infant prone (stomach) sleeping with an increased risk of SIDS, recommended that infants be placed on their back or side to reduce the risk of SIDS. In 1994, the NICHD joined the AAP and initiated the "Back to Sleep" campaign, which recommended placing healthy infants on their backs or sides to sleep to reduce the risk of SIDS.

Prior to the "Back to Sleep" campaign, nearly 70% of babies were stomach sleeping.

"Now, only about 21% of babies are stomach sleeping—and the SIDS death rate has dropped 38% between 1992 and 1996," reported NICHD Director Duane Alexander, M.D., at the AAP annual meeting in New Orleans on November 4, 1997.

The NICHD is joined by several federal agencies, including the Maternal and Child Health Bureau, the AAP, the SIDS Alliance, and the Association of SIDS and Infant Mortality Programs in spreading the word about the importance of back sleeping. To order "Back to Sleep" materials, write to NICHD/Back to Sleep, 31 Center Drive, Room 2A32, Bethesda, MD 20892-2425, or call toll-free, 1-800-505-CRIB. An Internet site providing the latest campaign information is also available at http://www.nih.gov/nichd.

Chapter 15

Apnea of Prematurity

What Is Apnea?

Apnea is a pause in breathing that has one or more of the following characteristics:

- lasts more than 15-20 seconds
- is associated with the baby's color changing to pale, purplish or blue
- is associated with bradycardia or a slowing of the heart rate

Is All Apnea Due to Prematurity?

No, apnea of prematurity is by far the most common cause of apnea in a premature infant. However, apnea can be caused or increased by many problems including infection, low blood sugar, patent ductusarteriosus, seizures, high or low body temperature, brain injury or insufficient oxygen.

Why Do Premature Babies Have Apnea?

Premature babies have immature respiratory centers in the brain. Preemies normally have bursts of big breaths followed by periods of shallow breathing or pauses. Apnea is most common when the baby is sleeping.

Reprinted with permission. © Jane E. Brazy, MD.

101

Will Apnea of Prematurity Go Away?

As your baby gets older, his/her breathing will become more regular. The time course is variable. Usually apnea of prematurity markedly improves or goes away by the time the baby nears his/her due date.

How Is Apnea Treated?

Several treatments are possible. Your baby may be treated with one or more of the following:

- Medications that stimulate breathing. Commonly used drugs include theophylline, aminophylline, or caffeine.

- CPAP or continuous positive airway pressure. This is air or oxygen delivered under pressure through little tubes into the baby's nose.

- Mechanical ventilation (breathing machine). If the apnea is severe, the baby may need a few breaths from the ventilator every minute. These might be given at regular intervals or only if apnea occurs.

- A rocking bed or periodic stimulation

How Do I Know if My Baby Has Apnea?

Your baby's respirations are monitored continuously if s/he is at risk for apnea. An alarm will sound if there is no breath for a set number of seconds.

What Happens if the Monitor Sounds?

- A nurse will observe your baby to see if s/he is breathing, if there is a change in color or if the heart rate is falling. False alarms occur often.

- The nurse may stimulate your baby if your baby needs a reminder to breathe.

- If there is a change in color, the nurse may give your baby extra oxygen.

- If your baby still doesn't breathe, s/he may give the baby a few breaths with a bag and mask, or extra breaths on the mechanical ventilator.

102

Does My Baby Have to Stay in the Hospital Until the Apnea Goes Away Completely?

Most infants are over their apnea completely when they go home; however, some babies reach all other criteria for discharge before their apnea is completely gone. Some babies are candidates for home apnea monitoring. Your baby may be a candidate for home apnea monitoring if :

- s/he has apnea that is short and s/he recovers without any stimulation

- s/he has no color change or bradycardia with the apnea

- the apnea is not expected to go away in the next several days

- your nursery has a home apnea program

- you have a phone and live near emergency help (if you would need it)

- you, and usually a second person, have completed home apnea training and a course in cardiopulmonary resuscitation of a baby

- your baby's doctor feels this is a good idea for your particular baby

Once Apnea Goes Away, Will it Come Back?

Apnea of prematurity is a result of immaturity. Once a baby matures and the apnea resolves, it will not return. If a baby should have breathing pauses after apnea goes away, it is not apnea of prematurity. It is due to some other problem and needs to be discussed with your baby's physician. This is very uncommon.

Is Apnea of Prematurity Related to Sudden Infant Death Syndrome(SIDS)?

No, these are two entirely different problems. Most babies who die of SIDS are born at term and have normal newborn stays. Babies who have needed newborn intensive care for any reason are at a slightly higher risk of SIDS than other babies. Apnea of prematurity does not determine this risk.

103

Chapter 16

Enuresis: Nighttime Urinary Incontinence in Children

In the United States, at least 13 million people have problems holding urine until they can get to a toilet. This loss of urinary control is called "urinary incontinence" or just "incontinence." Although it affects many young people, it usually disappears naturally over time, which suggests that incontinence, for some people, may be a normal part of growing up.

No matter when it happens or how often it happens, incontinence causes great distress. It may get in the way of a good night's sleep and is embarrassing when it happens during the day. That's why it is important to understand that occasional incontinence is a normal part of growing up and that treatment is available for most children who have difficulty controlling their bladders.

How Does the Urinary System Work?

Urination, or voiding, is a complex activity. The bladder is a balloonlike muscle that lies in the lowest part of the abdomen. The bladder stores urine, then releases it through the urethra, the canal that carries urine to the outside of the body. Controlling this activity involves nerves, muscles, the spinal cord, and the brain.

The bladder is made of two types of muscles: the detrusor, a muscular sac that stores urine and squeezes to empty, and the sphincter, a circular group of muscles at the bottom or neck of the bladder that

NIH Pub. No. 97-4095, January 1997

automatically stay contracted to hold the urine in and automatically relax when the detrusor contracts to let the urine into the urethra. A third group of muscles below the bladder (pelvic floor muscles) can contract to keep urine back.

A baby's bladder fills to a set point, then automatically contracts and empties. As the child gets older, the nervous system develops. The child's brain begins to get messages from the filling bladder and begins to send messages to the bladder to keep it from automatically emptying until the child decides it is the time and place to void.

Failures in this control mechanism result in incontinence. Reasons for this failure range from the simple to the complex.

What Causes Nighttime Incontinence?

After age 5, wetting at night—often called bedwetting or sleep-wetting—is more common than daytime wetting in boys. Experts do not know what causes nighttime incontinence. Young people who experience nighttime wetting tend to be physically and emotionally normal. Most cases probably result from a mix of factors including slower physical development, an overproduction of urine at night, a lack of ability to recognize bladder filling when asleep, and, in some cases, anxiety. For many, there is a strong family history of bedwetting, suggesting an inherited factor.

Slower Physical Development

Between the ages of 5 and 10, incontinence may be the result of a small bladder capacity, long sleeping periods, and underdevelopment of the body's alarms that signal a full or emptying bladder. This form of incontinence will fade away as the bladder grows and the natural alarms become operational.

Excessive Output of Urine During Sleep

Normally, the body produces a hormone that can slow the making of urine. This hormone is called antidiuretic hormone, or ADH. The body normally produces more ADH at night so that the need to urinate is lower. If the body doesn't produce enough ADH at night, the making of urine may not be slowed down, leading to bladder overfilling. If a child does not sense the bladder filling and awaken to urinate, then wetting will occur.

Anxiety

Experts suggest that anxiety-causing events occurring in the lives of children ages 2 to 4 might lead to incontinence before the child achieves total bladder control. Anxiety experienced after age 4 might lead to wetting after the child has been dry for a period of 6 months or more. Such events include angry parents, unfamiliar social situations, and overwhelming family events such as the birth of a brother or sister.

Incontinence itself is an anxiety-causing event. Strong bladder contractions leading to leakage in the daytime can cause embarrassment and anxiety that lead to wetting at night.

Genetics

Certain inherited genes appear to contribute to incontinence. In 1995, Danish researchers announced they had found a site on human chromosome 13 that is responsible, at least in part, for night time wetting. If both parents were bedwetters, a child has an 80 percent chance of being a bedwetter also. Experts believe that other, undetermined genes also may be involved in incontinence.

Structural Problems

Finally, a small number of cases of incontinence are caused by physical problems in the urinary system in children. Rarely, a blocked bladder or urethra may cause the bladder to overfill and leak. Nerve damage associated with the birth defect spina bifida can cause incontinence. In these cases, the incontinence can appear as a constant dribbling of urine.

Sometimes overly strenuous toilet training may make the child unable to relax the sphincter and the pelvic floor to completely empty the bladder. Retaining urine (incomplete emptying) sets the stage for urinary tract infections.

What Treats or Cures Incontinence?

Growth and Development

Most urinary incontinence fades away naturally. Here are examples of what can happen over time:

- Bladder capacity increases.
- Natural body alarms become activated.

- An overactive bladder settles down.
- Production of ADH becomes normal.
- The child learns to respond to the body's signal that it is time to void.
- Stressful events or periods pass.

Many children overcome incontinence naturally (without treatment) as they grow older. The number of cases of incontinence goes down by 15 percent for each year after the age of 5.

Medications

Nighttime incontinence may be treated by increasing ADH levels. The hormone can be boosted by a synthetic version known as desmopressin, or DDAVP. Users, including children, spray a mist containing desmopressin into their nostrils, where the drug enters the bloodstream. Researchers are developing a pill version of this drug.

Another medication, called imipramine, is also used to treat sleepwetting. It acts on both the brain and the urinary bladder. Unfortunately, total dryness with either of the medications available is achieved in only about 20 percent of patients.

If a young person experiences incontinence resulting from an overactive bladder, a doctor might prescribe a medicine that helps to calm the bladder muscle. This medicine controls muscle spasms and belongs to a class of medications called anticholinergics.

Table 16.1. Incontinence Is Also Called Enuresis

- Primary enuresis refers to wetting in a person who has never been dry for at least 6 months.

- Secondary enuresis refers to wetting that begins after at least 6 months of dryness.

- Nocturnal enuresis refers to wetting that usually occurs during sleep (nighttime incontinence).

- Diurnal enuresis refers to wetting when awake (daytime incontinence).

Bladder Training and Related Strategies

Bladder training consists of exercises for strengthening and coordinating muscles of the bladder and urethra, and may help the control of urination. These techniques teach the child to anticipate the need to urinate and prevent urination when away from a toilet.

Techniques that may help nighttime incontinence include:

- Determining bladder capacity
- Stretching the bladder (delaying urinating)
- Drinking less fluid before sleeping
- Developing routines for waking up.

Unfortunately, none of the above has demonstrated proven success.

Moisture Alarms

At night, moisture alarms can wake a person when he or she begins to urinate. These devices include a water-sensitive pad worn in pajamas, a wire connecting to a battery driven control, and an alarm that sounds when moisture is first detected. For the alarm to be effective, the child must awaken or be awakened as soon as the alarm goes off. This may require having another person sleep in the same room to awaken the bedwetter.

Table 16.2. Points to Remember.

- Urinary incontinence in children is common.

- Nighttime wetting occurs more commonly in boys.

- Daytime wetting is more common in girls.

- After age 5, incontinence disappears naturally at a rate of 15 percent of cases per year.

- Treatments include waiting, dietary modification, moisture alarms, medications, and bladder training.

Additional Resources

American Foundation for Urologic Disease
300 West Pratt Street
Suite 401
Baltimore, MD 21201
(Responds to written requests for patient information)

National Association For Continence
P.O. Box 8310
Spartanburg, SC 29305
(800) BLADDER or (864) 579-7900

National Kidney Foundation
30 East 33rd Street
New York, NY 10016
(800) 622-9010 or (212) 889-2210

The Simon Foundation for Continence
P.O. Box 835
Wilmette, IL 60091
(800) 23-SIMON

Society for Urologic Nurses and Associates
P.O. Box 56 East Holly Avenue
Pitman, NJ 08071
(609) 256-2335

Chapter 17

Common Bedtime Trauma

Description

Children who refuse to go to bed or stay in the bedroom often go to sleep while watching TV with a parent or they sleep in the parents' bed. In a milder form of bedtime refusal, a child stays in his bedroom but delays bedtime with ongoing questions, unreasonable requests, protests, crying, or temper tantrums. Such children are often tired in the morning and have to be awakened when it is time to get up.

These are manipulative behaviors, not fears. The child who occasionally comes to the parents' bed if he is frightened or not feeling well should be supported at these times. However, the child who postpones bedtime or tries to share your bed every night is taking advantage of your good nature.

Ending Bedtime Refusal

Establish a rule that your child can't leave the bedroom at night.

Enforce the rule that once your child is placed in the bedroom, she cannot leave that room, except to go to the bathroom, until morning.

Reprinted with permission from *Clinical Reference Systems*, December, 1997. © 1997 Barton Schmitt. The suggestions in this chapter were made by its author; please verify strategies with your child's pediatrician before implementing them.

Your child needs to learn to put herself to sleep for naps and at bedtime in her own bed. Do not stay in the room until she lies down or falls asleep. Establish a set bedtime and stick to it. Obviously, this change won't be accomplished without some crying or screaming for a few nights.

If your child has been sleeping with you, tell her "Starting tonight, we sleep in separate beds. You have your room and we have our room. You are too old to sleep with us anymore."

Ignore verbal requests.

Ignore ongoing questions or demands from the bedroom and do not engage in any conversation with your child. All requests should have been dealt with during your pre-bedtime ritual. Before you give your last hug and leave your child's bedroom, ask, "Do you need anything else?" Then don't return unless you think your child is sick. If your child says he needs to use the toilet, tell him to take care of it himself. If your child says his covers have fallen off, promise you will cover him up after he goes to sleep. (You will usually find him well covered.)

Close the bedroom door if your child is screaming.

Tell your child that you will open the door again when she stops screaming. If she pounds on the door, you can open it after 1 or 2 minutes and suggest that she go back to bed and stop screaming. If she doesn't, close the door again. If the screaming or pounding continues, open the door approximately every 15 minutes and remind your child that if she quiets down, the door can stay open. Never spend more than 30 seconds talking to her.

Close the door if your child is leaving the bedroom.

If your child comes out of the bedroom, return him immediately to his bed. Avoid any lectures and skip the hug and kiss. Get good eye contact and remind him again that he cannot leave his bedroom during the night. Warn him that if he comes out again you will need to close the door. If he does come out again, close the door for 2 or 3 minutes. If he continues to come out, close it for longer periods of time, up to 10 minutes. Open the door sooner if your child says he is in bed and promises to stay there.

Barricade the bedroom door if your child is repeatedly leaving the bedroom.

A helpful device is a half-door that you keep locked throughout the night. A heavy dresser, gate, or plywood plank may also work. If your child then screams at night, go to him and say, "Everyone is sleeping. I'll see you in the morning." If your child attempts to climb over the barricade, a full door may need to be kept closed until morning with a hook, piece of rope, or chain lock. Although this step seems extreme, it may be critical to protect children less than 5 years old who wander through the house at night without an understanding of dangers, such as fire, hot water, knives, or going outside.

Send your child back to her room if she comes into your bed at night.

Sternly order your child back to her own bed. If she doesn't move, escort her back immediately without any show of affection or pleasant conversation. If your child tries to leave her room again, temporarily close her door. If you are a deep sleeper, consider using some signaling device that will awaken you if your child enters your bedroom (such as a chair placed against your door or a loud bell attached to your doorknob). Some parents lock their bedroom door.

Remind your child that it is not polite to interrupt other people's sleep. Tell her that if she awakens at night and can't go back to sleep, she can look at books or play quietly in her room, but she is not to bother you.

Help siblings sleeping in the same bedroom.

If bedtime screaming wakes up a roommate, have the well-behaved sibling sleep in a separate room until the other child's behavior has improved. Tell the child who has the sleep problem that her roommate cannot return until she stays in her room quietly for three nights in a row. If you do not have a separate room available, have the sibling sleep in your room temporarily.

Praise appropriate sleeping behavior.

Praise your child in the morning if he stayed in his bedroom all night. Tell him that people are happier when they get a good night's sleep.

113

Call your child's physician during office hours if:

- Your child is not sleeping well after you try this program for 2 weeks.
- Your child is very frightened.
- Your child has lots of nightmares.
- Your child also has several discipline problems during the day.
- You have other questions or concerns.

— by B.D. Schmitt, M.D.

B.D. Schmitt, M.D. is the author of *Your Child's Health*, Bantam Books.

Chapter 18

Sleep Disorders in Childhood

Almost all children experience some type of sleep difficulty. Often, the problem is transient, with no long-lasting sequelae. For other children, however, sleep problems may have significant effects upon their behavior, level of functioning, and general well-being. These same sleep problems in children may affect others in the nuclear family. Historically, clinicians and researchers have tended to ignore childhood sleep disorders; parents rarely are concerned about an excessively sleepy child. Hence, the problem might not receive attention until the child's sleep difficulties begin to interfere with his or her waking function, primarily in school.

Recent surveys have found that approximately 25 percent of children between one and five years of age experience some type of sleep disturbance. Saizarulo and Chevalier (1983) interviewed the families of 218 children (2-15 years of age) who were referred for pediatric or child psychiatric consultation. Within this sample, sleep talking was quite common (32 percent), followed by nightmares (31 percent), waking at night (28 percent), trouble falling asleep (23 percent), bed wetting (17 percent), nocturnal teeth grinding (10 percent), sleep rocking (seven percent), and night terrors (seven percent). Dollinger (1982) surveyed mothers referring their children to a university health clinic.

From *Wake Up America: A National Sleep Alert*, Volume 1, Executive Summary and Executive Report, Report of the National Commission on Sleep Disorders Research, Submitted to the United States Congress and to the Secretary U.S. Department of Health and Human Services, January 1993.

Among 3-15 year old children and adolescents, the most common sleep problems noted were sleep talking (53 percent), restless sleep and refusing to go to bed (both 42 percent), and refusing to go to sleep without a night light (40 percent). Other sleep problems included bad dreams (35 percent), difficulty falling asleep (26 percent), crying out in sleep (16 percent), and nightmares (11 percent).

An added concern arises because research has suggested that childhood sleep disturbances tend to persist. Coterie et al. (1987) found that in their sample of children with sleep disturbances, 84 percent continued to experience these disturbances after three years. Bookseller and his colleagues (1976) found that sleep problems in older children often were associated with sleep-waking disorders in the first year of life. Furthermore, children who experienced disorders of the sleep-waking rhythm early in their lives often experienced a constellation of sleep problems in later years. In a third study, Zuckerman et al. (1987) found that 41 percent of children with sleep problems at eight months of age still had difficulties at three years of age. In contrast, only 26 percent of children who experienced no sleep problems at eight months were found to have a sleep problem at three years of age.

What Is Known

Childhood sleep disorders and problems have been aggregated and classified in the *International Classification of Sleep Disorders: Diagnostic and Coding Manual* (1990). Childhood diagnoses fall under the major categories of the dyssomnias and the parasomnias. Dyssomnias include those disorders either resulting in difficulty initiating or maintaining sleep, or disorders characterized by excessive sleepiness. On the other hand, parasomnias include disorders that disrupt sleep after it has been initiated.

A number of dyssomnias have been described in children. One such disorder is **narcolepsy**, characterized by excessive sleepiness that often presents itself as repeated episodes of naps or lapses into sleep of short duration throughout the day. Another common symptom of narcolepsy is cataplexy-the sudden loss of bilateral muscle tone following the experience of strong emotions such as laughter, elation, or anger. Treatment for this disorder often includes the use of prescription medications such as tricyclic antidepressants or stimulants (Wittig et al. 1983). Narcolepsy is a familial disorder that most frequently appears in the second decade of life, though it has been found in somewhat younger children as well.

A second dyssomnia often found in children is **obstructive sleep apnea syndrome** (OSAS). This disorder involves repetitive episodes of upper airway obstruction during sleep, often causing a reduction in blood oxygen saturation. These apneic episodes result in frequent brief awakenings throughout the night that are rarely remembered in the morning. The diagnosis of OSAS is somewhat more difficult in children than it is in adults. Children with this disorder may be excessively sleepy during the day, though the daytime disturbance often is not exhibited as sleepiness, but as behavior problems such as hyperactivity or acting out The mean age at diagnosis for children with sleep apnea is seven years; the disorder is more prevalent in boys than in girls (Mauer et al. 1983; Guilleminault and Anders 1976). The most common treatment for childhood OSAS is surgery to remove the airway obstruction. In about 70 percent of all cases, tonsillectomy or adenoidectomy relieves a child's symptoms of obstructive sleep apnea (Guilleminault and Demerit 1988).

Unlike narcolepsy or obstructive sleep apnea, both physiologically-based disorders, the other dyssomnias commonly seen in children often are environmentally-related. For example, **adjustment sleep disorder** is a form of insomnia related to emotional arousal caused by acute stress, conflict or environmental change. Children may experience this disorder following a move or before the first day of school. Another dyssomnia-**limit setting sleep disorder** involves difficulty falling asleep, typically characterized by stalling or refusing to go to bed. The problem may be as great for the parent or other caretaker as it is for the child. Five to ten percent of the childhood population experience this sleep disorder. Typically, limit-setting sleep disorder is alleviated once limits are established by the caretaker, the problem is highly amenable to behavioral mtmventions such as graduated extinction and the establishment of bedtime routines (Moniale 1990, Rohder and Van Houton 1984).

The parasomnias are distinct from the dyssomnias and are often quite dramatic, as well. **Sleep terrors** is reported to occur in about three percent of all children. This disorder is characterized by a sudden arousal from deep, slow-wave sleep with a piercing scream or cry, accompanied by physical and behavioral manifestations of intense fear. The child usually is unresponsive to attempts to soothe and may be confused and disoriented if awakened. Sleep terrors occur most commonly between the ages of four and 12; the problem tends to resolve during adolescence. Few broad-scale investigations have been undertaken to evaluate the treatment of sleep terrors, though a few case studies have been reported (Kellerman 1979; Kellerman 1980).

Other parasomnias experienced by children include **nightmares**, **sleep bruxism** (teeth grinding), and **sleep enuresis** (bed wetting). Nightmares are reported in approximately 10-50 percent of all children between the ages of three to six years (Diagnostic Classification Steering Committee 1990). Following a gradual onset, nightmares typically decrease in frequency over time. By adolescence, most children have stopped experiencing nightmares. Treatment strategies to control nightmares have focused on anxiety reduction, often combined with other behavioral strategies, such as systematic desensitization, flooding, and response prevention. No full-scale treatment studies of childhood nightmares have been performed, nor is it clear that treatment is necessary. Nightmares may reflect a developmental process for many children.

Bruxism occurs in over 50 percent of normal infants; the average age of onset is 10 months. Adult-related bruxism usually begins in the second decade of life. Bruxism may cause dental problems such as abnormal wear of the teeth or periodontal tissue damage; it also may be a cause of headache or jaw pain. Treatment with tooth guards, biofeedback, and other behavioral interventions has been evaluated intermittently.

The final common childhood parasomnia is sleep enuresis. Enuresis is diagnosed when persistent bed wetting occurs after the age of five. Estimates suggest that bed wetting occurs in 30 percent of four year olds, 10 percent of six year olds, five percent of 10 year olds, and three percent of 12 year olds. Several behavioral treatments have shown high success rates.

Several special subpopulations of children call for particular attention when considering sleep disorders. Mentally handicapped children, for example, experience higher rates of sleep disorders than found in the normal population and require special services. Bartlett et al. (1985) found that 80 percent of parents reported that their mentally handicapped child experienced sleep difficulties, difficulties that often cause undue stress for the care givers. Because behavioral interventions are highly successful in resolving sleep difficulties, appropriate intervention could reduce nocturnal stress and, therefore, improve the quality of life for the entire family.

A second population of concern are hospitalized children, a population that often suffers from sleep problems. Hagemann (1981) found that hospitalized children, ages three to eight years, lose one-fifth to one-fourth of their normal sleep time due to a delay in sleep onset. Several studies have explored means through which these sleep difficulties could be reduced; they found that hospitalized children may have more difficulty falling asleep at night when remembrances of home are present (White et al. 1988). Others have suggested that nursing staff should institute more structured bedtimes for the children or that the hospital should modify its environment at night (e.g., dimmed lights, reduced noise) to improve the capacity to initiate sleep.

Similarly, many children with chronic illness have difficulty with sleep. One study (Miser et al. 1987) found that nearly half of children presenting with newly diagnosed malignancy experience sleep disturbances due to pain. Mondale et al. (1990), however, found that while chronically ill children were not at greater risk of specific sleep disorders than healthy children, the chronically ill child generally gets less sleep altogether.

Sequelae of Childhood Sleep Disorders

A problem concomitant to childhood sleep disorders is the family stress that the child's problems can cause. Research has shown, for example, that parents of sleep disordered infants typically report more depressive symptomatology, decreased satisfaction in marriage, and greater anxiety (Damed and Mondale 1990).

Sleep problems in school-age children may begin to interfere with other aspects of the child's life. These children may have difficulty concentrating in school and may develop a secondary behavior problem in the classroom. Certain children misdiagnosed with hyperactivity or a learning disability actually may be suffering from primary sleep problems. An older child who continues to be enuretic often is embarrassed about the problem and will avoid situations in which the problem can be discovered by non-family members. For such children, sleep disorders have moved out of the bedroom and have become a problem of daily life.

An associated cause of concern, about which no information exists, is the impact of treatment for common pediatric medical conditions on the sleep/wake system. For example, treatments for asthma and allergies commonly involve drugs that alter neurotransmitter systems affecting sleeping and waking function. Dual emphasis on sleep and wakefulness is important because disturbed sleep—as caused by central nervous system and respiratory stimulants—can impair daytime functioning. Conversely, drugs such as antihistamines can impair alertness directly and can also affect sleep. Nevertheless, no research has examined whether such compounds impair sleep and wakeful function in children.

119

Given the widespread prevalence of sleep problems in infants and children, the relative paucity of research on mechanisms, treatments, and prevention is disturbing. Implementation of a national plan to attend to these issues holds great promise for immediate beneficial impact upon the lives of millions of Americans.

Chapter 19

How Much Sleep Does an Adolescent Need?

Parents are often concerned about the sleeping habits of their adolescent children. In my office, I commonly hear either "He sleeps past noon!" or "She's up all night!" (or both). Naturally, we want our children to be motivated and healthy. If it seems that they are sleeping their lives away, or that they are burning the candle at both ends, our parental instincts rise up.

The ideal amount of sleep at any given age varies widely between individuals, but adolescence is a particularly difficult age at which to pinpoint and ensure the proper amount of sleep.

Observations made in sleep laboratories (Carskadan, et al: Pubertal changes in daytime sleepiness. *Sleep* 2:453, 460, 1980) suggest that adolescents require more sleep than preteens. On the other hand, observations made in real life (Carskadan: Patterns of sleep and sleepiness in adolescents. *Pediatrician* 17:5, 1990) suggest that adolescents actually obtain much less sleep than they did during the preteen years.

This raises three important questions: First, is this data true? In other words, if researchers in a lab say one thing, and real life says another, are most teenagers really getting insufficient sleep? Second, if most teens do not get enough sleep, why? Are teens just short-sighted, stubborn and out of control? Third, what can be done to help teens get the sleep they need?

Reprinted with permission from *Dr. Greene's Housecalls*, June 24, 1996. © 1996 Dr. Greene's Housecalls. http//www.drgreene.com/adolescents.html

The contrast between ideal and actual sleep in teenagers is based on solid research. Its truth is bolstered by the additional observation that excessive sleepiness is a very common complaint among adolescents. Daytime sleepiness is the most common sleep-related disorder of adolescence.

For many years it was felt that the sleepiness of adolescents was their own fault. Their busy social agenda and burgeoning independence led to too many late nights. Recently, however, a different picture has emerged. Independent investigators in Brazil, Japan, and the United States (Andrade, et al; Ishihara, et al; and Carskadon, et al.) have suggested that the internal, biologic sleep-timing mechanism is reset along with the other changes of puberty. Their bodies signal them to go to sleep at a later hour and also to sleep later in the morning. They are often incapable of falling asleep earlier. Their school schedules, however, continue to force them out of bed at an early hour. This leads to a population of chronically sleep deprived adolescents.

Many teens are able to cope with chronic low-level sleep deprivation, often gaining some catch-up sleep by 'sleeping in' on the weekends. Others, however, fall asleep in school, have great difficulty getting out of bed in the morning, and/or experience great fatigue, emotional liability, irritability, poor impulse control, and poor decision making.

The average thirteen year old needs about 10 hours of sleep in a 24 hour period. However, adequacy of sleep should be determined by a careful evaluation of symptoms rather than by relying on numbers obtained from a large sample of adolescents.

If insufficient sleep is identified, telling the adolescent to "just go to bed earlier" is ineffective and alienating. Either the adolescent's schedule should be adjusted to complement his body's internal clock, or the internal clock can be gradually reset through a process called chronotherapy. This will only work if your child understands the problem and is a willing partner in the process.

Sudden changes in sleep schedule do not help to reset the body's circadian rhythm. Instead, begin by stabilizing bedtime at an hour when it is easy and natural to fall asleep. Then, make the bedtime earlier by about 15 minutes each day (any more than this is too long to lure the circadian rhythm to follow). During this process, naps must be avoided, and the procedure must be followed 7 nights a week. Upon awakening, exercise and exposure to bright light help to fix the new rhythm. (For children whose original bedtime is very late, it can be faster to move the bedtime later by 2 or 3 hours per night around the clock, rather than backward by 15 minutes,—the circadian rhythm will follow. This works extremely well, but requires a committed adult to help enforce waking at the proper time).

Once a new schedule appropriate to the individual is attained, bedtime and wake-up time should be rigidly maintained for 2 to 3 weeks. Later, occasionally staying up late on weekend nights will not reset the clock, as long as he doesn't sleep in more than 1 or 2 hours later than he would for school.

Some sleep experts recommend giving melatonin about 90 minutes before the desired bedtime as a way to reset the biologic clock. Melatonin is available in health food stores, and now in some drug stores, too. Preliminary studies in adults look exciting, but I'm still cautious about its use in children. Melatonin is a potent chemical which also affects the reproductive system. No one really knows what effects it might have on the reproductive system if given before or during puberty.

Many significant events in our recent history are at least partially attributable to sleep deprivation: The crash of the *Exxon Valdez*, the Union Carbide disaster in Bhopal, the explosion of the space shuttle *Challenger* (on the part of those responsible for the O-ring), and the nuclear disaster at Chernobyl. More automobile accidents are attributable to sleepiness than to any other single cause. Sleepiness robs more person-years through trauma than does any disease. While most teens handle chronic low-grade sleepiness well, I believe that starting high school an hour or two later would markedly improve the health and behavior of adolescents.

—by Alan Greene, M.D., F.A.A.P.,
Department of Pediatrics,
Stanford University
School of Medicine.
Author of The Parent's
Complete Guide to
Ear Infections
and DrGreene.com.

Chapter 20

Sleep in Women: A Woman's Guide to Her Unique Sleep Requirements

The quality of a woman's sleep is an important component of the quality of her life. For years, very little research was available concerning the sleep problems unique to women, and sleep complaints were not always taken seriously by healthcare providers. Recent studies, however, have paid more attention to the particular patterns, changing needs, and special problems associated with sleep throughout a woman's life. Notable among the findings is that women are twice as likely as men to have difficulties falling asleep or staying asleep.

In general, a woman's sleep is most sound and least prone to disturbances during young adulthood. The sleep disturbances most common to young women include those associated with the menstrual cycle, pregnancy, and motherhood. Also, many young women in today's fast-paced world cut back too often on their sleep, and ignore signs of fatigue, daytime sleepiness and other effects of insufficient sleep.

As a woman ages, physical and hormonal changes affect her sleep quality. Older women get less deep sleep and are more likely to wake up at night. Physical factors—such as arthritis, disorders of breathing, or hot flashes—may also disturb sleep.

A woman's feelings and concerns are also important components of sleep quality. Acute stress, depression, fear, and other emotional components can affect sleep patterns.

Getting enough sleep is enormously important to a woman's life, as it positively impacts her concentration, job performance, social interaction, and general well-being.

This chapter will describe some of the factors unique to women's sleep, and will provide suggestions and guidelines for overcoming these challenges.

The Menstrual Cycle

Distinct changes in sleep patterns accompany the changing phases of the menstrual cycle. An increased number of awakenings and more sleep disturbances occur during the premenstrual period in some women. Dreams are more frequent and more vivid during this phase of the cycle. Some women report excessive daytime sleepiness, fatigue, and longer sleeping hours during the premenstrual period.

Sleep changes are often associated with other premenstrual signs, such as abdominal cramping, irritability, food cravings, and emotional changes. These sleep problems generally disappear a few days after menstruation begins. For women who find these changes particularly disturbing, however, increased tension and irritability can result in lingering sleep problems and even to chronic insomnia.

Women who experience menstrual-related sleep disorders should pay careful attention to their sleep needs, maintain a regular sleep/wake schedule, eat a healthy diet, and try to reduce stress. If sleep problems interfere with daily functioning, medical advice should be sought.

Sleep During Pregnancy

Early in pregnancy, most women report feeling fatigued during the day and sleeping longer hours at night. This almost universal change in sleep requirement is probably caused by increasing levels of the hormone progesterone during pregnancy.

Later in pregnancy, particularly during the last trimester, women often note poor sleep quality. Certain changes in sleep patterns have been confirmed by studies: the amount of slow-wave sleep (deep stages of sleep) decreases, and the number of awakenings increases. Women may find it difficult to sleep in certain positions. Overall sleep efficiency and the proportion of time spent actually asleep begins to decrease by the second trimester, and continues to decrease in the third trimester.

There are many causes for sleep disruption in the late stages of pregnancy: leg cramps, backache, heartburn, movements of the fetus, general discomforts of pregnancy, and increased frequency of urination.

After the baby is born, the physical stresses of pregnancy on sleep may be replaced by the demands of the baby's feeding schedule and frequent awakenings at night.

Throughout pregnancy, women need to make sure they are getting enough sleep, maintaining regular sleep/wake schedules, and avoiding stress as much as possible. Because sleeping pills and alcohol should be avoided during pregnancy, other measures to improve sleep should be considered. Muscle relaxation techniques may be effective in promoting better sleep and reducing the discomforts of pregnancy. Maintaining a balanced diet and avoiding heavy meals and spicy foods within two or three hours of bedtime will help avoid provoking heartburn.

After delivery, getting enough rest continues to be very important, as severely disturbed sleep can be tied to postpartum depression and child abuse.

Menopause

Some natural changes in sleep accompany the aging process in women. The amount of deep sleep decreases, sleep becomes lighter, and more awakenings occur during the night.

In the years surrounding menopause, sleep disturbances occur with increased frequency. A gradual change in sex hormone levels impacts sleep directly and indirectly by affecting other important hormones that are related to sleep. Hot flashes and night sweats—associated with decreased levels of estrogen—may cause repeated awakenings associated with the sensation of heat and sweating, increased heart rate, and feelings of anxiety. Although hot flashes usually last only a few minutes, in severe cases a woman may wake up hundreds of times a night. The sleep disturbance and resultant sleep deprivation generated by these hot flashes may result in daytime fatigue, irritability and depression.

These measures may help alleviate the sleep disturbances associated with hot flashes:

- Control the bedroom temperature; use light and comfortable (preferably cotton) bed linen.

- Eliminate caffeine, sugar and alcohol from the diet. Increase vitamin E intake in the diet, or take a vitamin E supplement.

- Estrogen replacement therapy can be helpful in relieving severe hot flashes and resultant significant sleep loss. A physician can offer advice on this mode of treatment.

Postmenopausal Years

In the years following menopause, sleep grows lighter and more fragmented. It becomes more difficult to maintain long hours of uninterrupted sleep, and to maintain long hours of wakefulness during the day. An increase in daytime fatigue can be one result. Other physical factors can also disturb sleep: arthritis and other painful conditions, chronic lung disease, certain medications, heartburn, and increased frequency of urination.

Some sleep disorders occur more frequently in the postmenopausal years. For example, sleep-disordered breathing—uncommon in young women—is more common in postmenopausal women. This may be related to falling progesterone levels, since younger women who experience surgical menopause are also at increased risk of developing sleep-disordered breathing. Higher body weight and lower levels of physical activity are also risk factors for this syndrome. Signs of sleep-disordered breathing include loud snoring during sleep and excessive daytime sleepiness.

Other factors also influence the quality of sleep in postmenopausal women: psychosocial environment, physical health and emotional state. The connection between worry and insomnia may be obvious, but at times subtle signs and concerns can be less visible in their influence on tension and insomnia.

To promote better sleep during the postmenopausal years, women should follow these guidelines:

- Maintain a comfortable, safe environment in the bedroom: reduce disturbing noise and extreme temperature.

- Go to bed and get up at the same time every day.

- Avoid staying in bed late in the morning to make up for sleep loss.

- Get up early in the morning and maintain structured daily activity.

- Consider an afternoon nap at a regular time.

- Stay away from fatty, spicy foods that are likely to cause indigestion or heartburn.

- Seek medical advice if following these measures does not alleviate excessive daytime sleepiness.

Emotional issues continue to impact sleep in women of all age groups. Two conditions worthy of mention are depression and nocturnal eating syndrome.

Depression

Insomnia is one of the most common symptoms of depression at any age. Women who are depressed tend to fall asleep fairly quickly but often awaken in the middle of the night, unable to go back to sleep. The insomnia may be interpreted as the cause of the depression—"If I could just get more sleep I would not feel depressed"—but getting professional help and treatment for the depression can often solve the insomnia problem.

Nocturnal Eating Syndrome

Some women wake up in the middle of the night and feel that they are unable to go back to sleep until they eat. Unless there is a medical cause (such as an ulcer), this type of problem is typically associated with dieting during the day.

When to See a Healthcare Provider

Occasional disturbances in sleep can happen to anyone, and generally do not require medical intervention. Serious sleep problems, however, can affect a woman's daily functioning, her relationships, and her sense of well-being. When a sleep problem results in disruption in one of these areas, it may be wise to consult with a healthcare provider.

Women are particularly sensitive to sleep difficulties because they are affected by hormonal changes, family stresses and role conflicts, any of which can affect sleep quality.

The information in this article should help you cope with normal changes in sleep, and to decide when to seek medical attention.

Your healthcare provider will be able to refer you to a sleep disorders specialist for a comprehensive evaluation of your sleep difficulties. You may be asked to have your sleep monitored for a more detailed evaluation. At the sleep center, an accurate diagnosis will allow your healthcare practitioner to develop the right treatment plan for you.

Guidelines for Good Sleep

These guidelines can be helpful in alleviating all types of sleep problems, and will help most people sleep well:

- Get up about the same time every day.

- Go to bed only when sleepy.

- Establish relaxing pre-sleep rituals, such as a warm bath, light bedtime snack, or 10 minutes of reading.

- Exercise regularly. Consult a healthcare provider before beginning an exercise program. Confine vigorous exercise to early hours, at least six hours before bedtime, and do mild exercise—such as simple stretching or walking—at least four hours prior to bedtime.

- Keep a regular schedule. Regular times for meals, medications, chores, and other activities help keep the inner clock running smoothly.

- Avoid ingestion of caffeine within six hours of bedtime. Don't drink alcohol, especially when sleepy. Even a small dose of alcohol can have a potent effect when combined with being tired.

- Avoid smoking close to bedtime.

- Try to nap at the same time every day; mid-afternoon is the best time for most people.

- Avoid sleeping pills, or use them conservatively. Most doctors avoid prescribing sleeping pills for periods of longer than three weeks. Do not drink alcohol while taking sleeping pills.

Further Reading

Bodyrhythms: Chronobiology and Peak Performance by Lynne Lamberg (William Moffow and Company, Inc., 1994)

No More Sleepless Nights by Peter Hauri, PhD, and Shirley Linde, PhD (John Wiley and Sons, Inc. 1990)

Encyclopedia of Sleep and Dreaming edited by Mary A. Caskadon, PhD (New York: Macmillan, 1992)

Asleep in the Fast Lane: The Impact of Sleep On Work by Lydia Dotto (Stoddart Publishing Co. Limited, 1990)

Wide Awake at 3:00 a.m.: By Choice or By Chance? by Richard M. Coleman (W.H. Freeman and Company, New York, 1986)

Sleep, Dreaming, and Sleep Disorders, An Introduction by William H. Moorcraft (University Press of America, 1989, 2nd ed.)

Chapter 21

Sleep in Older Persons

Few things in life are as cherished as a good night's rest. Yet, for many older adults, bedtime is the hardest part of the day. Strong biological, clinical, and epidemiological evidence exists that indicates sleep is affected by the aging process. Moreover, changes in sleep are frequent concerns among older adults and their caregivers. The ongoing study of sleep in late life is vitally important for several reasons. First, a large proportion of elders suffer sleep disturbances. Older adults constitute the age group most severely affected by disorders of initiating and maintaining sleep and consume disproportionate quantities of sleeping pills and tranquilizers. Very often, nighttime insomnia (and/or the medication used to "relieve" it) leads to significant deterioration in daytime alertness and functioning, and a significant degree of distress is caused. Additionally, many daytime complaints and health problems seen in late life may be related to specific sleep disorders. Until recently, changes in sleep have been associated with the normal aging process. However, new research data indicate that many of the sleep changes in elders may be pathologic and amenable to intervention. Second, older persons who have sleep disturbances provide a sample that can be used to study aging effects in general, effects that are likely to be most clear-cut in the "old-old" and that may provide clues to improving the health and quality-of-life of all late-life age groups. In this context, the two most common

Excerpted from an undated document from the NIH, NINR, National Nursing Research Agenda, *Long Term Care for Older Adults*, Chapter 8 neuropsychiatric disorders of late life, depression and dementia of the Alzheimer's type, are both associated with profound disturbances in sleep and often with impaired alertness during the day. Further, many of the ills of old age (or their treatment) have a negative impact on the ability to achieve long uninterrupted periods of sleep and adequate depth of sleep, thus compounding the distress associated with chronic medical diseases. Third, studies have suggested that sleep-related behaviors often precipitate a family's decision to institutionalize an elderly relative. Any understanding that would help reduce the institutionalization rate would pay for itself many times over. The benefits that could accrue from understanding how the aging system mediates the deteriorations observed in the health and well-being of older adults, including sleep, would have an impact not only on older persons themselves but on society as a whole. The following discussion describes sleep and the measurement of sleep; provides a comprehensive review of sleep and aging research; and suggests directions for future research studies on sleep and older adults.

State of the Science

Sleep and Measurement

Sleep is a set of complete physiological processes involving a predictable sequence of operating states within the central nervous system identified by electroencephalographic (EEG) patterns and by specific behaviors. Sleep is measured objectively by EEG recordings or observational methods and subjectively through self-reports. EEG sleep is typically recorded in a laboratory during nocturnal and/or daytime sleep periods and requires a minimum of at least one full night of recording. Laboratory study provides objective and accurate data about sleep variables. These studies are limited, however, because of the necessity for expensive equipment and technical proficiency in obtaining and interpreting results, and because the person is removed from the normal sleep milieu. Portable recording methodologies are also available for use in community settings. Portable technologies provide accurate data but are restricted in number and type of EEG variables that can be recorded. EEG sleep recordings can be scored by hand or by automated computer analysis. Variables include measures of sleep continuity, sleep architecture (stages of non-rapid-eye-movement (NREM) sleep), and rapid-eye-movement (REM) sleep. Both REM sleep (dreaming sleep) and NREM sleep (quiet sleep) are part of the normal sleep cycle. Everyone has about four to five cycles of REM and NREM sleep per night. For older persons, the amount of time spent in the deepest stages of NREM sleep decreases. This may explain why older people are thought of as light sleepers. Additional variables generally recorded during nocturnal EEG monitoring are nocturnal myoclonus or periodic leg movements and measures of breathing including apnea, hypopneas, and oxygen desaturations. Observational methods are used in institutional settings. Periodic or continuous monitoring of sleep behaviors is done by direct personal observations or through video recordings. Observations are recorded on data forms and are typically categorical and descriptive. Observational study is less expensive than EEG recordings but yields less precise data and introduces questions of rater reliability and bias. Subjective self-report data is collected through questionnaires or interviews including sleep logs, post-sleep questionnaires, and surveys on sleep habits and sleep quality. Self-reports are valuable sources of information because they reflect an individual's attitudes, beliefs, and perceptions about his or her sleep and indicate problem areas. Data are, however, estimates.

Sleep and Aging Research

Sleep and aging research over the past decade has yielded many exciting and promising discoveries about sleep patterns, sleep structures, and subject sleep evaluations using methodologies described above. Several key areas of sleep research with older persons have emerged: 1) normal" or "healthy" aging; 2) pathologic aging (generally neuropsychiatric disorders of late life); 3) specific sleep disturbances (sleep-disordered breathing, nocturnal myoclonus, excessive daytime sleepiness, insomnia); 4)sleep problems in the nursing home; and 5) mortality.

Sleep and Healthy Aging. Research studies have consistently documented the following EEG sleep patterns among the healthy older adults: fragmented sleep with increased NREM Stages 1 and 2 sleep; decreased NREM Stage 4 (deep) sleep; and decreased absolute amounts of REM sleep. The nocturnal sleep of older persons is brittle and shallow; that is, it is characterized by numerous transient arousals (3-15 seconds) and by a loss of the deepest levels of NREM sleep. In addition, the sleep of older persons is often redistributed around the clock, as evidenced by both the fragmentation of nighttime sleep, the occurrence of daytime naps, and an advanced sleep phase (going to bed earlier and getting up earlier). Even if the ability to have slow-wave sleep and long noninterrupted sleep periods declines with age the issue of ability to sleep versus need for sleep is not settled. That is, do older people sleep less because they need less sleep, or because they cannot sleep as well as younger adults? Currently, research evidence favors the view that elders have less ability to sleep rather than less need for sleep. Hence, the occurrence of daytime sleepiness in many older people may be a manifestation of unmet sleep need. Yet, recent research also suggests that some aspects of age-related sleep deterioration are reversible. Thus, following sleep deprivation or sleep restriction (i.e., systematically spending less time in bed), older persons show an ability to generate recovery sleep with increased amounts of slow-wave sleep and improved sleep continuity. Gender-related differences also have been noted in the sleep of healthy older people. Elderly men show more impaired sleep maintenance and less slow-wave sleep than elderly women. However, older women are more likely than men to complain of sleep disturbance and to receive sleeping pills. An explanation of this paradox may lie in gender-related differences in sleep perception and effects of sleep disruption on mood. Research has shown that elderly women show higher and more stable correlations between estimates of sleep quality and objective laboratory measurements of sleep, and that elderly women find sleep deprivation to be a more mood-disturbing experience than elderly men. It is possible that elderly women may be more sensitive to sleep quality and sleep loss than elderly men. To determine if advancing age continues to affect the stability of sleep structure and reports of sleep quality, longitudinal studies of sleep in healthy elders have been initiated. Hoch and colleagues measured EEG sleep characteristics and perceptions of sleep quality of healthy elders at two-year intervals. In this study, most laboratory measures of sleep and measures of sleep quality were stable over two years. Both elderly men and women showed significantly more awakenings during the second recording series; however, there was no change in visual or computer-scored delta activity. Further, gender-dependent sleep changes were noted only in phasic REM measures. Activity, density, and intensity increased in men over time and decreased in women. Subjective estimates of sleep quality, although stable over time, showed gender-dependent differences with women reporting a lower sleep quality than men.

Sleep and Pathologic Aging. Depression and dementia are two of the most serious and prevalent neuropsychiatric disorders of old age. Sleep disturbances are among the most frequent and disturbing features of depressed and demented older adults. Sleep research in affective illness, particularly in late-life depression, has advanced over the past decade, resulting in a growing body of objective data concerning EEG sleep changes associated with depressive illness. The sleep of Alzheimer's patients in varying stages of the disease has been studied. Information concerning the specificity of EEG sleep changes in late-life depression, compared with other neuropsychiatric disorders such as probable Alzheimer's dementia as well as "healthy" (pathology-free) aging, is now available. Interactions between aging and illness determine the sleep characteristics of depression. The sleep changes that characterize depression also occur during the course of normal aging, but to a lesser extent. For instance, an age-dependent increase in wakefulness after sleep onset and decrease in slow-wave sleep characterize both normal aging and depressive illness. It is less clear whether REM sleep latency shortens during the course of normal aging (as it does to a considerable extent in depression) and if it does, how robust a trend this may be. However, it is recognized that the tendency for REM sleep periods to become progressively longer during the night is significantly less in older healthy persons than in young adults. Apparently, the capacity to sustain REM sleep inhibition during the first half of the night is diminished by advancing age and, to a greater extent, by the presence of depressive illness. Hence, abbreviation of REM sleep latency and alteration of intranight temporal distribution of REM sleep (with greater early REM sleep density) most specifically characterizes the sleep of older patients with major depressive disorders. These changes in REM sleep cycling and density are more marked in depressives in late-life than at any other age. It has been demonstrated that short REM latencies, prolonged first REM periods, and extreme sleep maintenance difficulty reliably characterize the EEG sleep of elderly unipolar, nondelusional, and endogenous depressed older adults. One of the findings from these studies has been the high frequency of sleep onset REM periods (SOREMP's) in elderly endogenous depressives, where approximately 45 percent of REM latency values are less than ten minutes as compared with less than two percent in healthy controls and 17 percent in nondepressed Alzheimer's patients. The sleep maintenance difficulties of depressed older people also correlated significantly with the severity of depression, as measured by Hamilton depression ratings. A concomitant finding was that the extent of cognitive impairment in depressed older adults, as measured by the Folstein mini-mental state, was significantly and positively correlated with the amount of Stage 1 sleep, another measure of sleep fragmentation.

The response characteristics and regulatory integrity of the sleep system in late-life depression have been elucidated further by the use of sleep deprivation research protocols as both clinical and physiologic probes. Sleep deprivation techniques have been used also to characterize the sleep of elderly depressives as compared with healthy controls and individuals with dementia of the Alzheimer's type. For example, during recovery sleep following a 36- to 40-hour total sleep deprivation procedure, time spent asleep and sleep efficiency were increased in depressed and demented patients as well as in healthy controls. However, neither of the patient groups achieved even baseline control levels of sleep efficiency or time spent in sleep. Further, the depressed patients had the lowest sleep efficiency throughout recovery sleep. Depressed patients also differed from the other groups with respect to the temporal distribution of delta wave activity, showing the greatest amount in the second NREM period. REM responses to sleep deprivation likewise differed among the three groups, with both depressed and demented patients experiencing increased REM latency during recovery sleep and healthy subjects experiencing decreased REM latency.

Self-reported measures of sleep disturbances and depressed feelings in community resident elders also support an interactive relationship between sleep regulation and depression. A recent longitudinal study examined the association between frequency of depressed mood and self-reports of sleep problems (difficulty falling asleep, waking up frequently in the night, early morning awakening, not feeling rested in the morning) in a group of community-residing elders over a three-year period. The investigators found that frequency of depressed feelings was related to moderate and severe levels of sleep disturbance, with early morning awakening emerging as the sleep problem most consistently associated with depressed affect over time. This finding is consistent with electroencephalographic investigations that have suggested the importance of early morning awakenings as a key sleep symptom among elderly depressives. Moreover, the presence of early morning awakenings has also been shown to correlate with severity of depression and to predict reversible dementia (pseudodementia) versus primary degenerative dementia with depressive features.

Disturbed sleep and sleep/wake cycles are common occurrences in individuals with Alzheimer's disease. These disturbances often result in disrupted nocturnal behaviors such as nighttime insomnia, wandering, and sundowning. The impaired sleep/wake patterns associated with Alzheimer's dementia may result from loss of or damage to

138

the neuronal pathways that initiate and maintain sleep. Brainstem regions and pathways that regulate sleep/wake cycles may undergo degenerative changes in Alzheimer's disease; similar changes also may occur in the cortical tissues that generate EEG slow-wave activity during sleep. Elderly individuals with dementia as compared with controls have exhibited greater disruption of sleep continuity, decreased REM sleep time and activity, decreased amounts of NREM Stages three and four sleep, frequent daytime naps with nighttime periods of wakefulness, and diminished delta activity. Some investigators reported that sleep measures in mildly demented Alzheimer's patients were minimally affected, but REM time and REM activity/density were significantly affected in later stages of dementia. Concurrent with advancing dementia, Alzheimer's patients show a gradual but progressive loss of phasic activity, both of rapid eye movements in dream sleep and of spindles and K-complexes in NREM sleep. In addition, the amount of slow-wave sleep and the number of delta waves diminish in dementia. Finally, Alzheimer's patients have significantly more sleep-disordered breathing than elderly controls or depressives. These sleep variables have been explored as potential biological markers for Alzheimer's disease. However, definitive markers in early or mild dementia have not been isolated yet.

Sleep Disturbances and Aging. Several sleep disturbances of considerable epidemiological and clinical interest have been studied in relation to advancing age including sleep-disordered breathing, nocturnal myoclonus, excessive daytime sleepiness, and insomnia. Each disturbance can be the result of pathology or may precipitate other significant sequelae among older adults.

Sleep-disordered breathing and its relation to advancing age is determined by nocturnal polysomnographic recordings. Sleep apnea occurs when there are at least five apneas (complete cessations of respiration) or hypopneas (partial cessation of respiration) per hour of sleep, with each event lasting a minimum of ten seconds. The apnea index (AI) is the number of apneas per hour of sleep; apnea-hypopnea index (AHI) is the number of apneas and hypopneas per hour of sleep. Apneic events are usually followed by an awakening or arousal and can be associated with many symptoms including decreased blood oxygen levels, cardiac arrhythmias, nocturnal hypertension, nighttime confusion, and neuropsychiatric impairment. Numerous studies have directly or indirectly examined the prevalence of sleep-disordered breathing (apneas, hypopneas, and oxygen desaturations) in healthy aging populations and in randomly selected community resident elders. Results consistently demonstrate age-related increases in the prevalence of sleep-disordered breathing. Estimates of AI and/or AHI of five or greater have been reported in one-fourth to one-third of older persons studied. Gender differences also have been noted with increased prevalence of sleep apnea in elderly men versus elderly women. However, the significance of the condition is not clear.

In studies with more medically and neuropsychiatrically compromised elders, the impact of sleep-disordered breathing may be differentially greater. Higher rates of sleep apneas have been found among nursing home residents and medical ward patients than in independently-living elderly. The higher rates of sleep apnea in randomly selected elderly medical ward patients were attributed to congestive heart failure. Other studies have reported significant associations between sleep-disordered breathing and substantial cardiovascular morbidity. Numerous investigators have examined cognitive impairment in patients with and without sleep apnea. All except one found a relationship between hypoxemia (caused by sleep apnea) and mental deterioration. In addition, impaired respiration has been linked to mortality. With respect to sleep-disordered breathing in elderly patients with neuropsychiatric impairment, the rate in elderly depressives does not appear to be significantly greater than that of age- and sex-matched controls. Studies have reported a 16 to 18 percent occurrence of sleep apnea in elderly depressives compared with four to six percent in healthy elders. However, a significantly higher prevalence of sleep-disordered breathing has been found in elderly patients with probable Alzheimer's disease than in age- and sex-matched controls by some but not all investigators. A few investigators also have examined the functional significance of sleep-disordered breathing in Alzheimer's disease. Severity of dementia has been correlated significantly with percent of indeterminate NREM sleep and severity of sleep apnea. Data also suggest that sleep-disordered breathing in nonmedicated Alzheimer's patients is relatively mild and is not a predictor of overnight changes in respiration, nocturnal oxyhemoglobin desaturation, overnight mental status, or nocturnal behavior. Finally, in elderly patients with mixed symptoms of depression and cognitive impairment who had died by 2-year followup, apnea-hypopnea indices (and REM latency) correctly predicted 77 percent of survivors.

Nocturnal myoclonus or periodic leg movement in sleep is a sleep disturbance in which people kick or jerk their legs every 20 to 40 seconds periodically throughout the night. It is measured by polysomnographic recordings of anterior tibalis muscle activity. Myoclonus index (MI) is calculated as the ratio of periodic leg movements associated with arousals to total sleep time in hours. Research has generally focused on prevalence rates. Few studies of nocturnal myoclonus have been reported specifically with regard to older adults. Among elderly with sleep complaints, the rates of nocturnal myoclonus range from four to 31 percent. However, in studies with healthy elderly people, rates range from 25 to 60 percent. Some investigators also have studied myoclonus in Alzheimer's patients but did not find associations between leg movements and diagnosis.

When nighttime sleep is reduced or disturbed, the result is increased sleepiness the next day. Excessive daytime sleepiness in older people may be indicative of an underlying sleep problem that results in a deterioration of the continuity of nocturnal sleep. Daytime sleepiness is measured objectively by the multiple sleep latency test (MSLT) using polysomnography during four or five daytime naps lasting 20 minutes. The MSLT measures how long it takes an individual to fall asleep during the daytime when given multiple opportunities to do so. Research has demonstrated that older adults consistently fall asleep in less than 15 minutes, more quickly than other age groups. When elders are asked to subjectively describe their sleep and daytime functioning, most report that their sleep is satisfactory, yet they also report daytime sleepiness. Investigations have shown also that older adults take more naps than younger people. MSLT data, in conjunction with nocturnal sleep studies, would be useful to determine the extent and severity of daytime sleepiness and to explore relationships with the nocturnal sleep of elders.

Studies suggest that older adults are the age group most affected by disorders of initiating and maintaining sleep. Insomnia refers to the perception of an individual that his/her sleep is inadequate or abnormal. Symptoms generally include both nocturnal symptoms (difficulty initiating sleep, frequent awakenings from sleep, short sleep time, "nonrestorative" sleep), and daytime symptoms (fatigue, sleepiness, depression, anxiety, other mood changes) that result from poor nighttime sleep. These symptoms are similar to those complaints most frequently offered by elders about their sleep: spending more time in bed; taking longer to fall asleep; awakening more often; being sleepy in the daytime; and needing longer to adjust to changes in the usual sleep-wake schedule. For transient insomnia among older persons, which lasts for three to four weeks and results from situational causes, medication is generally acceptable treatment. However, for prolonged or chronic geriatric insomnia, nonpharmacologic interventions are warranted. Improving sleep hygiene by promoting a safe and comfortable sleep environment, setting a regular time to go to bed, exercising, and avoiding alcohol and caffeine is essential. Overreliance on the use of over-the-counter drugs to treat symptoms of sleep disorders can be ineffective and make conditions worse. In addition, many cause side effects such as blurred vision, dry mouth, and drowsiness. Research protocols for geriatric insomnia, using sleep restriction and relaxation training methods, have had only limited success.

Sleep Problems in the Nursing Home. Disturbed sleep with nighttime wandering is one of the most frequent reasons why elderly individuals are institutionalized. Sleep disturbances and related behaviors and complaints are common among nursing home populations. Studies have estimated that 35 percent of nursing home residents receive tranquilizing medications. Observation, interview, and questionnaire measures are the most frequent methodologies used in studies of sleep in nursing home settings. Sleep patterns around the clock have been observed with increasing amounts of sleep in a 24-hour period usually resulting from increased daytime sleep rather than an increase in nocturnal sleep. Investigations also have demonstrated great individual variability in sleep patterns of nursing home patients. Objectively recorded sleep by portable nocturnal polysomnography was used in a randomly selected group of elderly nursing home patients. These patients averaged only 39.5 minutes of sleep per hour in any hour of the night, and 50 percent woke up at least two times per hour. When a subgroup of these nursing home residents were recorded for a full 24 hours, patients spent some portion of every hour asleep. In addition, their sleep was so fragmented that they rarely experienced even a single hour of consolidated sleep. As previously described, sleep-disordered breathing is also more prevalent among nursing home residents than community-residing elders.

Mortality. Mortality rates at various times during the night have been studied. Mortality rates from all causes are estimated to increase 30 percent during sleep. Excessive death between 2:00 a.m. and 8:00 a.m. has been found, with the peak being relatively specific to ischemic heart disease in persons over the age of 65 years. Studies have shown that people who report either sleeping less than seven hours or more than eight hours have a higher mortality rate, with 86 percent of these deaths among individuals over 60 years of age. It has been hypothesized that sleep apnea may be one cause of increased.

Research Needs and Opportunities

Research studies on sleep and older persons present a challenge for the next decade. Studies on sleep and older adults have focused primarily on observational and subjective methodologies, such as sleep patterns among institutionalized elders or sleep behaviors and routines, in a theoretical and empirical analysis of sleep disturbance patterns in aging, concluded that more research is needed to delineate specific assessment parameters and intervention techniques. We have yet to meet this goal.

Several research areas must be addressed with regard to sleep in healthy older adults. Because assessment of sleep is generally done with subjective data, it is imperative that a self-report or interview-administered instrument be developed that both accurately assesses sleep parameters and is validated by polysomnography. In addition, empirically-based sleep hygiene measures have to be developed and tested. Currently, elderly individuals are taught how to improve their sleep without the benefit of tested interventions. Although MSLT has been used with clinical populations of elderly, normative data about daytime sleepiness has not been established. Such information could enhance our understanding of nocturnal sleep changes associated with aging and their effects as well as provide a rationale for sleep hygiene interventions.

The sleep of depressed older persons has been well characterized by objective and subjective measures. It has yet to be determined, however, if these sleep markers occur with other mood-altering events such as retirement or bereavement. The intensity of such events can be measured using sleep parameters as well as other clinical instruments to develop models that characterize elders who become depressed in conjunction with mood-altering events.

Further exploration of sleep-disorder breathing in Alzheimer's disease and other dementias is warranted. This is a significant problem that may be related to disrupted nocturnal behaviors and overnight mental status changes. Once a firm knowledge base is established through research, intervention studies for sleep apnea should be developed for demented elders. The potential for keeping the dementia victim out of the institution will be reflected in decreased health care costs and may improve quality-of-life for patients and their significant others.

Because the use of prescribed and over-the-counter drugs is significantly increased in older persons (who are already at risk for sleep apnea), controlled studies of the effects of various medications on nocturnal respiratory function should be conducted. Studies could be conceptualized with chronically-ill older persons (medical as well as neuropsychiatric) in both acute-care settings and long-term care institutions. Careful attention should be directed toward changes in baseline respiratory function (such as oxygen desaturation) at selected intervals following medication administration. Perhaps links to disturbing behaviors, declining cognitive function, sleep fragmentation, and mortality will emerge. Interactions among sleep physiology, nocturnal respiration, illness, and medication must be explored. From this data, effective intervention protocols can be developed and tested.

Perhaps the elders most in need of sleep interventions are those in nursing homes who are at higher risk for sleep disturbances, sleep-disorder breathing, and mortality during sleep. Severe sleep fragmentation and disturbed sleep need examination. Biological, psychological, and environmental factors related to sleep disturbances and to disruptive nocturnal behaviors need characterization. Sleep intervention protocols that facilitate sleep consolidation such as sleep restriction or changing environmental routines should be developed and tested. These recommendations are in keeping with a recent NIH Consensus Development Conference that urged more research, education, and public awareness of sleep disorders in older persons. Research was recommended in the following areas: 1) classification and diagnostic criteria; 2) identification of appropriate animal models for studies on the basic mechanisms of sleep changes in aging; 3) identification of biological markers; 4) examination of the natural history of sleep disorders; 5) study of the disruption of normal circadian rhythms by dislocation (e.g., moving to a nursing home); and 6) examination of the benefits of treating these disorders.

Recommendations

Based on the foregoing assessment of research needs and opportunities in "Sleep and Older Persons," the Panel has made the following recommendations for research.

- Develop self-report or interview instruments to accurately assess sleep parameters in older persons.

- Establish normative data on daytime sleepiness in older persons.

- Determine the impact of mood-altering events on sleep in older persons (e.g., retirement, bereavement).

- Examine sleep-disordered breathing in Alzheimer's disease and other dementias.

- Conduct controlled studies on the effects of medications on nocturnal respiratory function in older persons.

- Test sleep interventions in the institutionalized elders.

Selected References

Ancoli-Israel, S. (1989). Epidemiology of sleep disorders. In T. Roth & T.A. Roehrs (Eds.), *Clinics in geriatric medicine.* (pp. 347-362). Philadelphia: W.B. Saunders.

Ancoli-Israel, S., Kripke, D.F., & Mason, W.J. (1984). Obstructive sleep apnea in a senior population. *Sleep Research*, 13, 130.

Ancoli-Israel, S., Kripke, D.F., Mason, W., & Kaplan, O.J. (1985). Sleep apnea and periodic movements in aging sample. *Journal of Gerontology*, 40, 419-425.

Ancoli-Israel, S. & Kripke, D.F. (1986). Sleep and aging. In E. Calkins, P.J. Davis, & A.B. Ford (Eds.), *The Practice of Geriatrics.* (pp. 240-247) Philadelphia: W.B. Saunders.

Ancoli-Israel, S., Kripke, D.F, & Mason, W., Gabriel, S., & Kaplan, O. (1986). Sleep apnea and period movements in a randomly selected elderly population: Final prevalence results. *Sleep Research,* 15, 101.

Ancoli-Israel, S., Parker, K., Sinaee, R., Fell, R.L., & Kripke, D.F. (1989). Sleep fragmentation in patients from a nursing home. *Journal of Gerontology*, 44, M18-21.

Berry, D.T.R., & Phillips, B.A. (1988). Sleep-disordered breathing in older persons: Review and methodological comment. *Clinical Psychology Review*, 8, 101-120.

Bixler, E.O., Kales, A., Cadieux, R.J., Vela-Bueno, A., Jacoby, J.A., & Soldaros, C.R. (1985). Sleep apneic activity in older healthy subjects. *Journal of Applied Physiology*, 58, 1597-1601.

Bliwise, D.L., Bevier, W.C., Bliwise, N.H., & Dement, W.C. (1987). Systematic behavioral observation of sleep/wakefulness in skilled care nursing home. *Sleep Research*, 16, 170.

Bliwise, D.L., Friedman, L. & Yesavage, J.A. (1988). A pilot study comparing sleep restriction therapy and relaxation training in geriatric insomniacs. *Sleep Research*, 17, 148.

Caplin-French, E. (1986). Sleep patterns for aged persons in long term care facilities. *Journal of Advanced Nursing,* 11, 57-66.

Dement, W.C., Miles, L.E. & Carskadon, M.A. (1982). "White paper" on sleep and aging. *Journal of the American Geriatric Society*, 30, 25-50.

Folstein, M.F., Folstein, S.E. & McHugh, P.R. (1975). Mini-mental state: A practical method for grading the cognitive state of patients for the clinician. *Journal of Psychiatric Research*, 12, 189.

Frommlet, M., Prinz, P., Vitiello, M.V., Ries, R., & Williams, D. (1986). Sleep hypoxemia and apnea are elevated in females with mild Alzheimer's disease. *Sleep Research*, 15, 189.

Hamilton, M. (1967). Development of a rating scale for primary depressive illness. British *Journal of Social and Clinical Psychiatry*, 6, 278.

Hayter, J. (1983). Sleep behaviors of older persons. *Nursing Research*, 32, 242-246.

Hoch, C.C., Reynolds, C.F., Kupfer, D.J., Houck, P.R., Berman, S.R., & Stack, J.A. (1986). Sleep-disordered breathing in normal and pathologic aging. *Journal of Clinical Psychiatry*, 133, 499-503.

Hoch, C.C., Reynolds, C.F., Kupfer, D.J., Berman, S.R., Houck, P.R., & Stack, J.A. (1987a). Empirical note: Self-report versus recorded sleep in healthy seniors. *Psychophysiology*, 24, 293-299.

Hoch, C.C., Reynolds, C.F., Kupfer, D.J., & Berman, S.R. (1988). Stability of EEG sleep quality in healthy seniors. *Sleep*, 11, 521-527.

Jacobs, D., Ancoli-Israel, S., Parker, L., & Kripke, D.F. (1989). Twenty-four hour sleep/wake patterns in a nursing home population. *Psychology and Aging*, 4(3), 352-356.

James, D.S. (1985). Survey of hypnotic drug use in nursing homes. *Journal of the American Geriatrics Society*, 33, 436-439.

Kripke, D.F. & Ancoli-Israel, S. (1983). Epidemiology of sleep apnea among the aged: Is sleep apnea a fatal disorder? In C. Guilleminault & E. Lagaresi (Eds.), *Sleep wake disorders: Natural history, epidemiology, and long-term evolution,* (pp. 137-142). New York: Raven Press.

Kripke, D.F., Ancoli-Israel, S., Mason, W., & Messin, S. (1983). Sleep-related mortality and morbidity in the aged. In M.H. Chase & D.E. Weitzman (Eds.), *Sleep disorders: Basic and clinical research.* (pp. 415-429). New York: SP Medical and Scientific Books.

Kripke, D.F., Ancoli-Israel, S., Mason, W.J., & Kaplan, O. (1986). Sleep apnea, long and short sleep. *Sleep Research,* 15, 139.

Kupfer, D.J., Reynolds, C.F., Ulrich, R., Shaw, D. & Coble, P. (1982). EEG sleep, depression, and aging. *Neurobiology of Aging: Experimental and Clinical Research,* 3, 351-360.

Lavie, P., Rachamin, B. & Rubin, A.E. (1984). Prevalence of sleep apnea syndrome among patients with essential hypertension. *American Heart Journal,* 108, 373-376.

Mitler, M.M., Hajdukovic, R.M., & Shafor, R. (1987). When people die: Cause of death versus time of death. *American Journal of Medicine,* 82, 266-274.

Mosko, S.S., Deckel, M.J., Paul, T., LaTour, T., Dhillon, S., Ghanim, A., & Sassin, J.F. (1988). Sleep apnea and sleep-related periodic leg movements in community resident seniors. *Journal of American Geriatric Society,* 36, 502-508.

National Institute on Aging. (1990). Age page: A good night's sleep. Washington, DC.

Pollak, C.P. & Perlick, D. (1987). Sleep problems and institutionalization of older persons. *Sleep Research,* 16, 407.

Rabins, P.V., Mace, N.L., & Lucas, M.J. (1982). The impact of dementia on the family. *Journal of the American Medical Association,* 248, 333-335.

Regenstein, Q.R., & Morris, J. (1987). Daily sleep patterns observed among institutionalized elderly. *Journal of the American Geriatrics Society,* 35, 767-772.

Reynolds, C.F., Kupfer, D.J., Taska, L.S., Hoch, C.C., Sewitch, D.E., Restifo, K., Spiker, D.G., Zimmer, B., Marin, R.S., Nelson, J., Martin, D., & Morycz, R. (1985a). Sleep apnea in Alzheimer's dementia: Correlation with mental deterioration. *Journal of Clinical Psychiatry,* 46, 257-261.

Reynolds, C.F., Kupfer, D.J., Taska, L.S., Hoch, C.C., Sewitch, D.E. & Spiker, D.G. (1985b). The sleep of healthy seniors: A revisit. *Sleep*, 8, 20-29.

Reynolds, C.F., Kupfer, D.J., Taska. L.S., Hoch, C.C., Spiker, D.G.,Sewitch, D.E., Zimmer, B., Marin, R.S., Nelson, J.P., Martin, D., & Morycz, R. (1985c). EEG sleep in healthy elderly, depressed, and demented subjects. *Biological Psychiatry*, 20, 431-442.

Reynolds, C.F., Kupfer, D.J., Hoch, C.C., Stack, J.A., Houck, P.R., Berman, S.R. (1986a). Sleep deprivation in healthy elderly men and women: Effects on mood and sleep during recovery. *Sleep*, 9, 492-501.

Reynolds, C.F., Kupfer, D.J., Hoch, C.C., Houck, P.R., Stack, J.A., Berman, S.R., Campbell, P.I., & Zimmer, B. (1987). Sleep deprivation as a probe in older persons. *Archives of General Psychiatry,* 44, 982-990.

Rodin, J., McAvay, G., & Timko, C. (1988). A longitudinal study of depressed mood and sleep disturbances in elderly adults. *Journal of Psychological Science*, 43, 45.

Part Three

The Major Sleep Disorders

Chapter 22

Abnormal Sleep

Like Faust, I would readily trade quite a few of my years, not to regain youth, but for the gift of normal, refreshing sleep.

—Witness, Commission Hearing, Washington, DC

Sleep disturbances range along a broad continuum from short-term, self-imposed sleep deprivation to serious sleep disorders that require medical attention. While everyone experiences an occasional night of insomnia, with its consequent poor judgment and coordination, irritability, and nausea, these symptoms diminish with successive nights of quality sleep. For many individuals, however, sleep is profoundly disturbed, as described by the witnesses in testimony before the Commission. More than 70 distinct sleep disorders affect both sexes and all ages and socioeconomic groups.

In its 1990 publication—International Classification of Sleep Disorders (ICSD)—the American Sleep Disorders Association (ASDA) divided sleep disorders into several groupings by possible cause:

Intrinsic sleep disorders are those that "either originate or develop within the body, or arise from causes within the body," and include, among others, narcolepsy, sleep apnea, restless legs syndrome, and certain forms of insomnia.

Excerpted from *Wake Up America: A National Sleep Alert*, Volume 1, Executive Summary and Executive Report, Report of the National Commission on Sleep Disorders Research, Submitted to the United States Congress and to the Secretary U.S. Department of Health and Human Services, January 1993.

Extrinsic sleep disorders are those that "originate or develop from causes outside of the body. External factors are integral in producing these sleep disorders, and removal of the external factors leads to resolution of the sleep disorder." These types of disorders range from alcohol-induced sleep disorders to disorders in sleep habits and practices.

Circadian rhythm sleep disorders include jet lag, shift work sleep disorder, and shifts in sleep phase. This cluster of disorders is characterized by a disruption in the biological clock in which there is a "misalignment between the patient's sleep pattern and that which is desired or regarded as the societal norm."

Parasomnias are "clinical disorders that are not abnormalities of the processes responsible for sleep...but rather are undesirable physical phenomena that occur predominantly during sleep," such as SIDS and infant sleep apnea, REM behavior disorder, sleepwalking, and sleep terrors.

In addition, the ICSD identifies a series of medical disorders, generally psychiatric, neurological, or cardiopulmonary in nature, that are associated with disturbances of sleep and wakefulness.

Chapter 23

Sleep Related Disorders and Their Treatment

Sleep is a state of being that every person experiences essentially every day of his or her life. In total, we spend one-third of our lives in this state, yet how little we understand it and how much we may yearn for it to be better than it is now

Studies on the epidemiology of insomnia show that 10% to 20% of randomly surveyed persons report either severe or constant sleep problems. Among a sample of older persons, the incidence of complaints would be substantially higher, apparently because of age-related changes in brain physiology as well as various pathological problems.

Women of all ages are more likely than men to report sleep difficulties. Among the many who report problems in sleeping, only one-third take their concern to a physician for help. That means the other two-thirds could be provided counsel for their sleep-related problems by a pharmacist who is well informed on the subject, sensitive to signs of a problem, and open to an opportunity to counsel.

"Asleep" is the antonym of "awake" wakeful or alert. The state of consciousness, i.e., being awake, is interrupted only by physiological sleep or pathological coma. Science has long sought an explanation of sleep, but only a few riddles of sleep physiology have been penetrated, and those successes came with great difficulty.

One recent writer stated that "the function of sleep is one of the remaining great mysteries of science." Currently, there is not even

Reprinted with permission from *Drug Topics*, Volume 139, Number 11, June 12, 1995. © 1995 Medical Economics Publishing.

unanimous agreement on the reason or reasons for sleep to be so necessary as it seems.

While many other researchers would hold a similar concept of sleep as having necessary restorative functions, some researchers place a distinctive added emphasis on thermoregulation. It has been suggested recently that sleep is a period devoted to removing cerebral free radicals, which accumulate to excess during wakefulness because of the high level of oxidative metabolism in brain tissue (E. Reimund, 1994). Thus, sleep is proposed to be a vital antioxidant defense mechanism.

Normal Sleep and Its Deviations

Sleep Stages

"Falling asleep" consists of a progression from awake to eyes-closed drowsiness to light sleep (stages 1 and 2) to deep sleep (stages 3 and 4). There are shifts in the electroencephalogram (EEG) corresponding to stages in this progression.

Researchers believe that it is the deep sleep for which the greatest physiological needs exist. This does not deny a lesser benefit from time spent in sleep stages 1 and 2; however, there is less evidence for their value or for any detrimental effect stemming from a deficit in these stages. And such a deficit is unlikely to occur except in total deprivation of sleep.

A phase of sleep that was first recognized only in the mid-twentieth century is known as REM (rapid eye movement) sleep. REM sleep usually follows a sleeper's progression into deep sleep; all other sleep stages (1 through 4) can be lumped as "non-REM sleep."

REM sleep has at times been dubbed "paradoxical sleep." This refers to the fact that the cerebrocortical EEG in REM sleep consists of fast, low-voltage waves like those of the waking state. However, the REM state is easily discriminated in sleep studies by using two other sets of electrodes, which provide: (1) an electro-oculogram (EOG) that records the distinctive rapid motion of the eyeballs, which are controlled by the external ocular muscles, and (2) an electromyogram (EMG) that displays electrical activity from the jaw muscles, which during REM sleep show a flaccidity characteristic of the musculature in general.

Dreaming

Another remarkable feature of REM sleep is the high proportion of all dreaming that occurs in that stage, although a smaller fraction does occur in "deep sleep," stages 3 and 4. The relationship between REM and dreaming suggests that dreamers in effect "watch" their dreams unfold like a scene in a play or movie. A physiological or even a psychological role for REM sleep has been inferred from the finding that persons selectively deprived of REM-stage sleep showed behavioral and mood changes not seen with selective deprivation of deep sleep.

Some see a needed psychodynamic role for dreaming and, thus, for REM sleep. For example, it is proposed that REM provides for much-needed affective information processing and affective discharge, especially for those in states such as bereavement, who show increased REM density.

For many persons, dreaming is an ordinary, every-night event. For some, however, it is a rare event to be aware, at waking, of having dreamed. Yet sleep researchers find that dreaming occurs in all of their subjects, probably on every night of observation. But for a dreamer to recall a dream, it is believed that at least a brief waking period must follow closely after the dream if the dream does not immediately precede the morning's awakening.

But why is it so rare for one and so common for another to have dream recall? What are the causes for such difference in awareness of dreams? Why do some have the frightening dreams that we call nightmares? Why do some persons dream "death dreams"? These are among the many sleep questions that remain to be answered.

Sleep in the Elderly

It might be helpful, however, to consider here a major characteristic of sleep—that it changes over the life span. The maximal length of daily sleep time occurs during infancy, followed by a strong downward trend in childhood. This trend continues to a lesser degree through adolescence and throughout most of adulthood, with the progressive changes in elder years all in an undesirable direction.

The high incidence of sleep problems in elderly persons encompasses the full range of conditions outlined in Lists 1 and 2. Thus, in addition to what seems to be a physiological aging-related increased frequency of awakenings, there are: (1) aging-related psychiatric illnesses, (2) myriad medical illnesses, especially arthritis and respiratory disorders, (3) primary sleep disorders (periodic leg movement disorder, REM sleep behavior disorders), and (4) poor sleep hygiene, arising especially from daytime napping and decreased daytime activity or exercise in retired persons.

Deviations from Normal Sleep

One of the greater sleep research advances appears to have been in defining the range of variation in "normal" sleep to permit a cataloging of its many deviations—how and why troubled sleep may differ from untroubled sleep.

Two "official" classifications of sleep disorders have been constructed: One is in the Diagnostic & Statistical Manual, 4th revision (DSM IV) of the American Psychiatric Association; the other is known as the International Classification of Sleep Disorders (ICSD), produced by sleep researchers worldwide. An outline combining useful features of the two can be found in Lists 1 and 2.

The scope of sleep disorders is too broad to allow us a complete treatment of every aspect. Thus, we shall select for discussion the more common, more serious, best-understood problems.

Primary/Intrinsic Dyssomnias

Breathing-Related Sleep Disorder

Intrinsic breathing-related disorders have been recognized only in recent decades as a major cause for the poor quality of sleep that leads to complaints of daytime drowsiness and fatigability. It has been estimated that five to 10 million Americans cannot breath normally during their sleep. Obstructive sleep apnea (OSA), a relatively common condition in middle-aged men, is the foremost of such respiratory conditions. It is aggravated by obesity and by alcohol consumption, and it is seldom found in premenopausal women. Besides being troubled by lowered daytime alertness, patients with OSA often have a history of exceptionally loud or strong snoring. Chronic OSA sufferers are at increased risk of hypertension, sudden death, and myocardial ischemic injury. Cognitive brain functions also may be injured, and there is an elevated risk for daytime automobile accidents.

Many serious nocturnal cardiac arrhythmias and conduction defects also are seen in the adult sleep apnea syndrome. The most striking is the great variability of the heart rate, which is cyclical in relation to apneic episodes: An initial bradycardia, dependent on the vagus, often is followed by a rebound tachycardia, which is believed to be secondary to a carotid chemoreceptor stimulation by hypoxemia.

While less common than conduction abnormalities, atrial arrhythmias—extrasystoles, flutter, fibrillation—are also possible complications of apnea. Most ominously, nocturnal ventricular hyperexcitability is sometimes observed, the probable mechanisms being the severe hypoxemia concurrent with an increase of sympathetic tone at the end of the apnea. However, all of these deviations can be reversed by relieving the inadequate O_2, by whatever means, or by opposing vagal hyperactivity by means of an antimuscarinic (atropinic) drug.

Mechanical obstruction of the upper airway may arise from excessive relaxation of muscles, so that there is "collapse" of the airway upon itself. When the airway is impeded, ventilation and oxygen exchange is impaired, resulting in lowered O_2 (hypoxemia) and elevated CO_2 (hypercapnia). These changes, detected by chemoreceptors in the medulla, carotid body, and aortic arch, trigger an upward discharge of impulses that evoke arousal through the reticular activating system of the brain stem. Increased activity of this system causes a "micro-awakening," an interruption of the normal pattern of sleep that may occur hundreds of times in the course of a night. In the move toward awakening, the muscles regain normal tone, and there is a relief of the obstruction. A 10-second or longer cessation of breathing and reduction by 30% of airflow are the criteria for apnea. The critical rate of apnea episodes for diagnosis of sleep apnea is five per hour.

The sleeper may not be aware of any of these arousals, because their short duration does not allow them to be established in memory that lasts to the morning. However, the consequence of this multitude of awakenings is a qualitative lack of restorative sleep despite the fact that there is not a striking reduction of total sleep time. Diagnosis of OSA requires the availability of a sleep laboratory (which may be a hospital unit under a pulmonologist), where patients spend one night of polysomnographic recording (PSG). This includes EEG, EOG, and EMG, plus other physiological measures during sleep: nasal airflow, ECG, breathing movements of the chest, leg movements, and blood oxygen through an external sensor on a digit or earlobe. When OSA is diagnosed, CPAP (continuous positive air pressure) is now commonly prescribed.

This treatment provides a "pneumatic splint" to the walls of the upper airway via an air pump connected to a nasal mask that patients wear when sleeping. Collapse and obstruction of the airway are prevented, as are hypoxemia and hypercapnia; thus, no reason exists for excess signals to awaken.

OSA patients commonly are improved so greatly in their daytime alertness and energy that any inconvenience of wearing the nasal mask is readily accepted. Nasal CPAP increases upper airway size and lowers edema of the upper airway. This therapy has reduced the use of a surgical procedure, known as uvulopalatopharyngoplasty, to remodel the upper airway so as to reduce physical blockage. Weight loss is also therapeutic for OSA patients, as it reduces upper airway collapsibility.

For some persons with concurrent sleep apnea and epilepsy, the former problem may aggravate the latter. Moreover, effective apnea therapy—using CPAP, tracheostomy, protriptyline, trazodone, or acetazolamide—gave improved seizure control in a 1994 study of patients with refractory partial seizures and OSA. The effect of sleep apnea on epilepsy may arise from the sleep deprivation, the hypoxemia leading to tissue hypoxia, and a reduced cerebral blood flow.

For some patients having a marginal evidence for OSA but showing "fragmented sleep," treatment with a tricyclic antidepressant is now favored by sleep lab physicians. Amitriptyline and protriptyline, which both have a considerable component of central anticholinergic activity, are favored for this indication. Reducing the intensity of the mechanism that is responsible for REM may be the basis for their benefit. Brain cholinergic activity favors the REM stage of sleep, which has been implicated as being excessive in persons troubled by fragmented sleep.

A rarer condition, central sleep apnea, found in the absence of obstruction, arises from a periodic deficit of ventilatory drive. It may arise from an elevation of the threshold of chemoreceptors to CO_2, but by another view there is a dysregulation of breathing, allowing hyperventilation during sleep and a consequent deficit of CO_2 (hypocapnia) so that the respiratory drive fails. In one recently reported case, effective treatment was achieved by the use of supplemental CO_2 inhalation.

Intrinsic Hypersomnia—Narcolepsy

Narcolepsy is a long-recognized primary sleep disorder reflective of a deviation of the neural mechanism(s) underlying sleep. The narcoleptic patient experiences irresistible daytime sleep as "attacks," which may interrupt common daily activities. There may also be feelings of being paralyzed while falling asleep or waking up, or the occurrence of vivid, hallucination-like dreams while still awake.

The classical psychomotor stimulant dexamphetamine, employed at dosages well above those used for appetite suppression, came into use early on as the first effective therapy. Patients show an intrinsic tolerance toward such stimulants and are clearly enabled to maintain a normal life that is so impaired by narcolepsy.

Polysomnographic research has shown that when this attack occurs, the narcoleptic is passing directly from wakefulness to REM sleep, a transition never seen in the normal sleep process. This also explains another feature, cataplexy, often associated with narcolepsy: This sudden weakness and general hypotonia of a person's voluntary muscles arises from the REM-induced skeletal muscle flaccidity. However, in narcolepsy, this phase may occur before the person has fallen asleep, adding greatly to his burdensome symptoms. While the use of stimulants has been effective, another possible approach would be to use tricyclics having a central anticholinergic effect against REM functions.

A 1991 report indicated that L-dopa effectively raised the vigilance level of narcoleptic patients. However, it seems unlikely that this approach will be accepted for broad use in narcolepsy therapy.

Sleep State Misperception

"I never get any sleep!" Results of some PSG studies for diagnosis of sleep complaints led to the recognition of a sleep-state misperception disorder. These studies gave no evidence for the insomnia of which some patients complained! Thus, these insomniacs are classified as having a perceptual disorder rather than a true insomnia. And their ability to receive treatment appears to be limited because of their skepticism about the PSG results.

Limb-Movements Syndromes

Restless legs syndrome (RLS) and periodic limb movement (PLM) disorder seem to be of higher frequency among the elderly. However, there is as yet little certainty about their etiologies and thus their rational therapy. For some patients, excessive intake of caffeine-containing beverages is thought to cause RLS; these patients obviously might benefit from abstinence. Alcohol intake has been found to aggravate the two periodic leg movement syndromes; thus, abstinence may be helpful.

Another idea is that "restless legs" may be an early manifestation of iron deficiency anemia or magnesium deficiency. One such report in 1994 found that serum ferritin was negatively correlated with degree of RLS symptoms in elderly subjects and that supplemental iron over a two-month period lowered the severity of symptoms. Furthermore, several recent studies claim that these conditions may arise from a dopaminergic D-2 receptor deficit; L-dopa therapy was shown effective for some patients. Lastly, a 1993 study with PSG and placebo controls found a dose of 15 mg oxycodone effective in reducing leg movements and associated arousals as well as increasing sleep efficiency.

Pickwickian Syndrome

This disorder, also known as hypersomnia, is one among a select group of diseases that take their name from literature. Some bear names of fictional characters, but in this case it is the name of the work wherein the relevant character appears. In Dickens' *Pickwick Papers*, Fat Boy's corpulence was associated with a remarkable tendency to fall asleep in the midst of considerable activity. Thus, a Pickwickian syndrome is defined as extreme obesity with somnolence and polycythemia related to hypoventilation, which produces also arterial O_2 unsaturation, hypercapnia, and pulmonary hypertension.

This state of hyperphagic obesity and another eating disorder, bulimia, share the common feature of hypersomnia. It is hypothesized that the two aspects of both disorders may arise from a yet undefined dysfunction of the hypothalamus that affects regulatory mechanisms for feeding and sleep.

Circadian Rhythm-Associated Disorders

The normal state of various body functions is one of synchronization to a 24-hour day-night rhythm. Persons who rapidly travel through several time zones may experience rhythm desynchronization, which has an adverse impact on sleep.

Until resynchronization of the daily pattern can occur within the new environment, sleep will be disturbed in what is commonly called jet-lag syndrome. Some improvement of adjustment has been seen by the use of benzodiazepines.

In 1984, experimental data were published on triazolam and flurazepam versus placebo in regard to sleep after a 12-hour shift of sleep schedule—like that of a flight halfway around the world. That study indicated that both medications reduced sleep loss, but that only triazolam enabled subjects to be less impaired than placebo. However, some problems have been reported with triazolam use. In one instance of triazolam-associated amnesia, a physician who took triazolam (with ethanol) while flying to Europe experienced a "blackout" or anterograde amnesia; the traveler "lost" a period of time between deplaning

160

and later waking from sleep at her hotel. Furthermore, there are indications that disinhibition of violent behavior may occur often enough after triazolam to mitigate against its use for such purposes, or at least to require careful patient selection.

It has long been recognized that persons differ in their capacity to adapt to fluctuating shift work—primarily changing to the night shift (commonly midnight to 8:00 A.M.). Personnel of the military and merchant marine had long experienced such problems before industrial and business activities began to operate around the clock.

It is fully documented that alertness and cognition can be impaired to a dangerous degree under the adverse effects of shift-work sleep disorder. No real remedy—but for use of a stimulant drug—has been discovered. While military forces have employed amphetamine-type stimulants at times, such usage is fraught with risks of adverse psychological changes, including dependence. The medical literature describes cases of disastrous paranoid schizophrenia-like reactions in persons misusing dexamphetamine or like agents. Even the use of caffeine for all-night activities is not without some risks of adverse effects.

Sleep researchers have identified two states of rhythm-associated sleep disorders: non-24-hour rhythm sleep disorder and delayed sleep phase syndrome, both of which are the consequence of being out of synchrony with one's environment. That state occurs when the person's daily physiological rhythms (e.g., body temperature, cortisol secretion by the adrenal cortex, and melatonin secretion by the pineal gland) do not run on a 24-hour basis.

Because of this desynchronization with the day-night cycle, the person experiences both poor daytime alertness and difficulty in sleeping at night. A current approach to treatment is to expose the patient to bright light upon awakening at a standard time to help establish synchronization of the person's internal clock to a 24-hour cycle.

Melatonin, a pineal gland hormone rather similar in chemical structure to serotonin, has been implicated in the physiological regulation of 24-hour rhythmicity. For some years, there has been speculation that supplementing melatonin levels could be helpful in human adjustment to a sleep-schedule shift. Studies in the past several years tested the effect of melatonin on workers' tolerance of and adjustment to a night shift and on jet-lag adjustment by airline cabin crews after multiple time-zone crossing on long international flights. Reports indicate positive, but limited, effects of oral melatonin (5 mg/day).

Self-medication with melatonin to improve sleep is being practiced via an over-the-counter "dietary supplement" preparation now being marketed. However, use among a general array of insomnia sufferers is unwarranted by the data now at hand. Persons whose sleep problem is not responsive to this agent may obtain only a placebo effect.

Another drug treatment for the desynchronization disorders described above has been advocated by a group of Japanese clinical researchers. In the early 1990s, they reported finding their patients improved with treatment consisting of oral vitamin B_{12} in a dosage of 3 mg per day. For those who were not synchronized by the vitamin alone, a combination with bright light was found to be successful. However, a paucity of evidence regarding a mechanism for such supposed benefits may retard acceptance of the data, especially until other research groups have succeeded in replicating them.

A possible mode of action for oral B_{12} is suggested by one report: When nine healthy subjects were given oral B_{12} for four weeks, it phase-advanced the 24-hour rhythm of melatonin secretion by 1.1 hours, perhaps by enhancing the response to bright light exposure. The area of work seems very promising.

Primary Intrinsic Parasomnias

The category known as parasomnias consists of neither insomnia nor hypersomnia but of qualitatively deviant occurrences in conjunction with sleep. Some are of no great significance and are merely annoyances, whereas others are so severe as to entail fatal outcomes. For few of these is reliable treatment available.

Sleepwalking and Night Terrors

Sleepwalking, or somnambulism, involves leaving one's bed and performing complex behaviors while outside a state of normal, conscious awareness. Sleepwalkers enter into activities such as strolling about with eyes open while in, or not fully removed from, non-REM (rarely REM) sleep and have no later recall of events while in this behavioral state. There may be, among other actions, moaning, talking that is either sensible or nonsensical, handling and examining of objects, gesturing, grabbing at apparently hallucinated objects.

The sleep terrors of childhood, similar to sleepwalking, comprise an abnormal state of apparent but not real arousal. The child leaves the bed and walks about the house crying in what seems to be a terror-stricken emotional state. Any efforts of the parents to calm, comfort, and communicate with the child prove fruitless, as if the child is neither seeing, even with eyes open, nor hearing.

Preferred current treatment for both sleepwalking and night terrors, as well as for nightmares, is imipramine. Imipramine also is favored for another parasomnia, sleep enuresis.

Nocturnal (sleep-related) Eating Disorders

Although the ICSD lists this diagnosis as extrinsic, it is difficult not to see it as being of an intrinsic nature; at least one of its types is so closely associated with sleepwalking as to suggest that it is only a variant of it.

A sleep-related eating disorder was first described in 1955 as night-eating syndrome, based on the finding that 80% of patients with treatment-refractory cases of obesity had nocturnal hyperphagia, insomnia, and morning-after anorexia.

There have been some reports of awareness and later memory of this behavior. However, patients of another type, described in a 1991 paper by Schenck et al., lacked awareness of and suffered amnesia after such an event.

Of the 19 cases in five years at the Minnesota Regional Sleep Disorders Center, 14 were female, their ages ranging from 18 to 54 years with an average age of 37. Seven had concurrent psychiatric diagnoses, and two more were in remission. Twelve definitely, and four probably, were sleepwalkers; of the remaining three, one had the problem only after onset of triazolam abuse and was cured of it by abstinence, while the other two had a motor deviation other than sleepwalking (PLM syndrome).

Most nocturnal eaters (58%) had amnesia regarding the night eating but were later aware of it as evidenced by the messy preparation areas and the burns/injuries incurred. That night eaters were uncustomarily sloppy is not surprising, since their actions were unconscious automatisms.

Eleven of 14 (74%) patients for whom outcome of treatment was known showed remission of the nocturnal eating after treatment with clonazepam at 0.5-1.0 mg hs. For some patients, addition of codeine, carbidopa/L-dopa, or bromocriptine was required to gain full remission of symptoms. Four patients experienced substantial and sustained weight loss after cessation of their nocturnal eating. Thus, a highly optimistic prognosis was presented for this problem of sleep disorder-related obesity.

By 1993, the Schenck team had seen another 19 patients and found sleep-eating in conjunction with other sleep disorders—confusional arousals, OSA, and RLS. Onset of sleep-related eating was also closely associated with: (1) acute stress involving reality-based concerns about the safety of family members or relationship problems, (2) abstinence from alcohol and opiate or cocaine abuse, and (3) cessation of cigarette smoking. Clearly, this disorder is not an extremely rare occurrence.

Enuresis

Sleep studies indicate that enuretic patients are normal sleepers and that enuresis can occur during all stages of sleep whenever the bladder is filled to the equivalent of maximal daytime capacity. These sleepers exhibit voiding characteristics similar to those of daytime voiding, and reservoir capacity of the bladder appears normal, with bladder instability unimportant.

However, enuretics were found to lack the normal nocturnal rise in secretion of antidiuretic hormone; they were also found to experience nocturia, or urine production up to four times the functional bladder capacity. Such findings explain the need for bladder emptying and suggest a new approach to enuresis via antidiuretic therapy in addition to the current use of imipramine.

Sleep Bruxism

This condition consists of teeth grinding and/or clenching during sleep. This can be severe enough that dental health is threatened, and tenderness of teeth may be a daytime symptom. It is said to occur in about 15% of children and over 90% of adults. The etiology of bruxism is unclear, but it is associated with stress, occlusal disorders, allergies, and sleep positioning.

Because of its nonspecific pathology, bruxism may be difficult to diagnose. In addition to complaints from sleep partners, signs of bruxism may include pain or fatigue upon chewing, headaches, tooth sensitivity/attrition, oral infection, and temporomandibular joint disorders. Adults may be managed with stress-reduction therapy, modification of sleep position, biofeedback training, physical therapy, and dental evaluation. One approach is to wear a bruxism brace—a plastic device comparable to the mouthpiece or tooth guard worn in competitive team sports.

Sudden Death in Sleep

Unresolved mystery persists regarding the cause of sudden, unexpected fatalities of adults or infants in sleep; these are classified as distinct entities. There are many etiologic theories, especially for the sudden infant death syndrome (SIDS). However, where there are too many hypotheses, one must conclude either that none is verifiable or that the condition may not be as homogeneous as it is regarded to be. When there is no understanding of etiology and pathogenesis, little progress can be expected for prophylaxis or therapy.

Secondary Sleep Disorders

The universal importance of sleep can readily be appreciated when we consider the great number of medical circumstances that comprise a hindrance to the normal quantity and/or quality of sleep (List 2).

Extrinsic Sleep Disorders

Inadequate sleep hygiene disorder encompasses a wide variety of environmental, ingestive, habitual, and lifestyle factors to which insomnia may be attributed. Rather than be given a prescription for a hypnotic drug, such persons need counseling about making adjustments in their environment and in their personal habits.

Intake of ethanol and caffeine should be reduced or avoided altogether. Use of ear plugs or a masking-sound generator device can resolve problems based on noise, while window darkeners and/or use of an eyeshade can remedy light-hindered daytime sleeping.

A favorable alternative is available over the counter in products derived from the antihistaminics. Diphenhydramine, 25 or 50 mg hs, for example, provides sedation with minimal risk of adverse responses. But while physical dependence is not known to occur, undesirable habituation is possible. Therefore, only occasional use, or nightly use over short periods of time, should be encouraged.

Hypnotic-induced physical dependence can lead to a withdrawal syndrome in which sleep disturbance plays a prominent role. When CNS depressants of this type are used to combat insomnia or anxiety long enough to induce dependence, withdrawal involves a high level of that condition against which they were used. This, in turn, discourages the person from maintaining abstinence, and a vicious cycle can begin. Misuse tends to continue despite the fact that the best hypnotics do not induce a normally patterned sleep; their use is therefore widely discouraged by sleep researchers.

In the case of stimulant dependence, there surely is great damage to normal sleep during steady drug intake. When the drug regimen is interrupted, there tends to be a withdrawal in which hypersomnia prevails for several days concurrently with a depressed mood. Both for this and for hypnotic dependency, psychotherapy supporting abstinence may be the most needed and successful approach.

Sleep Disorders in Psychiatric Conditions

List 2 shows that a variety of psychiatric states can be the context of secondary sleep problems. Obviously, the foremost need is for effective therapy of the primary psychiatric problem, therapy with antipsychotics, lithium, antidepressants, or the new SSRIs—selective serotonin reuptake inhibitors. Mania comprises the most extreme condition of insomnia among these conditions.

Sleep Disorders in Neurological Conditions

Sleep disturbance, common in many neurological diseases, can be caused by the underlying CNS pathology, medication effects, altered motor system function, associated cognitive and psychiatric disorders, and/or secondary effects of the disease, such as pain and immobility.

This category includes problems arising from the cerebral dysfunctions seen in dementias and other degenerative brain diseases. A 1993 review on Alzheimer's disease (AD) suggested that not only brain acetylcholine but also catecholamines and serotonin are dysfunctional. Whereas the cholinergic deficit is blamed for failure of cognitive activity, deficits of the monoamines are blamed for affective and psychotic aspects along with sleep impairment. Therapies to enhance/restore monoamine functions that may alleviate insomnia or perturbed sleep-wake cycles of AD patients could be quite valuable. Disordered sleep often is the reason the demented patient becomes unmanageable for the family. Thus, nocturnal wandering is a major factor in institutionalizing AD patients.

Sleep Problems and Pharmaceutical Care

List 2 shows a wide variety of other diseases, beyond our space to comment, that may severely disturb or hinder sleep. Adequate relief of pain or of other symptoms specific to each condition—in order to minimize the stress of inadequate rest—is essential for the well-being of the patient. Equal attention to sleep problems is needed whatever their origin, either primary or secondary in nature. Pharmacists need to be mindful of this when they are in a position to monitor drug response.

If a patient fails to obtain relief of symptoms sufficient to permit restful sleep, his or her illness may be aggravated.

166

*List 1—Primary Sleep Disorder Diagnoses**

<u>Intrinsic sleep deficiency disorders</u>

- Breathing-related disorders:
    Obstructive sleep apnea
    Central sleep apnea

- Restless legs syndrome

- Periodic limb movement syndrome

- Sleep state misperception

<u>Intrinsic sleep excess disorders</u>

- Narcolepsy

- Pickwickian syndrome

- Bulimia nervosa

<u>Circadian rhythm-associated sleep disorders</u>

- Delayed sleep phase syndrome

- Jet-lag sleep disorder

- Shift-work sleep disorder

- Non-24-hour rhythm sleep-wake disorder

<u>Intrinsic parasomnias (qualitative deviations)</u>

- Arousal-associated disorders
    Sleepwalking
    Sleep terrors
    Confusional arousals

- Waking-transition-associated disorders
    Sleep talking (somniloquy)
    Sleep starts (startles)
    Nocturnal leg cramps

- REM-associated disorders
    Nightmares
    Sleep paralysis

- Other parasomnias

    Sleep bruxism
    Sleep enuresis
    Sudden unexplained nocturnal death syndrome (adult)
    Sudden infant death syndrome
    Infant sleep apnea

*This list is shortened and modified from the International Classification of Sleep Disorders and DSM IV.

*List 2—Secondary sleep deficit disorder diagnosis**

Extrinsic sleep disorders

- Inadequate sleep hygiene insomnia

- Nocturnal eating/drinking disorder

- Hypnotic-dependent sleep disorder

- Stimulant-dependent sleep disorder

Sleep problems associated with mental conditions

- Psychoses

- Mood disorders, (e.g., mania, hypomania, neurotic [but not major] depressions)

- Anxiety disorders (including sleep-related phobias)

- Panic disorder

- Alcoholism

Sleep problems associated with neurological disorders

- Cerebral degenerative disease

- Dementias (including Alzheimer's disease)

- Parkinsonism

- Sleep-related epilepsy

- Fatal familial insomnia

Sleep problems associated with other medical conditions

- Sleeping sickness
- Nocturnal myocardial ischemia
- Respiratory disorders
    - Gross obesity—dyspnea when reclining
    - Coughing—also worse when reclining
    - Acute impairment of breathing
        - nocturnal asthma
        - severe nasal congestion
    - Chronic impairment of breathing
        - chronic obstructive pulmonary disease
        - mandibular abnormalities
        - upper airway resistance
- Gastric disorders
    - Gastroesophageal reflux in sleep
    - Peptic ulcer disease
- Endocrine disorders
    - Endometriosis, PMS, menopausal, post-menonopausal symptoms
    - Adrenocortical hypersecretion
- Pain states not listed above
    - Postsurgical pain
    - Traumatic injury, (e.g., low back pain, fractures)
    - Rheumatoid arthritis
    - Osteoarthritis
    - Fibrositis (fibromyalgia) syndrome
    - Myofascial pain syndrome
- Nonpain sensory problems
    - Pruritus/itching
    - Dermatitis (e.g., eczema, ivy poisoning)

*This list is shortened and modified from the International Classification of Sleep Disorders and DSM IV.

Chapter 24

Sleep Apnea: Breathing Disorders during Sleep

Habitual loud snoring is the most common symptom of breathing disorders that occur during sleep. The person who snores not only sleeps restlessly, but also is at risk for serious disorders of the heart and lungs. Snoring can therefore be life-threatening because it can lead to high blood pressure, irregular heart beats, heart attacks, and sudden death.

Normal breathing must continue at all times whether awake or asleep. The act of breathing is an automatic, highly regulated mechanical function of the body. In healthy sleeping individuals, most muscular and neural activities will slow or even shut down but respiration goes on under a neuromuscular "auto pilot." However, if something goes wrong with the auto pilot during sleep, breathing may become erratic and inefficient.

Understanding Sleep

Sleep is a complex neurological state. Its primary function is rest and restoring the body's energy levels. Repeated interruption of sleep by breathing abnormalities such as cessation of breathing (apnea) or heavy snoring, leads to fragmented sleep and abnormal oxygen and carbon dioxide levels in the blood. Excessive daytime sleepiness and various disorders of the heart, lungs, and the nervous system result.

In the 1950's scientists realized that sleep is not just a quiet state of rest. In fact, two types of sleep occur with distinct physiological

National Heart, Lung, and Blood Institute, August 1994

patterns—rapid-eye-movement sleep (REM), and non-rapid-eye-movement sleep (NREM) or deep sleep. In normal sleep, REM occurs about 90 minutes after a person falls asleep. The REM and NREM recur in cycles of about 90 minutes each, with three non-REM stages (light to deep slumber) at the beginning and REM towards the end. The amount of sleep needed by each person is usually constant although there is a wide variation among some individuals.

How sleep occurs and how it restores the body are not well understood. Scientists originally believed that sleep occurs because the brain lapses into a passive resting state from lack of stimulation. Another theory proposed that sleep occurs when the body generates and accumulates sufficient amounts of a "sleep-inducing substance." However, research now suggests that sleep results when specific changes in brain function occur. By studying the brain waves, scientists can define and measure various degrees, levels, and stages of sleep.

Sleep consists of a rhythmic combination of changes in physiological, biochemical, neurophysiological and psychological processes. When the rhythm is disturbed or the individual processes are abnormal during sleep, a variety of sleep-related disorders may result.

Sleep-Related Disorders

Sleep-related complaints appeared regularly in medical literature in the beginning of the 19th century. However, from 1900 to the mid-1960's little was published in scientific journals about the "sleepy patient" except for an occasional report on the normal or abnormal aspects of sleep physiology. Recent developments of research techniques in neurobiology, molecular biology, molecular genetics, physiology, neuropsychiatry, internal medicine, pulmonary medicine, and cardiology have allowed scientists to study the details of sleep. As a result, there has been an explosion in interest in understanding sleep and "sleep disorders."

Some sleep-related disturbances are simply temporary inconveniences while others are potentially more serious. Sleep apnea is the most common sleep disorder. Other serious sleep-related disorders are narcolepsy and clinical insomnia. "Jet lag syndrome," caused by rapid shifts in the biological sleep-wake cycle, is also an example of a temporary sleep-related disorder. So are the sleep problems experienced by shift workers.

Sleep apnea is the condition of interrupted breathing while asleep. "Apnea" is a Greek word meaning "want of breath." Clinically, sleep apnea, first described in 1965, means cessation of breathing during sleep.

Narcolepsy is a neurological disorder whose main symptom is uncontrollable, excessive sleep, regardless of the time of day or whether the person has had enough sleep during the previous night. The other features of this disorder can include brief episodes of muscle weakness or paralysis caused by laughter and anger (cataplexy), paralysis for brief periods upon awakening from sleep (sleep paralysis), and dreamlike images at sleep onset (hypnagogic hallucinations). Narcolepsy, which may affect several members of the same family, is a lifelong condition. Medications help to reduce the symptoms but do not cure the disease.

Insomnia is the commonly experienced difficulty in falling asleep, remaining asleep throughout the night, and the inability to return to sleep once awakened. Its causes may be physical or psychological and it may occur regularly or only occasionally

Even a partial list of all the disorders caused by or associated with disturbed sleep adds up to some 70 items. The costs to society due to loss of productivity, industrial accidents and medical bills are estimated to be over $60 billion. These staggering statistics led to the creation by the U.S. Congress in 1988 of a National Commission on Sleep Disorders Research. This group is charged with the task of developing a blueprint for a national effort to reduce the medical and economic consequences of sleep disorders.

Likely Candidates for Sleep-Related Disorders

Some of the people most likely to have or to develop a sleep-related disorder include:

- adults who fall asleep at inappropriate times and places (e.g., during conversation, lecturing, driving) and who exhibit night-time snoring

- elderly men and women

- postmenopausal women

- people who are overweight, or have some physical abnormality in the nose, throat, or other parts of the upper airway

- night-shift workers

- people who habitually drink too much alcohol

- blind individuals who tend to develop impaired perception of light and darkness and have disturbed circadian rhythms, the

cycles of biologic activities that occur at the same time during
each 24 hours

• people with depression and other psychotic disorders.

Sleep and Breathing Disorders

In 1944, the important observation was made that ventilation (exchange of air between the lung and environment) normally decreases
during sleep. Even in "normal" people, breathing patterns during sleep
may show a few irregularities. For example, a person might experience an average of seven breathing pauses of up to 10 seconds per
night without any associated symptoms or problems. However if the
breathing irregularities are accompanied by reduced oxygen supply
to tissue (hypoxia) and fragmented sleep, these people are at risk of
developing more serious problems.

Sleep Apnea

Sleep apnea is the most common sleep disorder in terms of mortality and morbidity, especially in middle-age men. Perhaps the best
known sleep apnea "patient" is Charles Dickens' Fat Joe in *The Post-
humous Papers of the Pickwick Club*, the overweight, red-faced boy
in a permanent state of sleepiness, who snored and breathed heavily.
The term "Pickwickian" syndrome has been used to describe patients
with the most severe form of sleep apnea that is associated with reduced levels of breathing even during the day.

Sleep apnea occurs in all age groups and both sexes, but seems to
predominate in males (it may be underdiagnosed in females) and in
African Americans. The Associated Professional Sleep Societies estimates that as many as 20 million Americans have this condition. The
conditions associated with sleep apnea are a cascade: apnea, arousal,
sleep deprivation, and excessive daytime sleepiness. Each is related
to the frequency of the prior condition.

Like obesity with which it is often associated, the clustering of sleep
apnea in some families suggests a genetic abnormality. Ingestion of
alcohol And sleeping pills increases the frequency and duration of
breathing pauses during sleep in people with sleep apnea.

Because of serious disturbances in their normal sleep patterns,
patients with sleep apnea feel sleepy during the day and their concentration and daytime performance suffer. The common consequences of sleep apnea range from annoying to life-threatening. They

include personality changes, sexual dysfunction and falling asleep at work, on the phone, or driving.

Symptoms of Sleep Apnea

Patients with sleep apnea have many repeated involuntary breathing pauses during sleep. The length of the breathing pause can vary within a patient, and among patients, and can last from 10 seconds to 60 seconds. Fewer than 30 such breathing pauses during a 7-hour sleep, or shorter breathing pauses, are not considered indicative of sleep apnea. Most sleep apnea patients experience 20 to 30 "apneic events" per hour, more than 200 per night. These pauses may occur in clusters.

The breathing pauses are often accompanied by choking sensations which may wake up the patient, intermittent snoring, nighttime insomnia, early morning headaches, and excessive daytime sleepiness, although not all patients, for some reason, complain of daytime sleepiness. During the apneic events, a person may turn blue from low blood oxygen levels.

Other features of sleep apnea include slowing down of heart beat below 60 beats per minute (bradycardia), irregular heart beat (cardiac arrhythmias), high blood pressure (both systemic and pulmonary artexial), increase in red cells in the blood polycythemia), and obesity. The absence of restful sleep may cause deterioration of performance, depression, irritability, sexual dysfunction, and defects in attention and concentration.

Types of Sleep Apnea

Scientists have distinguished three types of sleep apnea: obstructive, central, and mixed. However, since all three types may have similar symptoms and signs, a sleep evaluation is needed to tell the difference among them.

Obstructive Sleep Apnea (OSA) is the most common type. During OSA efforts to breath continue but air cannot flow in or out of the patient's nose or mouth. The patient snores heavily and has frequent arousals (abrupt changes from deep sleep to light sleep) without being aware of them.

OSA occurs when the throat muscles and tongue relax during breathing and partially block the opening of the airway. When the muscles of the soft palate at the base of the tongue and the uvula (the small conical fleshy tissue hanging from the center of the soft palate) relax and sag, the airway becomes obstructed making breathing labored and noisy. Airway narrowing may also occur due to overweight, possibly because of the associated increases in the amount of tissue in the airway.

The reduction in oxygen and increase in carbon dioxide which occur during apnea cause arousals. With each arousal, a signal is sent to the upper airway muscles to open the airway; breathing is resumed with a loud snort or gasp. Although arousals serve as a rescue mechanism and are necessary for a patient with apnea, they interrupt sleep, and the patient ends up with less restorative and deep sleep than normal individuals. Central apnea occurs less frequently than obstructive apnea. There is no airflow in or out of the airways because efforts to breathe have stopped for short periods of time. In central apnea, the brain temporarily fails to send the signals to the diaphragm and the chest muscles that maintain the breathing cycle. It is present more often in the elderly than in younger people but often goes unrecognized. In central apnea, there is periodic loss of rhythmic breathing movements. The airway remains open but air does not pass through the nose or mouth because activity of the diaphragm and the chest muscles stops. Patients with central apnea may not snore and they tend to be more aware of their frequent awakenings than those with obstructive apnea.

In mixed apnea, a period of central apnea is followed by a period of obstructive apnea before regular breathing resumes. People with mixed apnea frequently snore.

Snoring and Sleep Apnea

Snoring is a sign of abnormal breathing. It typically occurs when physical obstruction causes vibration of the soft palate and the adjacent soft tissues.

Snoring always occurs with obstructive sleep apnea. When diagnosing sleep disorders, obstructive sleep apnea is excluded if snoring is not a symptom. All snorers do not necessarily have sleep apnea; however, because they almost certainly have some physical obstruction in their airways, they may develop sleep apnea.

The prevalence of snoring is greater in the older population and apparently peaks in 60-year-old men and women, declining in older individuals. Men seem to snore more than women. Men also are more likely to develop sleep-disordered breathing. It is estimated that nearly half of all males over 40 snore habitually. Snoring is also more common in overweight people.

A visit to the doctor is not necessary when a person snores unless some of the other symptoms of sleep disordered breathing also occur. However, since snoring is an annoying or irritating symptom with some negative social aspects, many people have sought a "cure" for it. More than 300 devices have been patented in the U.S. which claim to control snoring. Many of these devices were developed even before medical scientists found out that heavy snoring is a potential marker of sleep apnea.

Sleep Apnea and the Heart

Sleep apnea with snoring seems to increase the likelihood of having a variety of cardiovascular diseases. These include high blood pressure, ischemic heart disease (a condition caused by reduced blood supply to the heart muscle), cardiac arrhythmias (abnormal heartbeat rhythm), and cerebral infarction (blood clot in the brain). It is not unusual for patients with sleep apnea to be mistakenly treated for primary heart disease because cardiac arrhythmias may be more prominent than the breathing disturbances.

Nearly 50 percent of sleep apnea patients have high blood pressure. Patients with the most severe sleep apnea seem to have the highest blood pressure levels and are also more likely to have trouble controlling their blood pressure than patients who do not have sleep apnea. No one knows whether a cause and effect relationship exists between high blood pressure and sleep apnea. If it does exist, the ways these conditions interact is unknown.

Snoring alone does not appear to be a risk factor for heart disease. Only when snoring occurs with sleep apnea or obesity does it seem to be associated with these conditions.

Sleep Apnea in Infants

Before a baby is born, the mother's breathing takes care of its respiratory needs. Although the unborn baby's lungs are filled with fluid and are not ready to take in air, its respiratory muscles make breathing motions, as if "training" to take on the responsibilities of breathing after birth.

As soon as birth occurs, the normal newborn baby begins a continuous pattern of periodic breathing characterized by a succession of apneas followed by regular breathing. Apneas occasionally lasting longer than 10 to 15 seconds are common during the newborn period. Apneas are more frequent and longer in premature newborns than in full-term infants. The frequency of apnea decreases with age during the first 6 months of life.

Babies who turn blue during sleep and appear limp may be undergoing episodes of insufficient breathing. They should be checked for a sleep-related disorder.

Sleep Apnea and Sudden Infant Death Syndrome

Sleep apnea is sometimes implicated in sudden infant death syndrome (SIDS), also called crib death. About 10,000 infants die every year in this country from SIDS. Scientists do not know the reasons for these deaths but sleep apnea may play a role because these babies die when they are asleep and show no evidence of trauma. On autopsy, pinpoint hemorrhages are sometimes noted in the thoracic cavity which may be caused by lack of oxygen prior to cardiac arrest and vigorous respiratory movements.

Diagnosis of Sleep Apnea

The general physician may sometimes recognize sleep apnea, but specialists in neurology, psychiatry, pulmonary medicine and cardiology may be needed for accurate diagnosis and management. Diagnosis of sleep apnea is difficult because disturbed sleep can cause various other diseases or make them worse. Several major medical centers now have pulmonologists, neurologists, and psychiatrists with specialty training in sleep disorders on their staff Although an evaluation for sleep apnea can sometimes be done at home, it is more reliable if it is done in a sleep laboratory.

A variety of tests can be used to diagnose sleep apnea. These include pulmonary function tests, polysomnography, and the multiple sleep latency test. Physicians continue to try to develop other simple and economic procedures for the early diagnosis of sleep apnea.

Pulmonary function tests taken by sleep apnea patients may show normal results unless the patient has a coexisting lung disease. To make a definitive diagnosis of sleep apnea, the physician may order an all-night evaluation of the patient's sleep stages, and of the status of breathing and gas exchange during sleep.

Polysomnography is a group of tests that monitors a variety of functions during sleep. These include sleep state, electrical activity of the brain (EEG), eye movement (EOG), muscle activity (EMG), heart rate, respiratory effort, airflow, blood oxygen and carbon dioxide levels. Other tests may be ordered depending on a particular patient's needs.

Polysomnography sometimes helps to distinguish between different sleep disorders. These tests are used both to diagnose sleep apnea and to determine its severity.

The Multiple Sleep Latency Test is done during normal working hours. It consists of observations, repeated every 2 hours, of the time taken to reach various stages of sleep. In this test, people without sleep apnea take more than 10 minutes to fall asleep. On the other hand, patients with sleep apnea or narcolepsy fall asleep fairly rapidly. When it takes the patient an average of less than 5 minutes to fall asleep, it is considered pathological sleepiness. There is thus some uncertainty in the diagnosis if the sleep latency period (speed of falling asleep) is between 5 and 10 minutes. This test is important because it measures the degree of excessive daytime sleepiness and also helps to rule out narcolepsy, which is associated with the onset of REM sleep (dream sleep) in many of the naps.

Treatment of Sleep Apnea

More than 50,000 patients are treated each year for breathing disorders of sleep. Physicians tailor therapy to the individual patient based on medical history, physical examination, and the results of laboratory tests and polysomnography. Patients with sleep apnea can help themselves by trying to avoid doing anything that can worsen the disease. Sleeping in improper positions can increase the frequency of apnea. Use of alcohol suppresses the activity of the upper airway muscles so that the airway is more likely to collapse. Sleeping pills and sedative-hypnotic drugs suppress arousal mechanisms and prolong apneas. Moving to high altitudes may aggravate the condition because of low oxygen levels. Overweight sleep apnea patients should lose weight.

Because the exact mechanism responsible for obstructive sleep apnea is not known, there is still no treatment that directly addresses the underlying problem. In most cases, medications have not proved successful. Some surgical procedures are effective approximately 50 percent of the time because the exact location of the airway obstruction is usually unclear.

Since patients with sleep apnea usually have significant family and work problems, the treatment should include strategies that will help them cope with these problems. Education of the patient, family, and employers is sometimes needed to help the patient return to an active normal life.

Position Therapy

In mild cases of sleep apnea, breathing pauses occur only when the individual sleeps on the back. Thus using methods that will ensure that patients sleep on their side is often helpful.

Nasal Continuous Positive Airway Pressure (CPAP)

CPAP is the most common effective treatment for sleep apnea. In this procedure, the patient wears a mask over the nose during sleep and pressure from an air compressor forces air through the nasal passages. The air pressure is adjusted so that it is just enough to hold the throat open when it relaxes during sleep. The pressure is constant and continuous. Nasal CPAP prevents obstruction while in use but apneas return when CPAP is stopped.

The major disadvantage of CPAP is that about 40 percent of patients have difficulty using it for long periods of time. Irritation and drying in the nose occur in some patients. Facial skin irritation, abdominal bloating, mask leaks, sore eyes, and headaches are some of the other problems. Because many patients stop using nasal CPAP due to the discomfort arising from exhaling against positive pressure, the search goes on for more comfortable devices. Modifications of CPAP in the treatment of sleep apnea are currently ongoing.

One device, which some patients find more comfortable, is the bilevel positive airway pressure. Unlike CPAP where the pressure is equal during inhalation and exhalation, bilevel devices are designed to follow the patient's breathing pattern. It lowers the pressure during expiration and maintains a constant inspiratory pressure.

The ramp system, a modification of CPAP, allows the pressure to be applied only when the patient goes to sleep, increasing pressure slowly over a preset period of time (usually 15 to 30 minutes). The purpose of the ramp system is to make CPAP more comfortable for the patient.

Nocturnal Ventilation

Patients can be ventilated noninvasively during sleep with positive pressure ventilation through a CPAP mask. This involves use of a machine other than regular CPAP to provide cyclic ventilation to the patient. This technique is now used in patients whose breathing is impaired to the point that their blood carbon dioxide level is elevated, as happens in patients with obesity-hypoventilation syndrome, certain neuromuscular diseases, and central apnea.

Pharmacologic Therapies

No medications are effective in the treatment of sleep apnea. However some physicians believe that mild cases of sleep apnea respond to drugs that either stimulate breathing or suppress deep sleep. Acetazolamide has been used to treat central apnea. Tricyclic antidepressants inhibit deep sleep (REM) and are useful only in patients who have apneas in the REM state.

Oxygen administration sometimes benefits patients without any side effects. However, the role of oxygen in the treatment of sleep apnea is controversial and it is difficult to predict which patients will respond to oxygen therapy.

Dental Appliances

Dental appliances which reposition the lower jaw and the tongue have been helpful to some patients with mild obstructive sleep apnea. Possible side effects include damage to teeth, soft tissues, and the jaw joint.

Surgery

Some patients with sleep apnea may require surgical treatment. Useful procedures include removal of adenoids and tonsils, nasal polyps or other growths, or other tissue in the airway, or correction of structural deformities. Younger patients seem to benefit from surgery better than older patients.

Tracheostomy

Tracheostomy is used only in patients with severe, life-threatening obstructive sleep apnea. In this procedure a small hole is made in the windpipe (trachea) below the Adam's apple. A tube is inserted into the opening. This tube stays closed during waking hours and the person breathes normally. It is opened for sleep so that air flows directly into the lungs, bypassing any upper airway obstruction. Its major drawbacks are that it is a disfiguring procedure and the tracheostomy tube requires proper daily care to keep it clean.

Uvulopalatopharyngoplasty (UPPP)

UPPP is a procedure used to remove excess tissue at the back of the throat (tonsils, adenoids, uvula, and part of the soft palate). This technique probably helps only half of the patients who choose it. Its negative effects include nasal speech and backflow (regurgitation) of liquids into the nose during swallowing in some cases. UPPP is not considered as universally effective as tracheostomy but does seem to be a cure for snoring. It does not appear to prevent mortality from cardiovascular complications of severe sleep apnea.

Other Surgical Procedures

Some patients whose sleep apnea is due to deformities of the lower jaw (mandible) benefit from reconstruction or surocal advancement of the mandible. Gastric stapling procedures to treat obesity are sometimes recommended for sleep apnea patients who are morbidly obese.

Treatment of Patients with Coexisting Lung Diseases

Asthma, chronic bronchitis, emphysema, or other lung diseases can cause breathing problems during sleep. Patients with these diseases may be frequently awakened by cough, aspiration of secretions, choking sensations, and apnea-like sleep disturbances. The treatment in these cases depends on whether the sleep disturbances are due to lung disease or sleep apnea.

Pathophysiology of Sleep and Breathing: Highlights of the National, Heart, Lung, and Blood Institute Programs

Sleep

The modem era of sleep research started in the mid-1950's with the discovery that sleep is not a homogeneous phenomenon. Rather, it fluctuates cyclically between two distinct sequential stages of sleep.

The first sleep stage is variously called synchronized sleep, slow sleep, slow-wave sleep, quiet sleep, or non-rapid-eye-movement (NREM) sleep. In this state the EEG is dominated by large-amplitude slow waves; body functioning generally slows; there are slow, rolling eve movements; the pupils constrict; the respiratory and heart rates decline; blood pressure decreases; and total body oxygen consumption is reduced. It is believed that NREM sleep is a recuperative state.

The second state of sleep is called synchronized sleep, fast sleep, fast-wave sleep, dream sleep, or rapid-eye-movement (REM) sleep. The EEG is synchronized, with low-voltage fast waves and there are intermittent eve movements. It is also called paradoxical sleep because of the paradox that the EEG in this sleep stage is similar to that in wakefulness or light sleep, although this is deep sleep in terms of arousability. During REM sleep, central-nervous-system (CNS) activity, generally increases, and body systems are variously activated and inactivated in a complex physiological pattern. The normal adult spends some 15 to 20 percent of the sleeping hours in REM sleep; this percentage decreases with aging. In contrast, the human fetus of 30 weeks spends 80 percent of its sleep in REM sleep. This declines to 50 percent at term. The amount of quiet sleep (NREM) increases from 50 to 60 percent by 3 months and to 70 percent between 6 and 23 months.

At the biochemical level, hormone-like prostaglandins and cytokines, which are intercellular messengers found in the brain, are implicated in the mechanisms that control sleep. Some speculate that a balance between prostaglandin D2 which increases sleep, and prostaglandin E2 which increases wakefulness, may be involved in the controlling mechanism. The prostaglandins produce their effects when injected into the preoptic area of the hypothalamus, an area responsible for temperature regulation. This may explain the link between sleep and fall in temperature, and also may unify the neurophysiological and biochemical mechanisms of sleep.

Interleukin- I is localized in the brain in areas associated with control of sleep, and is believed to play a sleep regulatory role. The amount of interleukin-I in cerebrospinal fluid fluctuates in parallel with the normal sleep/wake cycle.

There is no clear biological answer to the fundamental question of why we sleep, A wide variety of medical and psychiatric illnesses and factors related to age and gender can interfere with falling and staying asleep, with a multitude of pathophysiological sequelae. A major goal of sleep research is the characterization of the etiology and pathophysiology of the causes and effects of disturbed sleep.

Breathing

The two major components of breathing are inspiration and expiration. Inspiration is an active process involving contraction of the diaphragm, external intercostal, and in certain circumstances, accessory muscles. It serves to increase intrathoracic volume, decrease intrapleural pressure and allow exchange of air and carbon dioxide within the alveoli of the lungs. Oxygen is transported from the alveoli to the pulmonary, bloodstream by passive diffusion and is made available to tissues. Expiration, on the other hand, is a relatively passive process, requiring little or no contraction of the muscles during quiet breathing. A main function of the breathing process is to bring about the exchange of oxygen and carbon dioxide and other gaseous products from biological systems.

At birth, the baby switches from dependence on placental gas exchange to air breathing. At the moment of birth there is also a switch from intermittent breathing efforts of the fetal stage to sustained breathing efforts. Since the infant's respiratory muscles are not well-equipped to sustain high workloads, respiratory muscle fatigue is a problem for premature infants, and apneic episodes requiring intervention occur in at least 50 percent of surviving infants weighing less than 1,500 grams.

Breathing disorders during sleep occur either when there are deficiencies in neurally generated rhythmic respiratory efforts or when there is normal generation of rhythmic efforts but mechanically impeded airflow in upper airways. Metabolic and behavioral control systems in the brain are believed to be the control mechanisms for sleep and breathing. The metabolic system that responds to changes in carbon dioxide and oxygen seems to exert its major influence over NREM sleep. On the other hand, the behavioral control system is involved in voluntary respiratory activities and appears to influence REM sleep; many of the ventilatory changes that occur in REM sleep are similar to the behavioral ventilatory activities such as swallowing, voluntary breath holding, and hyperventilation.

Subjects without any clinical problems may exhibit obstructive or central apnea during periods of REM sleep. Although severe changes in respiratory behavior often occur during the REM sleep, sleep apnea can occur in both NREM and REM sleep. However, sleep staging in patients with severe sleep apnea syndrome is difficult because of severe sleep fragmentation. Thus it is difficult to define the relative importance of abnormal respiration detected during REM or NREM sleeps.

Research Highlights

A recent basic research advance of potential clinical implication relates to the application of modem three-dimensional medical imaging techniques to the study of pathogenesis of sleep apnea. Magnetic resonance imaging (NM) and ultrafast x-ray computed tomography (CT) of the upper airways, combined with computer graphics and reconstructions, gave begun to provide exquisite details of the geometry of the upper airway. These approaches now permit identification of the precise anatomical sites of collapse or areas of abnormal compliance to determine if the problem is in a specific area or is a more generalized multifocal abnormality. This information ill impact on the treatment options, particularly if there is more diffuse involvement since this would predict failure of localized surgical procedures.

Only 50 percent of patients with sleep apnea undergoing uvulopalatopharyngoplasty benefit from this procedure. Investigators are exploring ways to identify those patients most likely to benefit from this procedure. A small scale clinical trial conducted to determine predictors of success for UPPP revealed that 86 percent of patients who had documented (by fiberoptic endoscopy) preoperative nasopharyngeal obstruction at the level of the soft palate, showed significant improvement in the number of apneas, arousals and in the cumulative time in apnea-hypopnea following surgery. In contrast, only 18 percent of the patients who had a collapsing segment in regions of the pharynx other than the soft palate showed any improvement following UPPP. This is the first prospective clinical study to demonstrate that closure of the passive pharynx at the level of the soft palate predicts a favorable surgical outcome.

An important opportunity for research on the pathophysiology and treatment of sleep apnea has opened up with the finding that the English bulldog seems to be a suitable animal model of sleep apnea. This model is permitting the study of the regularly occurring periodicities in neural activity of the upper airways and the inspiratory muscles, and the role of neural mechanisms in the genesis of sleep apnea. Studies with this model revealed that the consequences of intermittent apnea (sleepiness or hypoxemia) serve to increase the magnitude and frequency of neural inhibitory activity, thereby worsening the apnea.

Other studies exploring new treatments for obstructive sleep apnea in animals and humans have identified buspirone, a hypnotic agent as a potentially effective drug for sleep apnea. Buspirone seems to increase ventilation in both anesthetized and awake rats and cats without producing the traditional respiratory depressive effects. In a small scale, controlled clinical trial, this drug decreased sleep apnea and improved respiratory status in the patients receiving the drug.

Associations between snoring, hypertension, heart disease, and stroke raise the possibility of common factors and/or causal relationships between sleep apnea and cardiovascular disorders. Such links may be related to biochemical factors such as insulin, catecholamine, or cortisol that are increased in stress. Sleep apnea may itself be a stress that produces hormonal imbalances that lead to the hytertensive state. Alternately obesity, sleep apnea, and other cardiovascular risk factors may share common metabolic pathways and therefore may be genetically determined. These relationships are being explored by studying families with a history of sleep apnea and/or sudden infant death syndrome as well as by studying racial and genetic differences in the prevalence of sleep apnea-related illnesses.

Research Opportunities

Since 1986, the Division of Lung Diseases, National Heart, Lung, and Blood Institute, has been engaged in a concerted national program in cardiopulmonary disorders in sleep designed to fill critical gaps in the understanding of the pathogenesis, diagnosis, treatment, and prevention of sleep-disordered breathing. Some research areas of current emphasis include the following:

1. Natural history of sleep apnea with the goal of determining the magnitude of the problem and designing the most effective therapy

2. Scientific basis for the influence of age, gender, ethnicity, smoking, obesity, and snoring on the development of sleep apnea.

3. Assessment of the severity of sleep apnea and defining the relationships of disease severity, response to treatment and prognosis.

4. Cellular and molecular basis of the role of hypoxia in excessive daytime sleepiness and sleep apnea.

5. Cardiovascular consequences of sleep apnea and the underlying neural cellular and respiratory mechanisms.

6. Improved therapeutic modalities for sleep apnea when associated with blood pressure, asthma. chronic heart failure, angina pectoris, chronic pulmonary disease and stroke.

For More Information

Additional information about breathing-related sleep disorders and other disorders of sleep can be obtained from your local sleep disorders center and the following sources:

American Sleep Apnea Association
334 Pleasant Street, Suite D
Belmont, MA 02178

The American Sleep Disorders Association
1610 14th Street, NW
Suite 300
Rochester, MN 55901

Narcolepsy Network
Box 1365
FDR Station
New York, NY 10150

National Center on Sleep Disorders Research
31 Center Drive, MSC 2490
National Heart, Lung, and Blood Institute
Bethesda, MD 20892-2490

National Heart, Lung, and Blood Institute (NBLBI)
Communications and Public Information Branch
31 Center Drive, MSC 2470
Bethesda, NM 20892-2470

Other institutes at NIH that have information about sleep disorders include the National Institute of Neurological Disorders and Stroke, National Institute of Child Health and Human Development, National Institute of Mental Health, National Institute on Aging. The address for each is 9000 Rockville Pike, Bethesda, MD 20892.

National Sleep Foundation
122 South Robinson Boulevard
Third Floor
Los Angeles, CA 90048

Restless Legs Syndrome Foundation, Inc.
1904 Banbury Road
Raleigh, NC 27608

Glossary

Adenoids: Gland-like tissue growths in the nose above the throat which obstruct breathing when swollen.

Airway obstruction: Narrowing, clogging or blocking of the air passages to or in the lung.

Apnea: Cessation of breathing.

Arousal: An abrupt change from deep sleep to a lighter stage of sleep which may or may not lead to awakening.

Cardiac arrest: Sudden cessation of cardiac function.

Cardiac arrhythmia: Variation in the normal rhythm of the heart-beat.

Circadian rhythm: Natural daily fluctuation of physiological and behavioral functions.

Corpulmonale: Heart disease secondary to lung disease.

CPAP: A mechanical device used to deliver continuous positive airway pressure.

Dyspnea: Difficult or labored breathing.

Diaphragm: The major respiratory muscle that participates in the act of breathing. The diaphragm separates the chest and abdominal areas.

Edema: Abnormal amount of fluid in body tissues.

Hemorrhage: Escape of blood from blood-carrying tissue.

Hypoxia: A state in which there is oxygen deficiency.

Hyperventilation: A state in which abnormally fast and deep respiration results in the intake of excessive amount of oxygen into the lung and reduced carbon dioxide levels in the blood.

Hypoventilation: A state in which there is an insufficient amount of air entering and leaving the lung to bring oxygen to the tissues and eliminate carbon dioxide.

Ischemic heart disease: Heart disease from restricted blood supply due to obstruction in blood vessels.

Nares: Openings in the nasal cavities—nostrils.

NONREM sleep: A nonuniform series of four stages of sleep which occur early in the night and are characterized by the absence of movement and slow wave brain activity. NREM generally preceded the first REM period.

Polysomnography: The continuous recording of a number of physiological functions and events during sleep.

Prostaglandins: A group of fat-delived chemicals involved in the regulation of a number of body functions.

Pulmonary function tests: Tests to measure the degree of damage to the lung; the most common tests measure, using a devise called the spirometer, the ability of the lung to move air into and out of the lung.

Rapid eye movement: A stage of sleep in which dreaming is associated with mild involuntary muscle movements. Adults cycle in and out of REM at about 90 minute intervals. REM occupies about 20 percent of total sleep.

Sleep fragmentation: Interruption of a sleep stage by awakening, arousal or appearance of another sleep stage.

Sleep hygiene: Conditions and practices that promote effective and continuous sleep, e.g., regular bedtime and arise time; restriction of alcohol, coffee etc.

Sleep latency: Time measured from "lights out" or bedtime to actually falling asleep.

Tracheostomy: Surgical insertion of a tube into the airway through the neck to maintain an opening for the outside air to enter the lungs.

Ventilation: The process of exchange of air between the lungs and the atmospheric air leading to exchange of gases with blood.

Chapter 25

Being Evaluated for Sleep Apnea

If you suspect that you have sleep apnea and need to see a doctor about your symptoms, we suggest that you first check your insurance policy before making any appointments. You may be required to get a referral to a sleep specialist from your primary care physician and/ or you may be required to go to a certain testing facility. (Keep in mind that you may be tested in a sleep center or laboratory or in your own home.) In some cases, your primary care physician orders the tests and receives the results for you.

Doctors who work in sleep medicine may be pulmonologists (specializing in lungs), neurologists (the brain), otolaryngologists (the ears, nose, and throat), psychiatry (mental health), or primary care physicians such as internists or family practitioners. Their expertise in the field of sleep may come from having trained with other sleep specialists and/or having studied sleep medicine through a residency program, continuing medical education (CME) courses, and scientific meetings. Some are certified by the American Board of Sleep Medicine (ABSM) as well. In any case, a sleep doctor may hold one of many degrees that meet the requirements of the ABSM: an MD, DO, MB (the European equivalent of an MD), or a PhD or a PsyD in a health-related field.

In addition, some dentists have studied sleep and, when appropriate, treat sleep apnea patients by fitting them with an oral appliance.

You should feel free to ask any doctor or dentist about his/her credentials and experience. You should also be satisfied with the explanations of what sleep apnea is and how it is diagnosed and treated in your particular case.

If you do have a choice of doctors and sleep testing facilities, you can find a referral from a few different sources. There is currently no one complete. list of all such facilities, and as a non-profit organization, the American Sleep Apnea Association (ASAA) does not endorse or recommend any company, product, or health care provider. However, there is a list of sleep centers and laboratories accredited by the American Sleep Disorders Association that pay their ASDA membership dues. (The ASDA is the professional society in the field of sleep medicine that accredits such facilities; accreditation implies adherence to a certain set of standards.) The most up-to-date list of accredited member sleep centers and laboratories appears on the ASDA's web site: www.asda.org, if you have access to the Internet. You can request a list from the ASAA as well. Remember that other centers are in the process of being accredited, have chosen not to be accredited, or do not qualify for accreditation.

You can also check with local hospitals, home health care companies, health care professionals to find a testing facility. The telephone directory for businesses can be helpful in this regard. Neighbors, friends, and family members may have further suggestions.

Sleep apnea also occurs in children. If you suspect your child has sleep apnea, you can bring this to the attention of your pediatrician.

For more information on the difference between a home study and a in-laboratory study, you can order the reprint from the April-May 1997 issue of the newsletter. "Home Tests or In-Laboratory Studies" by sending $2 per reprint with your request and mailing address to the ASAA. You may also want to order the reprint "Understanding a Sleep Study" (also $2) to learn more about what information is gathered in a sleep study and what the findings mean. For information about sleep apnea and insurance coverage, contact the ASAA.

Chapter 26

Lessening the Effects of Sleep Apnea

Breathing disorders during sleep can lead to disturbances as commonplace as snoring. In more extreme cases, they may cause daytime hypersomnolence—the inability to stay awake during the day. The term apnea is used to describe a pause in breathing of 10 or more seconds. Sleep apnea is defined as having 30 or more apneic episodes per 8 hours of sleep. Sleep Apnea Syndrome (SAS) is characterized by numerous apneic episodes along with loud snoring and daytime sleeping.

Daytime sleeping is a real problem on the job or while driving. Falling asleep at the wheel is a common problem for SAS patients and the cause of numerous accidents. Falling asleep at work frequently results in injury and/or job loss.

Believe it or not, SAS can also lead to memory problems as well as difficulty concentrating and thinking. Anxiety and/or depression are frequent symptoms, as is irritable and aggressive behavior. Physically, a person with SAS may experience early morning headaches, sexual dysfunction, chronic tiredness, high blood pressure, and swelling of the extremities.

Treatment

There are numerous treatment possibilities available for people experiencing sleep apnea. Obese patients must lose weight. There is very little risk associated with medically supervised weight-loss programs, and the weight loss may offer additional physical benefits.

Sleeping on your side may reduce the number of apneic episodes you experience by nearly 50%.

If you have sleep apnea, do not drink alcoholic beverages or take sleeping pills before bedtime. This will make your condition worse by depressing your respiratory system's drive to breathe.

Nonsurgical treatments for SAS include supplemental oxygen and continuous positive airway pressure (CPAP). CPAP is effective but it is uncomfortable, and wearing a mask while sleeping is inconvenient. Bilevel positive airway pressure (BIPAP®) also provides noninvasive ventilatory support through a nasal mask offering alternated levels of gas flow.

Sometimes surgery will be required. There may be an obstruction that has to be removed or the situation may warrant a tracheostomy. A tracheostomy requires the surgical insertion of a tube into the trachea. This procedure is intended for people with severe symptoms.

Patient history and a physical exam may indicate the need for a polysomnogram (a formal sleep study) to confirm a diagnosis of SAS. It will document the number and length of each apneic episode and help to determine the severity of the breathing disorder. A polysomnogram is only one of a series of tests that will probably include an electrocardiogram (ECG), a chest x-ray, a pulmonary function test, and arterial blood gas analysis.

Polysomnography requires the attachment of sensors to various parts of the body. These sensors provide signals that are amplified and recorded on a printout. The printout can be analyzed to determine how severe the condition is as well as what therapy is most desirable.

Chapter 27

Choosing a Continuous Positive Pressure Airway Machine, a Mask, and Headgear

Choosing a CPAP

CPAP, or Continuous Positive Airway Pressure, therapy is the most common form of treatment for sleep apnea. There are several CPAP manufacturers that offer different types of machines with different features. Once you have been diagnosed with sleep apnea and have been prescribed CPAP therapy, you may be able to choose one machine among the many offered.

Talk to your doctor and your home care company representative about which machine is best for you, and keep in mind any restrictions on cost and/or provider which your insurance company may impose. In deciding which CPAP machine to use, think about what features you want or need. Current options include a carrying case, the ability to convert to foreign currents, an attached heated humidifier, ramping (which allows for a gradual increase in pressure), DC (direct current) operations via a car or boat battery, and the capability to adjust for different altitudes. Bi-level devices with two different pressures—one for inhalation and one lower pressure for exhalation—are also available. In addition, the Food and Drug Administration has approved a few autoadjusting devices for the market; these machines are to change the pressure automatically as needed.

Reprinted with permission. © 1997, 1998 American Sleep Disorders Association, 1610 14th Street NW, Suite 300, Rochester, MN. 55901. Telephone 202/293-3650 Web site - http://www.sleepapnea.org

The mask fit will also be critical to you. Again, talk to your doctor and home care company representative about your choices, and keep in mind that the mask may be manufactured by one company and the CPAP by another.

To obtain a current list of CPAP manufacturers with their address and phone number and to contact them directly for more information about their products, contact the American Sleep Apnea Association.

Choosing a Mask and Headgear

Once you have been prescribed Continuous Positive Airway Pressure (CPAP) therapy, you will need to be fitted for a mask and headgear that is both comfortable and that provides a proper seal for the airflow. In fact, the proper air pressure level cannot be established unless the mask and headgear fit is correct. Thus to obtain the optimal benefits of CPAP treatment, it is essential that both mask and headgear fit well. Moreover, a comfortable mask that fits well will make using CPAP easier.

The hard plastic body and softer silicon seal of the mask are worn over your nose while the adjustable straps of the headgear hold the mask in place. Straps that are too loose will permit air to leak. In some cases, straps that are too tight can break the seal and create leaks; any strap pulled too tightly can cause pain. Headgear straps must be tight enough for a good fit in all sleeping positions (back, side, and front) but no tighter.

CPAP machines compensate for the "built-in leak" in the mask system that is necessary to keep the air supply fresh. However, too much leaking from the mask itself may reduce the set pressure. Masks that are too large tend to leak more easily than those that are snug, so as a rule of thumb, select the smaller size. If you extend your hosing, be sure the total length is less than twelve feet as longer hoses generally will not maintain the proper pressure. If you must use one that is longer, measure the pressure at the mask, not at the machine.

Dry skin and facial hair can compromise the effectiveness of CPAP masks. Skin moisturizers may help with the problem of dry skin, and although they slightly reduce the life of the mask, an improved facial seal may very well be worth it. Some moisturizers are manufactured specifically for CPAP users and can be used inside the nose as well. As for facial hair, some masks are made with moustache and beard wearers in mind, and masks with a lower profile can typically accommodate eyeglasses better. Varying the style or type of mask can reduce chronic nose, lip, or facial discomfort caused by repeated nightly use of the same mask. However, some insurance carriers resist paying for more than one CPAP mask, so additional masks may be an out-of-pocket expense for you.

An allergic reaction to mask materials can also be a problem. If you are allergic to the silicone, ask for a mask made from synthetic rubber or vinyl. The nasal pillows may also be a solution to this problem as the pillows fit directly to the nostrils. and do not rest on the nose, upper lip, or cheeks. Some people, especially people with a beard or moustache, simply prefer nasal pillows to a mask.

As of this writing, the newest type of mask to receive approval by the Food and Drug Administration is one made out of gel-like material. These masks are intended to mold to each person's face in order to alleviate pressure points and to be more comfortable. However, because these masks tend to be larger than other types, some people may be less comfortable with them. In addition, the FDA recently approved a thin seal, also made out of a gel-like material with wound-healing promotion characteristics as well, that can be attached to many different sizes and types of masks. The seal usually lasts two to four weeks, depending upon the care of the seal. Again, it is intended to alleviate pressure points and to be more comfortable.

Just as there are several CPAP manufacturers that offer different types of machines with different features, there are different masks and headgear styles within manufacturers' lines. The mask may be manufactured by one company and the CPAP by another as virtually any mask will fit the standard air hose size (or can be adapted easily). It is also possible to have masks custom-made, so ask your doctor or home care company's representative about all options. Before selecting a mask, try using it with the CPAP machine and under the most realistic conditions possible (for example, turn from side to side while wearing the mask). You, as the wearer, should be happy with it. However, as with any medical expense, keep in mind any restrictions on cost and/or provider your insurance company may impose.

As new masks and headgear come on the market, information is updated. For the most current publication contact the ASAA.

If you have difficulty using CPAP that may be unrelated to the mask fit (such as nasal congestion), you may be interested in obtaining a reprint of the article "CPAP and the Nose" from the October-November 1995 *WAKE-UP CALL The Wellness Letter for Snoring and Apnea*. Contact the ASAA for ordering information, but don't hesitate to talk to your doctor about your situation.

Chapter 28

Snoring:
Not Funny, Not Hopeless

Forty-five percent of normal adults snore at least occasionally, and 25 percent are habitual snorers. Problem snoring is more frequent in males and overweight persons, and it usually grows worse with age.

More than 300 devices are registered in the U.S. Patent and Trademark Office as cures for snoring. Some are variations on the old idea of sewing a sock that holds a tennis ball on the pajama back to force the snorer to sleep on his side. (Snoring is often worse when a person sleeps on his back). Some devices reposition the lower jaw forward; some open nasal air passages; a few others have been designed to condition a person not to snore by producing unpleasant stimuli when snoring occurs. But, if you snore, the truth is that it is not under your control whatsoever. If anti-snoring devices work, it is probably because they keep you awake.

What Causes Snoring?

The noisy sounds of snoring occur when there is an obstruction to the free flow of air through the passages at the back of the mouth and nose. This area is the collapsible part of the airway where the tongue and upper throat meet the soft palate and uvula. Snoring occurs when these structures strike each other and vibrate during breathing.

199

People who snore may suffer from:

- Poor muscle tone in the tongue and throat. When muscles are too relaxed, either from alcohol or drugs that cause sleepiness, the tongue falls backwards into the airway or the throat muscles draw in from the sides into the airway. This can also happen during deep sleep.

- Excessive bulkiness of throat tissue. Children with large tonsils and adenoids often snore. Overweight people have bulky neck tissue, too. Cysts or tumors can also cause bulk, but they are rare.

- Long soft palate and/or uvula. A long palate narrows the opening from the nose into the throat. As it dangles, it acts as a noisy flutter valve during relaxed breathing. A long uvula makes matters even worse.

- Obstructed nasal airways. A stuffy or blocked nose requires extra effort to pull air through it. This creates an exaggerated vacuum in the throat, and pulls together the floppy tissues of the throat, and snoring results. So, snoring often occurs only during the hay fever season or with a cold or sinus infection.

Also, deformities of the nose or nasal septum, such as a deviated septum (a deformity of the wall that separates one nostril from the other) can cause such an obstruction.

Is Snoring Serious?

Socially, yes. It can be, when it makes the snorer an object of ridicule and causes others sleepless nights and resentfulness.

Medically, yes. It disturbs sleeping patterns and deprives the snorer of appropriate rest. When snoring is severe (see below), it can cause serious, long-term health problems, including obstructive sleep apnea.

Obstructive Sleep Apnea

When loud snoring is interrupted by frequent episodes of totally obstructed breathing, it is known as obstructive sleep apnea. Serious episodes last more than ten seconds each and occur more than seven times per hour. Apnea patients may experience 30 to 300 such events per night. These episodes can reduce blood oxygen levels, causing the heart to pump harder.

The immediate effect of sleep apnea is that the snorer is forced to sleep lightly and keep his muscles tense in order to keep airflow to the lungs. Because the snorer does not get a good rest, he may be sleepy during the day, which impairs job performance and makes him a hazardous driver or equipment operator. After many years with this disorder, elevated blood pressure and heart enlargement may occur.

Remember, snoring means obstructed breathing, and obstruction can be serious. It's not funny, and not hopeless.

Self-Help for the Light Snorer

Adults who suffer from mild or occasional snoring should try the following self-help remedies:

1.   Adopt a healthy and athletic lifestyle to develop good muscle tone and lose weight.

2.   Avoid tranquilizers, sleeping pills, and antihistamines before bedtime.

3.   Avoid alcohol for at least four hours and heavy meals or snacks for three hours before retiring.

5.   Establish regular sleeping patterns

6.   Sleep on your side rather than your back.

7.   Tilt the head of your bed upwards four inches.

Can Heavy Snoring be Cured?

Heavy snorers, those who snore in any position or are disruptive to the family, should seek medical advice to ensure that sleep apnea is not a problem. An otolaryngologist will provide a thorough examination of the nose, mouth, throat, palate, and neck. A sleep study in a laboratory environment may be necessary to determine how serious the snoring is and what effects it has on the snorer's health.

Treatment

Treatment depends on the diagnosis. An examination will reveal if the snoring is caused by nasal allergy, infection, deformity, or tonsils and adenoids. Snoring/sleep apnea may respond best to surgery on the throat and palate that tightens flabby tissues and expands air passages, an operation known as uvulopalatopharyngoplasty (UPPP). If surgery is too risky or unwanted, the patient may sleep every night with a nasal mask that delivers air pressure into the throat (CPAP).

A chronically snoring child should be examined for problems with his or her tonsils and adenoids. A tonsillectomy and adenoidectomy may be required to return the child to full health.

Chapter 29

Putting Snoring to Bed

"Until now, the only other remedy for snoring was staying awake," claims a full-page ad for Breathe Right nasal strips—small plastic strips that hug the top of the nostrils and pull open nasal passages. But while the Food and Drug Administration has approved the devices as aids to quell snoring, they're certainly not the only potential remedy for nightly noise—which most commonly comes from men over the age of 40 and wreaks havoc on their bed partners' ability to get a good night's sleep.

For quieting a snorer, weight loss is by far the most effective treatment. Consider a study of 19 overweight male snorers put on a 6-month weight-loss program at the University of Florida. For the most part, men who lost weight decreased their number of snores per hour. Several who lost more than 13 pounds were down to only about a dozen snores each hour. While the researchers also gave the men nasal decongestants and sandbags to help them sleep on their sides—2 aids that can help decrease snoring—the amount of weight the men lost appeared to play the biggest role.

Obesity seems to promote snoring by adding to the tissue around the neck. Even people who are relatively lean yet have thick neck or double chins are likely to snore. That's because the extra tissue in the neck area narrows the upper airway at the back of the throat. With the airway constricted, air that flows into the lungs when a sleeper

Reprinted with permission. © 1997 *Tufts Health & Nutrition Letter*, telephone: 1-800-274-7581.

inhales must be sucked in harder than usual, at high pressure, to get through the narrow passage. This creates a wind tunnel, so to speak, and the strong current blowing in causes tissues at the back of the throat to vibrate—hence, the snoring sound.

In addition to losing excess weight, snorers can try the following strategies to lessen nightly noise:

- *Sleep on Your Side.* Lying on your back causes the tongue to fall backward and partially block narrow airways, which in turn aggravates the "wind tunnel" effect. Instead of relying on a bed partner to roll snorers over, experts recommend sewing a tennis ball into the breast pocket of a T-shirt and wearing the shirt backwards at night.

- *Get Plenty of Sleep.* Sleep deprivation aggravates snoring by causing the muscles of the throat to relax greatly during the better portion of the night. The "loose" muscle tissues are much more likely to vibrate and make snoring noises.

- *Avoid Alcohol and Cigarettes.* One of the ways alcohol contributes to snoring is that it leads to swelling of throat tissue, which contributes to narrowing of the upper airways. Cigarette smoke, which irritates the nose and throat tissues, also causes swelling.

- *If Snoring Persists, See a Physician.* Snoring can be caused by a number of medical conditions, including hypothyroidism, allergies (which cause throat and nose tissues to swell), or conditions involving the structure of the nasal cavities, such as a deviated nasal septum.

Snorers who are consistently tired during the day should also check with a physician to see whether they have a condition called sleep apnea. What distinguishes apnea is that during the "snore," breathing stops for short periods, usually because airways have narrowed to the point at which they are temporarily blocked. This can occur hundreds of times throughout the night, interfering with normal sleep patterns and often leading to extreme sleep deprivation.

The repeated breaks in breathing may also make the oxygen in the blood drop to dangerously low levels. That places stress on the heart, which can increase the risk of heart rhythm problems, heart attack, and stroke: Fortunately, once diagnosed, sleep apnea can usually be successfully treated.

Chapter 30

What Is Narcolepsy?

Narcolepsy is a chronic sleep disorder with no known cause. The main characteristic of narcolepsy is excessive and overwhelming daytime sleepiness, even after adequate nighttime sleep. A person with narcolepsy is likely to become drowsy or to fall asleep, often at inappropriate times and places. Daytime sleep attacks may occur with or without warning and may be irresistible. These attacks can occur repeatedly in a single day. Drowsiness may persist for prolonged periods of time. In addition, nighttime sleep may be fragmented with frequent wakenings.

Three other classic symptoms of narcolepsy, which may not occur in all patients, are:

- *Cataplexy:* sudden episodes of loss of muscle function, ranging from slight weakness (such as limpness at the neck or knees, sagging facial muscles, or inability to speak clearly) to complete body collapse. Attacks may be triggered by sudden emotional reactions such as laughter, anger, or fear and may last from a few seconds to several minutes. The person remains conscious throughout the episode.

- *Sleep paralysis:* temporary inability to talk or move when falling asleep or waking up. It may last a few seconds to minutes.

- *Hypnagogic hallucinations:* vivid, often frightening, dream-like experiences that occur while dozing or falling asleep.

NIH Pub. No. 96-3649, October, 1996.

Daytime sleepiness, sleep paralysis, and hypnagogic hallucinations can also occur in people who do not have narcolepsy.

In most cases, the first symptom of narcolepsy to appear is excessive and overwhelming daytime sleepiness. The other symptoms may begin alone or in combination months or years after the onset of the daytime sleep attacks. There are wide variations in the development, severity, and order of appearance of cataplexy, sleep paralysis, and hypnagogic hallucinations in individuals. Only about 20 to 25 percent of people with narcolepsy experience all four symptoms. The excessive daytime sleepiness generally persists throughout life, but sleep paralysis and hypnagogic hallucinations may not.

The symptoms of narcolepsy, especially the excessive daytime sleepiness and cataplexy, often become severe enough to cause serious disruptions in a person's social, personal, and professional lives and severely limit activities.

When Should You Suspect Narcolepsy?

You should be checked for narcolepsy if:

- you often feel excessively and overwhelmingly sleepy during the day, even after having had a full night's sleep;

- you fall asleep when you do not intend to, such as while having dinner, talking, driving, or working;

- you collapse suddenly or your neck muscles feel too weak to hold up your head when you laugh or become angry, surprised, or shocked;

- you find yourself briefly unable to talk or move while falling asleep or waking up.

How Common Is Narcolepsy?

Although it is estimated that narcolepsy afflicts as many as 200,000 Americans, fewer than 50,000 are diagnosed. It is as widespread as Parkinson's disease or multiple sclerosis and more prevalent than cystic fibrosis, but it is less well known. Narcolepsy is often mistaken for depression, epilepsy, or the side effects of medications.

Who Gets Narcolepsy?

Narcolepsy can occur in both men and women at any age, although its symptoms are usually first noticed in teenagers or young adults.

There is strong evidence that narcolepsy may run in families; 8 to 12 percent of people with narcolepsy have a close relative with the disease.

What Happens in Narcolepsy?

Normally, when an individual is awake, brain waves show a regular rhythm. When a person first falls asleep, the brain waves become slower and less regular. This sleep state is called non-rapid eye movement (NREM) sleep. After about an hour and a half of NREM sleep, the brain waves begin to show a more active pattern again, even though the person is in deep sleep. This sleep state, called rapid eye movement (REM) sleep, is when dreaming occurs.

In narcolepsy, the order and length of NREM and REM sleep periods are disturbed, with REM sleep occurring at sleep onset instead of after a period of NREM sleep. Thus, narcolepsy is a disorder in which REM sleep appears at an abnormal time. Also, some of the aspects of REM sleep that normally occur only during sleep—lack of muscle tone, sleep paralysis, and vivid dreams—occur at other times in people with narcolepsy. For example, the lack of muscle tone can occur during wakefulness in a cataplexy episode. Sleep paralysis and vivid dreams can occur while falling asleep or waking up.

How Is Narcolepsy Diagnosed?

Diagnosis is relatively easy when all the symptoms of narcolepsy are present. But if the sleep attacks are isolated and cataplexy is mild or absent, diagnosis is more difficult.

Two tests that are commonly used in diagnosing narcolepsy are the polysomnogram and the multiple sleep latency test. These tests are usually performed by a sleep specialist. The polysomnogram involves continuous recording of sleep brain waves and a number of nerve and muscle functions during nighttime sleep. When tested, people with narcolepsy fall asleep rapidly, enter REM sleep early, and may awaken often during the night. The polysomnogram also helps to detect other possible sleep disorders that could cause daytime sleepiness.

For the multiple sleep latency test, a person is given a chance to sleep every 2 hours during normal wake times. Observations are made of the time taken to reach various stages of sleep. This test measures the degree of daytime sleepiness and also detects how soon REM sleep begins. Again, people with narcolepsy fall asleep rapidly and enter REM sleep early.

How Is Narcolepsy Treated?

Although there is no cure for narcolepsy, treatment options are available to help reduce the various symptoms. Treatment is individualized depending on the severity of the symptoms, and it may take weeks or months for an optimal regimen to be worked out. Complete control of sleepiness and cataplexy is rarely possible. Treatment is primarily by medications, but lifestyle changes are also important. The main treatment of excessive daytime sleepiness in narcolepsy is with a group of drugs called central nervous system stimulants. For cataplexy and other REM-sleep symptoms, antidepressant medications and other drugs that suppress REM sleep are prescribed. Caffeine and over-the-counter drugs have not been shown to be effective and are not recommended.

In addition to drug therapy, an important part of treatment is scheduling short naps (10 to 15 minutes) two to three times per day to help control excessive daytime sleepiness and help the person stay as alert as possible. Daytime naps are not a replacement for nighttime sleep.

Ongoing communication among the physician, the person with narcolepsy, and family members about the response to treatment is necessary to achieve and maintain the best control.

What Is Being Done To Better Understand Narcolepsy?

Studies supported by the National Institutes of Health (NIH) are trying to increase understanding of what causes narcolepsy and improve physicians' ability to detect and treat the disease. Scientists are studying narcolepsy patients and families, looking for clues to the causes, course, and effective treatment of this sleep disorder. Recent discovery of families of dogs that are naturally afflicted with narcolepsy has been of great help in these studies. Some of the specific questions being addressed in NIH-supported studies are the nature of genetic and environmental factors that might combine to cause narcolepsy and the immunological, biochemical, physiological, and neuromuscular disturbances associated with narcolepsy. Scientists are also working to better understand sleep mechanisms and the physical and psychological effects of sleep deprivation and to develop better ways of measuring sleepiness and cataplexy.

How Can Individuals and Their Families and Friends Cope With Narcolepsy?

Learning as much about narcolepsy as possible and finding a support system can help patients and families deal with the practical and emotional effects of the disease, possible occupational limitations, and situations that might cause injury. A variety of educational and other materials are available from sleep medicine or narcolepsy organizations. Support groups exist to help persons with narcolepsy and their families.

Individuals with narcolepsy, their families, friends, and potential employers should know that:

- Narcolepsy is a life-long condition that requires continuous medication.

- Although there is not a cure for narcolepsy at present, several medications can help reduce its symptoms.

- People with narcolepsy can lead productive lives if they are provided with proper medical care.

- If possible, individuals with narcolepsy should avoid jobs that require driving long distances or handling hazardous equipment or that require alertness for lengthy periods.

- Parents, teachers, spouses, and employers should be aware of the symptoms of narcolepsy. This will help them avoid the mistake of confusing the person's behavior with laziness, hostility, rejection, or lack of interest and motivation. It will also help them provide essential support and cooperation.

- Employers can promote better working opportunities for individuals with narcolepsy by permitting special work schedules and nap breaks.

For More Information

For additional information on sleep and sleep disorders, contact the following offices of the National Heart, Lung, and Blood Institute of the National Institutes of Health:

National Center on Sleep Disorders Research (NCSDR)

The NCSDR supports research, scientist training, dissemination of health information, and other activities on sleep and sleep disorders. The NCSDR also coordinates sleep research activities with other Federal agencies and with public and nonprofit organizations.

National Center on Sleep Disorders Research
Two Rockledge Centre
Suite 7024
6701 Rockledge Drive, MSC 7920
Bethesda, MD 20892-7920
301) 435-0199
(301) 480-3451 (fax)

National Heart, Lung, and Blood Institute Information Center

The Information Center acquires, analyzes, promotes, maintains, and disseminates programmatic and educational information related to sleep and sleep disorders. Write for a list of available publications or to order additional copies of this fact sheet.

NHLBI Information Center
P.O. Box 30105
Bethesda, MD 20824-0105
(301) 251-1222
(301) 251-1223 (fax)

For more information about narcolepsy and patient support groups, contact the Narcolepsy Network at P.O. Box 42460, Cincinnati, OH 45242.

Chapter 31

What Is Restless Legs Syndrome?

Restless legs syndrome (RLS) is a sleep disorder in which a person experiences unpleasant sensations in the legs described as creeping, crawling, tingling, pulling, or painful. These sensations usually occur in the calf area but may be felt anywhere from the thigh to the ankle. One or both legs may be affected; for some people, the sensations are also felt in the arms. These sensations occur when the person with RLS lies down or sits for prolonged periods of time, such as at a desk, riding in a car, or watching a movie. People with RLS describe an irresistible urge to move the legs when the sensations occur. Usually, moving the legs, walking, rubbing or massaging the legs, or doing knee bends can bring relief, at least briefly.

RLS symptoms worsen during periods of relaxation and decreased activity. RLS symptoms also tend to follow a set daily cycle, with the evening and night hours being more troublesome for RLS sufferers than the morning hours. People with RLS may find it difficult to relax and fall asleep because of their strong urge to walk or do other activities to relieve the sensations in their legs. Persons with RLS often sleep best toward the end of the night or during the morning hours. Because of less sleep at night, people with RLS may feel sleepy during the day on an occasional or regular basis. The severity of symptoms varies from night to night and over the years as well. For some individuals, there may be periods when RLS does not cause problems, but the symptoms usually return. Other people may experience severe symptoms daily.

NIH Pub. No. 96-3645, October 1996.

211

Many people with RLS also have a related sleep disorder called periodic limb movements in sleep (PLMS). PLMS is characterized by involuntary jerking or bending leg movements during sleep that typically occur every 10 to 60 seconds. Some people may experience hundreds of such movements per night, which can wake them, disturb their sleep, and awaken bed partners. People who have RLS and PLMS have trouble both falling asleep and staying asleep and may experience extreme sleepiness during the day. As a result of problems both in sleeping and while awake, people with RLS may have difficulties with their job, social life, and recreational activities.

Common Characteristics of Restless Legs Syndrome

Some common symptoms of RLS include:

- Unpleasant sensations in the legs (sometimes the arms as well), often described as creeping, crawling, tingling, pulling, or painful;

- Leg sensations are relieved by walking, stretching, knee bends, massage, or hot or cold baths;

- Leg discomfort occurs when lying down or sitting for prolonged periods of time;

- The symptoms are worse in the evening and during the night.

Other possible characteristics include:

- Involuntary leg (and occasionally arm) movements while asleep;

- Difficulty falling asleep or staying asleep;

- Sleepiness or fatigue during the daytime;

- Cause of the leg discomfort not detected by medical tests;

- Family members with similar symptoms.

What Causes It?

Although the cause is unknown in most cases, certain factors may be associated with RLS:

- *Family history.* RLS is known to run in some families—parents may pass the condition on to their children.

- *Pregnancy.* Some women experience RLS during pregnancy, especially in the last months. The symptoms usually disappear after delivery.

- *Low iron levels or anemia.* Persons with these conditions may be prone to developing RLS. The symptoms may improve once the iron level or anemia is corrected.

- *Chronic diseases.* Kidney failure quite often leads to RLS. Other chronic diseases such as diabetes, rheumatoid arthritis, and peripheral neuropathy may also be associated with RLS.

- *Caffeine intake.* Decreasing caffeine consumption may improve symptoms.

Who Gets RLS?

RLS occurs in both sexes. Symptoms can begin any time, but are usually more common and more severe among older people. Young people who experience symptoms of RLS are sometimes thought to have "growing pains" or may be considered "hyperactive" because they cannot easily sit still in school.

How Is It Diagnosed?

There is no laboratory test that can make a diagnosis of RLS and, when someone with RLS goes to see a doctor, there is usually nothing abnormal the doctor can see or detect on examination. Diagnosis therefore depends on what a person describes to the doctor. The history usually includes a description of the typical leg sensations that lead to an urge to move the legs or walk. These sensations are noted to worsen when the legs are at rest, for example, when sitting or lying down and during the evening and night. The person with RLS may complain about trouble sleeping or daytime sleepiness. In some cases, the bed partner will complain about the person's leg movements and jerking during the night.

To help make a diagnosis, the doctor may ask about all current and past medical problems, family history, and current medications. A complete physical and neurological exam may help identify other conditions that may be associated with RLS, such as nerve damage (neuropathy or a pinched nerve) or abnormalities in the blood vessels. Basic laboratory tests may be done to assess general health and to rule out anemia. Further studies depend on initial findings. In some cases, a doctor may suggest an overnight sleep study to determine whether PLMS or other sleep problems are present. In most people with RLS, no new medical problem will be discovered during the physical exam or on any tests, except the sleep study, which will detect PLMS if present.

How Is It Treated?

In mild cases of RLS, some people find that activities such as taking a hot bath, massaging the legs, using a heating pad or ice pack, exercising, and eliminating caffeine help alleviate symptoms. In more severe cases, medications are prescribed to control symptoms. Unfortunately, no one drug is effective for everyone with RLS. Individuals respond differently to medications based on the severity of symptoms, other medical conditions, and other medications being taken. A medication that is initially found to be effective may lose its effectiveness with nightly use; thus, it may be necessary to alternate between different categories of medication in order to keep symptoms under control.

Although many different drugs may help RLS, those most commonly used are found in the following three categories:

- Benzodiazepines are central nervous system depressants that do not fully suppress RLS sensations or leg movements, but allow patients to obtain more sleep despite these problems. Some drugs in this group may result in daytime drowsiness. Benzodiazepines should not be used by people with sleep apnea.

- Dopaminergic agents are drugs used to treat Parkinson's disease and are also effective for many people with RLS and PLMS. These medications have been shown to reduce RLS symptoms and nighttime leg movements.

- Opioids are pain-killing and relaxing drugs that can suppress RLS and PLMS in some people. These medications can sometimes help people with severe, unrelenting symptoms.

Although there is some potential for benzodiazepines and opioids to become habit forming, this usually does not occur with the dosages given to most RLS patients.

A non-drug approach called transcutaneous electric nerve stimulation may improve symptoms in some RLS sufferers who also have PLMS. The electrical stimulation is applied to an area of the legs or feet, usually before bedtime, for 15 to 30 minutes. This approach has been shown to be helpful in reducing nighttime leg jerking.

Due to recent advances, doctors today have a variety of means for treating RLS. However, no perfect treatment exists and there is much more to be learned about the treatments that currently seem to be successful.

Where Can I Get More Information?

For additional information on sleep and sleep disorders, contact the following offices of the National Heart, Lung, and Blood Institute of the National Institutes of Health:

National Center on Sleep Disorders Research (NCSDR)

The NCSDR supports research, scientist training, dissemination of health information, and other activities on sleep and sleep disorders. The NCSDR also coordinates sleep research activities with other Federal agencies and with public and nonprofit organizations.

National Center on Sleep Disorders Research
Two Rockledge Centre, Suite 7024
6701 Rockledge Drive, MSC 7920
Bethesda, MD 20892-7920
(301) 435-0199
(301) 480-3451 (fax)

National Heart, Lung, and Blood Institute Information Center

Information Center acquires, analyzes, promotes, maintains, and disseminates programmatic and educational information related to sleep and sleep disorders. Write for a list of available publications or to order additional copies of this fact sheet.

NHLBI Information Center
P.O. Box 30105
Bethesda, MD 20824-0105
(301) 251-1222
(301) 251-1223 (fax)

To learn more about RLS, contact the Restless Legs Syndrome Foundation, Inc., a nonprofit organization dedicated to helping the public, patients, families, and physicians better understand RLS. The Foundation can be reached by mail at 514 Daniels Street, Box 314, Raleigh, NC 27605-1317, or on the World Wide Web at http://www.rls.org.

Chapter 32

What Is Insomnia?

Insomnia is the perception or complaint of inadequate or poor-quality sleep because of one or more of the following:

- difficulty falling asleep

- waking up frequently during the night with difficulty returning to sleep

- waking up too early in the morning

- unrefreshing sleep

Insomnia is not defined by the number of hours of sleep a person gets or how long it takes to fall asleep. Individuals vary normally in their need for, and their satisfaction with, sleep. Insomnia may cause problems during the day, such as tiredness, a lack of energy, difficulty concentrating, and irritability.

Insomnia can be classified as transient (short term), intermittent (on and off), and chronic (constant). Insomnia lasting from a single night to a few weeks is referred to as transient. If episodes of transient insomnia occur from time to time, the insomnia is said to be intermittent. Insomnia is considered to be chronic if it occurs on most nights and lasts a month or more.

NIH Pub. No. 95-3801, October 1995

What Causes It?

Certain conditions seem to make individuals more likely to experience insomnia. Examples of these conditions include:

- advanced age (insomnia occurs more frequently in those over age 60)
- female gender
- a history of depression

If other conditions (such as stress, anxiety, a medical problem, or the use of certain medications) occur along with the above conditions, insomnia is more likely.

There are many causes of insomnia. Transient and intermittent insomnia generally occur in people who are temporarily experiencing one or more of the following:

- stress
- environmental noise
- extreme temperatures
- change in the surrounding environment
- sleep/wake schedule problems such as those due to jet lag
- medication side effects

Chronic insomnia is more complex and often results from a combination of factors, including underlying physical or mental disorders. One of the most common causes of chronic insomnia is depression. Other underlying causes include arthritis, kidney disease, heart failure, asthma, sleep apnea, narcolepsy, restless legs syndrome, Parkinson's disease, and hyperthyroidism. However, chronic insomnia may also be due to behavioral factors, including the misuse of caffeine, alcohol, or other substances; disrupted sleep/wake cycles as may occur with shift work or other nighttime activity schedules; and chronic stress.

In addition, the following behaviors have been shown to perpetuate insomnia in some people:

- expecting to have difficulty sleeping and worrying about it

- ingesting excessive amounts of caffeine

- drinking alcohol before bedtime

- smoking cigarettes before bedtime

- excessive napping in the afternoon or evening

- irregular or continually disrupted sleep/wake schedules

These behaviors may prolong existing insomnia, and they can also be responsible for causing the sleeping problem in the first place. Stopping these behaviors may eliminate the insomnia altogether.

Who Gets Insomnia?

Insomnia is found in males and females of all age groups, although it seems to be more common in females (especially after menopause) and in the elderly. The ability to sleep, rather than the need for sleep, appears to decrease with advancing age.

How Is It Diagnosed?

Patients with insomnia are evaluated with the help of a medical history and a sleep history. The sleep history may be obtained from a sleep diary filled out by the patient or by an interview with the patient's bed partner concerning the quantity and quality of the patient's sleep. Specialized sleep studies may be recommended, but only if there is suspicion that the patient may have a primary sleep disorder such as sleep apnea or narcolepsy.

How Is It Treated?

Transient and intermittent insomnia may not require treatment since episodes last only a few days at a time. For example, if insomnia is due to a temporary change in the sleep/wake schedule, as with jet lag, the person's biological clock will often get back to normal on its own. However, for some people who experience daytime sleepiness and impaired performance as a result of transient insomnia, the use of short-acting sleeping pills may improve sleep and next-day alertness. As with all drugs, there are potential side effects. The use of over-the-counter sleep medicines is not usually recommended for the treatment of insomnia.

Treatment for chronic insomnia consists of:

- First, diagnosing and treating underlying medical or psychological problems.

- Identifying behaviors that may worsen insomnia and stopping (or reducing) them.

- Possibly using sleeping pills, although the long-term use of sleeping pills for chronic insomnia is controversial. A patient taking any sleeping pill should be under the supervision of a physician to closely evaluate effectiveness and minimize side effects. In general, these drugs are prescribed at the lowest dose and for the shortest duration needed to relieve the sleep-related symptoms. For some of these medicines, the dose must be gradually lowered as the medicine is discontinued because, if stopped abruptly, it can cause insomnia to occur again for a night or two.

- Trying behavioral techniques to improve sleep, such as relaxation therapy, sleep restriction therapy, and reconditioning.

  Relaxation Therapy. There are specific and effective techniques that can reduce or eliminate anxiety and body tension. As a result, the person's mind is able to stop "racing," the muscles can relax, and restful sleep can occur. It usually takes much practice to learn these techniques and to achieve effective relaxation.

  Sleep Restriction. Some people suffering from insomnia spend too much time in bed unsuccessfully trying to sleep. They may benefit from a sleep restriction program that at first allows only a few hours of sleep during the night. Gradually the time is increased until a more normal night's sleep is achieved.

  Reconditioning. Another treatment that may help some people with insomnia is to recondition them to associate the bed and bedtime with sleep. For most people, this means not using their beds for any activities other than sleep and sex. As part of the reconditioning process, the person is usually advised to go to bed only when sleepy. If unable to fall asleep, the person is told to get up, stay up until sleepy, and then return to bed. Throughout this process, the person should avoid naps and wake up and go to bed at the same time each day. Eventually the person's body will be conditioned to associate the bed and bedtime with sleep.

Other sleep publications available from the National Heart, Lung, and Blood Institute Information Center:

- *Facts About Sleep Apnea*—A four-page brochure that discusses sleep apnea and how it is treated. (NIH Publication No. 95-3798)

- *Test Your Sleep I.Q.*—This quiz tests your knowledge about sleep and sleep-related disorders. (NIH Publication No. 95-3797)

Where to Get More Information

Talk to your doctor if you are having trouble getting good, refreshing sleep each night. Together you can identify possible reasons for your sleeping difficulty and then try appropriate measures to correct the problem. For additional information on sleep and sleep disorders, contact the following offices of the National Heart, Lung, and Blood Institute of the National Institutes of Health.

National Center on Sleep Disorders Research (NCSDR)

The NCSDR, located within the National Heart, Lung, and Blood Institute, supports research, scientist training, dissemination of health information, and other activities on sleep disorders and related concerns. The NCSDR also coordinates sleep research activities with other Federal agencies and with public and nonprofit organizations.

National Center on Sleep Disorders Research
Two Rockledge Centre
Suite 7024
6701 Rockledge Drive, MSC 7920
Bethesda, MD 20892-7920
(301) 435-0199
(301) 480-3451 (FAX)

National Heart, Lung, and Blood Institute Information Center

The Information Center acquires, analyzes, promotes, maintains, and disseminates programmatic and educational information related to sleep disorders and sleep-disordered breathing. Write for a list of available publications or to order additional copies of this fact sheet.

NHLBI Information Center
P.O. Box 30105
Bethesda, MD 20824-0105
(301) 251-1222
(301) 251-1223 (FAX)

Chapter 33

Hypnotics and Behavioral Therapies for Insomnia

When are sleep problems part of the human experience, and when are they pathological? Can hypnotics help chronic insomnia? Do patients develop tolerance and dependence? Which behavioral strategies work best, and what improves patient compliance? These and other clinical controversies in insomnia kept audiences wide awake at this year's joint annual meeting of the American Sleep Disorders Association and Sleep Research Society in San Francisco, Calif.

Some 27% of 26,000 primary care patients in 15 countries reported that they experienced persistent insomnia in a recent World Health Organization study. Insomnia is a broad term that encompasses trouble falling asleep or staying asleep and the perception that sleep is not refreshing or restorative. Its daytime consequences include diminished alertness, concentration, and memory, as well as depressed mood. About 1 in 10 persons claims to have suffered insomnia most nights or every night for 1 month or longer, and thus is said to have chronic insomnia. Long-term poor sleepers often blame insomnia for spoiling the quality of their lives (*Sleep*. 1996;19:412-416).

Insomnia has substantial associated morbidity, according to a recent epidemiologic survey of more than 10,000 adults in the United States. Even in the absence of pain and other medical conditions, depression and other psychiatric disorders, use of medications, and

Reprinted with permission from the *Journal of the American Medical Association*, Volume 271, Number 20, November 26, 1997. © 1997 American Medical Association.

alcohol and other drug abuse, insomnia is linked with increased use of general medical and mental health treatment for emotional problems and, in the year after it starts, the first onset of major depression, panic disorder, and alcohol abuse (*Gen Hosp Psychiatry*. 1997;19:245-250). The Johns Hopkins Precursors Study, a long-term prospective study of more than 1000 male medical students, found that insomnia in young men predicts a higher likelihood of subsequent clinical depression and psychiatric distress (*Am J Epidemiology*. 1997;146:105-114).

Insomnia is a symptom of 60 discrete disorders listed in the *International Classification of Sleep Disorders* (Rochester, Minn: American Sleep Disorders Association; 1997). Yet in 29% of persons complaining of chronic insomnia, no underlying cause can be determined, even after a comprehensive workup, Meir Kryger, MD, professor of medicine at the University of Manitoba Faculty of Medicine and director of the sleep disorders center at St Boniface Hospital Research Center, both in Winnipeg, reported at the sleep meeting. "Physicians find this frustrating," observed Kryger, who is chief editor of *Principles and Practice of Sleep Medicine*, the sleep field's leading text (Philadelphia, Pa: WB Saunders Co; 1994). "With no apparent etiology," he said, "they are forced to treat symptoms."

Of the remaining 71% of chronic insomniacs, the following are characteristic:

- 34% have primary psychiatric disorders, such as depression or anxiety. Ideally, Kryger said, the insomnia will subside when the illness is treated. Some selective serotonin reuptake inhibitors used to treat psychiatric disorders, however, may themselves disrupt sleep.

- 29% have movement disorders such as restless legs syndrome and periodic leg movements. Medications such as carbidopa-levidopa and pergolide may relieve these conditions, Kryger said, although patients also may need hypnotics to reduce their arousability.

- 11% have circadian rhythm disorders, often caused by shiftwork and jet lag. The key to successful treatment, Kryger said, is good lifestyle management, seldom fully achieved.

- 9% have respiratory disorders, for which hypnotics usually are contraindicated, as they may further depress respiration. Continuous positive airway pressure may benefit those with obstructive sleep apnea and upper airway resistance syndrome, a variant of sleep apnea.

- 9% have arthritis or other illnesses causing pain. The sleep complaint usually abates when the condition improves.

- 8% have primary insomnia, which is not caused by any of the above disorders or use of medications or other drugs. Also sometimes called psychophysiological, conditioned, or learned insomnia, it may be related to poor sleep hygiene and/or may reflect trouble sleeping that was triggered by a loss of a job, death in the family, or other situational crisis, and that persists long afterward.

Agreement on Treatment

Both primary care physicians and sleep specialists discriminate between subtypes of insomnia and generally agree in their treatment recommendations, according to findings from a field trial of the American Psychiatric Association (APA) Diagnostic and Statistical Manual of Mental Disorders, Fourth Edition, conducted by the APA and the National Institute of Mental Health. "This counters the popular misconception by the general public and even by some physicians that insomnia is a final diagnosis," noted Daniel Buysse, MD, associate professor of psychiatry, University of Pittsburgh School of Medicine, Pittsburgh, Pa, and first author of the field trial report (*Sleep.* 1997; 20:542-552).

"The findings imply," Buysse said in an interview, "that troubled sleepers do not need to see a sleep specialist right off the bat. The nonspecialist can make key decisions and initiate treatment. Treatment-resistant patients are the ones who most need a specialist's care."

Despite the ubiquity of sleep complaints and the availability of effective treatment, 7 of 10 poor sleepers have not discussed their difficulties with a physician or other health care professional, believing that it is not a "big enough" problem or assuming that little can be done about it, a Gallup survey conducted for the National Sleep Foundation (NSF) shows. Most tried a variety of self-help strategies, including reading, taking hot baths, and self-medication (*Sleep in America.* Washington, DC: National Science Foundation; 1995).

Indeed, about 25% of the American population took a chemical last year to help them sleep, Thomas Roth, PhD, professor of psychiatry at the University of Michigan School of Medicine, Ann Arbor, and chief of the division of sleep medicine at Henry Ford Hospital, Detroit, Mich, said in an interview. Most used alcohol and over-the-counter sleep aids. Only 5% used prescription hypnotics. Current guidelines for the use of hypnotics call for using the lowest effective dose for the shortest possible time. For short-term insomnia—lasting less than 2 weeks—the benefits of hypnotics are clear, Roth said at a sleep meeting symposium he chaired on the chronic use of hypnotics. It generally is assumed that hypnotics rapidly lose their efficacy, he noted, but few studies have been conducted on the use of these drugs for chronic insomnia.

According to Wallace Mendelson, MD, professor of psychiatry and medicine and director of the sleep research laboratory at the University of Chicago, Chicago, Ill, some evidence suggests that tolerance may not be inevitable with long-term nightly use. One study, he said, looked at the use of zolpidem by 14 elderly psychiatric patients for 90 days, finding that arousals declined and total sleep time increased as the study progressed.

Mendelson conducted a 1-month study of triazolam, finding a disparity between what the polygraph showed and subjects' own impressions. The laboratory studies indicated that latency to sleep onset fell from 54 minutes to 27 minutes by week 4, on average, and total sleep time increased by nearly 1 hour over the month. The subjects initially described better sleep, but starting at the third week reported that they took longer to fall asleep while using the medication. "It suggests to me," Mendelson said, "that objective and subjective measures of tolerance may have different time courses" (Clin Drug Invest. 1995:10:276-279).

'Insomnophobia'

Malcolm Lader, MD, professor of clinical psychopharmacology at the University of London, London, England, said that persons with chronic difficulty sleeping sometimes develop "insomnophobia." Fear of trouble sleeping comes to dominate their lives. A nightly hypnotic, he said, thus may serve a prophylactic purpose. This benefit must be balanced, however, against the risk of further escalating sedation in persons who already experience daytime fatigue or depression and increased motor vehicle crashes. Sedation also is a concern in the elderly and physically ill, who often get out of bed at night and are at high risk for falls. Drug interactions also are a higher risk in these populations.

Even therapeutic doses, Lader said, sometimes cause dependence. Some people can go on and off hypnotics with impunity, he added, while others have difficulty stopping their use. The commonly prescribed benzodiazepines are seldom abused by those who take them for insomnia, he said, but the drugs do have an often-overlooked potential for abuse. Some people use them to counteract overstimulation, potentiate alcohol, or even as their main drug of abuse. Flunitrazepam (Rohypnol), a benzodiazepine hypnotic not licensed in the United States, although smuggled into the country from Mexico, has become a major problem worldwide, he said, as it is used intravenously, snorted, and smoked.

Given the uncertainties about the effectiveness and safety of long-term hypnotic use, the physician must make hard choices, Manitoba's Kryger said. "Denying a patient symptomatic relief," he quipped, "may mean that the clinician sleeps well, while the patient suffers. Giving a patient symptomatic relief may make the physician toss and turn."

Some patients with primary insomnia may benefit from using hypnotics a few nights a week on an ongoing basis, Kryger said, much as those with headaches or arthritis use analgesics or anti-inflammatory agents. Whether intermittent use promotes inappropriate pill-taking behavior in insomniacs is unknown. The physician must balance the amount of nighttime distress, "which can be terrible," he said, with the impact of the medications and of the insomnia itself on daytime alertness and performance. Some patients, he said, elect not to use medication and can tolerate not being champion sleepers.

Behavioral interventions can offer lasting benefits to chronic insomniacs, according to Richard Bootzin, PhD, professor of psychology and psychiatry and codirector of the insomnia clinic at the University of Arizona College of Medicine, Tucson. "Pharmacological treatment works faster," Bootzin said, "but nonpharmacological treatment works better in the long run." Two meta-analyses of outcome studies comparing treated subjects and untreated controls, he said, show that psychological treatment significantly shortens time to fall asleep, improves sleep maintenance, and enhances patient satisfaction with sleep. Benefits usually become apparent in about 3 weeks and continue to accrue over time. Studies show that patients maintain improvements 6 months or longer (*J Consult Clin Psychol.* 1995; 63:79-89; *Am J Psychiatry.* 1994;151:1172-1180). Although counseling patients about behavioral strategies takes more time than writing a prescription for a hypnotic, Bootzin said, recent studies show that effective instruction can be given by a nurse-educator, in group sessions, and even via a televised sleep education program.

The most effective behavioral strategies are stimulus control and sleep restriction, the meta-analyses found. Stimulus control, devised by Bootzin 25 years ago, aims to strengthen the bed and bedroom as cues for sleep and to weaken their association with insomnia. It directs patients to reserve the bed and bedroom for sleep, using other rooms for all other activities such as television viewing, reading, snacking, and work. Sex is the only exception.

Sleep restriction acknowledges insomniacs' tendency to spend more time in bed, hoping, usually in vain, to get more sleep. Devised in 1987 by Arthur Spielman, PhD, director of the sleep disorders center at the City College of New York, New York, NY, this strategy asks patients to start by limiting their hours in bed to the amount of time they currently sleep, or 4.5 hours at minimum. Once sleep solidifies, time in bed is increased in 15- to 30-minute increments.

Stimulus control addresses problems in both falling and staying asleep, Bootzin said, while sleep restriction is particularly useful for trouble sustaining sleep, the most common complaint in older adults.

Progressive muscle relaxation, biofeedback, breathing exercises, and other relaxation techniques are only mildly effective in relieving insomnia, Bootzin said at a course he chaired on behavioral strategies, but they are useful in managing the daytime anxiety that insomniacs often manifest. Counting sheep is not in the "top 10" list, Bootzin said in an interview, as it is too slow a method of distraction. "A person can count sheep and still worry," he said, adding, "It's better for someone beset by worries to get out of bed, jot down some notes, and think about the problem in the morning, when problems seldom loom as large." Trouble falling asleep and early morning awakenings may reflect disturbances in biological rhythms, according to Leon Lack, PhD, director of the sleep research laboratory at Flinders University, Adelaide, South Australia. Sleep comes most easily when body temperature is falling, he noted, and it is hardest to sustain when temperature is rising. In good sleepers, body temperature rhythms are appropriately aligned with desired sleep onset and wake-up times: the daily minimum occurs about 4 hours after sleep begins.

In sleep-onset insomniacs, he said, rhythms often are phase delayed, so that the daily minimum does not occur until 6 hours after sleep onset. This fact also makes it hard to get up in the morning. In contrast, some people who awaken early, particularly older adults, may experience their temperature minimum only 2 hours after they fall asleep. Therefore, they also are more likely to become excessively sleepy early in the evening.

Both trouble falling asleep and early morning awakening may respond to appropriately timed exposure to daylight-intensity artificial lights, Lack's studies show. For sleep onset problems, light in the morning will advance the temperature minimum, while for problems with early awakening, light in the late afternoon or early evening will help delay it (Sleep. 1993;16:436-443). It is essential to first determine the temperature rhythm, Lack stressed, before instituting light therapy.

Whether hypnotics and behavioral therapy work better in tandem or separately is not known. Theoretically, Bootzin said, one might start with hypnotics and at the same time teach behavioral strategies to sustain improvements. According to Roth, only 3 studies have evaluated the effects of using the 2 approaches alone and together, and the findings are inconsistent. "It's hard to imagine that combining them would not be advantageous," Roth said. "No one should get a hypnotic," he asserted, "without being instructed in the need to keep regular hours, limit use of alcohol and caffeine, exercise regularly, and observe other universal principles of good sleep hygiene."

—by Lynne Lamberg, JAMA *contributor*

Chapter 34

Differing Approaches to Insomnia and Chronic Pain

What Behavioral and Relaxation Approaches Are Used for Conditions Such as Chronic Pain and Insomnia?

Pain

Pain is defined by the International Association for the Study of Pain as an unpleasant sensory experience associated with actual or potential tissue damage or described in terms of such damage. It is a complex, subjective, perceptual phenomenon with a number of contributing factors that are uniquely experienced by each individual. Pain is typically classified as acute, cancer- related, and chronic non-malignant. Acute pain is associated with a noxious event. Its severity is generally proportional to the degree of tissue injury and is expected to diminish with healing and time. Chronic nonmalignant pain frequently develops following an injury but persists long after a reasonable period of healing. Its underlying causes are often not readily discernible, and the pain is disproportionate to demonstrable tissue damage. It is frequently accompanied by alteration of sleep; mood; and sexual, vocational, and avocational function.

Insomnia

Insomnia may be defined as a disturbance or perceived disturbance of the usual sleep pattern of the individual that has troublesome

Integration of Behavioral and Relaxation Approaches into the Treatment of Insomnia and Chronic Pain, *NIH Technical Statement Online*, October 1995.

consequences. These consequences may include daytime fatigue and drowsiness, irritability, anxiety, depression, and somatic complaints. Categories of disturbed sleep are (1) inability to fall asleep, (2) inability to maintain sleep, and (3) early awakening.

Selection Criteria

A variety of behavioral and relaxation approaches are used for conditions such as chronic pain and insomnia. The specific approaches that were addressed in this article were selected using three important criteria. First, somatically directed therapies with behavioral components (e.g., physical therapy, occupational therapy, acupuncture) were not considered. Second, the approaches were drawn from those reported in the scientific literature. Many commonly used behavioral approaches are not specifically incorporated into conventional medical care. For example, religious and spiritual approaches, which are the most commonly used health-related actions by the U.S. population, were not considered in this article. Third, the approaches are a subset of those discussed in the literature and represent those selected by the contributors as most commonly used in clinical settings in the United States. Several commonly used clinical interventions such as music, dance, recreational, and art therapies were not addressed.

Relaxation Techniques

Relaxation techniques are a group of behavioral therapeutic approaches that differ widely in their philosophical bases as well as in their methodologies and techniques. Their primary objective is the achievement of nondirected relaxation, rather than direct achievement of a specific therapeutic goal. They all share two basic components: (1) repetitive focus on a word, sound, prayer, phrase, body sensation, or muscular activity and (2) the adoption of a passive attitude toward intruding thoughts and a return to the focus. These techniques induce a common set of physiologic changes that result in decreased metabolic activity. Relaxation techniques may also be used in stress management (as self-regulatory techniques) and have been divided into deep and brief methods.

Deep Methods

Deep methods include autogenic training, meditation, and progressive muscle relaxation (PMR). Autogenic training consists of imagining a peaceful environment and comforting bodily sensations. Six basic focusing techniques are used: heaviness in the limbs, warmth in the limbs, cardiac regulation, centering on breathing, warmth in the upper abdomen, and coolness in the forehead. Meditation is a self-directed practice for relaxing the body and calming the mind. A large variety of meditation techniques are in common use; each has its own proponents. Meditation generally does not involve suggestion, autosuggestion, or trance. The goal of mindfulness meditation is development of a nonjudgmental awareness of bodily sensations and mental activities occurring in the present moment. Concentration meditation trains the person to passively attend to a bodily process, a word, and/or a stimulus. Transcendental meditation focuses on a "suitable" sound or thought (the mantra) without attempting to actually concentrate on the sound or thought. There are also many movement meditations, such as yoga and the walking meditation of Zen Buddhism. PMR focuses on reducing muscle tone in major muscle groups. Each of 15 major muscle groups is tensed and then relaxed in sequence.

Brief Methods

The brief methods, which include self-control relaxation, paced respiration, and deep breathing, generally require less time to acquire or practice and often represent abbreviated forms of a corresponding deep method. For example, self-control relaxation is an abbreviated form of PMR. Autogenic training may be abbreviated and converted to a self-control format. Paced respiration teaches patients to maintain slow breathing when anxiety threatens. Deep breathing involves taking several deep breaths, holding them for 5 seconds, and then exhaling slowly.

Hypnotic Techniques

They are often used to induce relaxation and also may be a part of CBT. The techniques have pre- and postsuggestion components. The presuggestion component involves attentional focusing through the use of imagery, distraction, or relaxation, and has features that are similar to other relaxation techniques. Subjects focus on relaxation and passively disregard intrusive thoughts. The suggestion phase is characterized by introduction of specific goals; for example, analgesia may be specifically suggested. The postsuggestion component involves continued use of the new behavior following termination of hypnosis. Individuals vary widely in their hypnotic susceptibility and suggestibility, although the reasons for these differences are incompletely understood.

Biofeedback Techniques

BF techniques are treatment methods that use monitoring instruments of various degrees of sophistication. BF techniques provide patients with physiologic information that allows them to reliably influence psychophysiological responses of two kinds: (1) responses not ordinarily under voluntary control and (2) responses that ordinarily are easily regulated, but for which regulation has broken down. Technologies that are commonly used include electromyography (EMG BF), electroencephalography, thermometers (thermal BF), and galvanometry (electrodermal-BF). BF techniques often induce physiological responses similar to those of other relaxation techniques.

Cognitive-Behavioral Therapy

CBT attempts to alter patterns of negative thoughts and dysfunctional attitudes in order to foster more healthy and adaptive thoughts, emotions, and actions. These interventions share four basic components: education, skills acquisition, cognitive and behavioral rehearsal, and generalization and maintenance. Relaxation techniques are frequently included as a behavioral component in CBT programs. The specific programs used to implement the four components can vary considerably. Each of the aforementioned therapeutic modalities may be practiced individually, or they may be combined as part of multimodal approaches to manage chronic pain or insomnia.

Relaxation and Behavioral Techniques for Insomnia

Relaxation and behavioral techniques corresponding to those used for chronic pain may also be used for specific types of insomnia. Cognitive relaxation, various forms of BF, and PMR may all be used to treat insomnia. In addition, the following behavioral approaches are generally used to manage insomnia:

- Sleep hygiene, which involves educating patients about behaviors that may interfere with the sleep process, with the hope that education about maladaptive behaviors will lead to behavioral modification.

234

- Stimulus control therapy, which seeks to create and protect conditioned association between the bedroom and sleep. Activities in the bedroom are restricted to sleep and sex.

- Sleep restriction therapy, in which patients provide a sleep log and are then asked to stay in bed only as long as they think they are currently sleeping. This usually leads to sleep deprivation and consolidation, which may be followed by a gradual increase in the length of time in bed.

- Paradoxical intention, in which the patient is instructed not to fall asleep, with the expectation that efforts to avoid sleep will in fact induce it.

How Successful Are These Approaches?

Pain

A plethora of studies using a range of behavioral and relaxation approaches to treat chronic pain is reported in the literature. The measures of success reported in these studies depend on the rigor of the research design, the population studied, the length of followup, and the outcome measures identified. As the number of well-designed studies using a variety of behavioral and relaxation techniques grows, the use of meta-analysis as a means of demonstrating overall effectiveness will increase.

One carefully analyzed review of studies on chronic pain, including cancer pain, was prepared under the auspices of the U.S. Agency for Health Care Policy and Research (AHCPR) in 1990. A great strength of the report was the careful categorization of the evidential basis of each intervention. The categorization was based on design of the studies and consistency of findings among the studies. These properties led to the development of a 4-point scale that ranked the evidence as strong, moderate, fair, or weak; this scale was used by the contributors to evaluate the AHCPR studies.

Evaluation of behavioral and relaxation interventions for chronic pain reduction in adults found the following:

- *Relaxation:* The evidence is strong for the effectiveness of this class of techniques in reducing chronic pain in a variety of medical conditions.

- *Hypnosis:* The evidence supporting the effectiveness of hypnosis in alleviating chronic pain associated with cancer seems strong. In addition, information was provided suggesting the effectiveness of hypnosis in other chronic pain conditions, which include irritable bowel syndrome, oral mucositis, temporomandibular disorders, and tension headaches.

- *CBT:* The evidence was moderate for the usefulness of CBT in chronic pain. In addition, a series of eight well-designed studies found CBT superior to placebo and to routine care for alleviating low back pain and both rheumatoid arthritis and osteoarthritis-associated pain, but inferior to hypnosis for oral mucositis and to EMG BF for tension headache.

- *BF:* The evidence is moderate for the effectiveness of BF in relieving many types of chronic pain. Data were also reviewed showing EMG BF to be more effective than psychological placebo for tension headache but equivalent in results to relaxation. For migraine headache, BF is better than relaxation therapy and better than no treatment, but superiority to psychological placebo is less clear.

- *Multimodal Treatment:* Several meta-analyses examined the effectiveness of multimodal treatments in clinical settings. The results of these studies indicate a consistent positive effect of these programs on several categories of regional pain. Back and neck pain, dental or facial pain, joint pain, and migraine headaches have all been treated effectively.

Although relatively good evidence exists for the efficacy of several behavioral and relaxation interventions in the treatment of chronic pain, the data are insufficient to conclude that one technique is usually more effective than another for a given condition. For any given individual patient, however, one approach may indeed be more appropriate than another.

Insomnia

Behavioral treatments produce improvements in some aspects of sleep, the most pronounced of which are for sleep latency and time awake after sleep onset. Relaxation and BF were both found to be effective in alleviating insomnia. Cognitive forms of relaxation such as meditation were slightly better than somatic forms of relaxation such as PMR. Sleep restriction, stimulus control, and multimodal treatment were the three most effective treatments in reducing insomnia. No data were presented or reviewed on the effectiveness of CBT or hypnosis. Improvements seen at treatment completion were maintained at followups averaging 6 months in duration. Although these effects are statistically significant, it is questionable whether the magnitude of the improvements in sleep onset and total sleep time are clinically meaningful. It is possible that a patient-by-patient analysis might show that the effects were clinically valuable for a special set of patients, as some studies suggest that patients who are readily hypnotized benefited much more from certain treatments than other patients did. No data were available on the effects of these improvements on patient self-assessment of quality of life.

To adequately evaluate the relative success of different treatment modalities for insomnia, two major issues need to be addressed. First, valid objective measures of insomnia are needed. Some investigators rely on self-reports by patients, whereas others believe that insomnia must be documented electrophysiologically. Second, what constitutes a therapeutic outcome should be determined. Some investigators use time until sleep onset, number of awakenings, and total sleep time as outcome measures, whereas others believe that impairment in daytime functioning is perhaps another important outcome measure. Both of these issues require resolution so that research in the field can move forward.

Critique

Several cautions must be considered threats to the internal and external validity of the study results. The following problems pertain to internal validity: (1) full and adequate comparability among treatment contrast groups may be absent; (2) the sample sizes are sometimes small, lessening the ability to detect differences in efficacy; (3) complete blinding, which would be ideal, is compromised by patient and clinician awareness of the treatment; (4) the treatments may not be well described, and adequate procedures for standardization such as therapy manuals, therapist training, and reliable competency and integrity assessments have not always been carried out; and (5) a potential publication bias, in which authors exclude studies with small effects and negative results, is of concern in a field characterized by studies with small numbers of patients.

With regard to the ability to generalize the findings of these investigations, the following considerations are important:

- The patients participating in these studies are usually not cognitively impaired. They must be capable not only of participating in the study treatments but also of fulfilling all the requirements of participating in the study protocol.

- The therapists must be adequately trained to competently conduct the therapy.

- The cultural context in which the treatment is conducted may alter its acceptability and effectiveness.

In summary, this literature offers substantial promise and suggests a need for prompt translation into programs of health care delivery. At the same time, the state of the art of the methodology in the field of behavioral and relaxation interventions indicates a need for thoughtful interpretation of these findings. It should be noted that similar criticisms can be made of many conventional medical procedures.

How Do These Approaches Work?

The mechanism of action of behavioral and relaxation approaches can be considered at two levels: (1) determining how the procedure works to reduce cognitive and physiological arousal and to promote the most appropriate behavioral response and (2) identifying effects at more basic levels of functional anatomy, neurotransmitter and other biochemical activity, and circadian rhythms. The exact biological actions are generally unknown.

Pain

There appear to be two pain transmission circuits. Some data suggest that a spinal cord-thalamic-frontal cortex-anterior cingulate pathway plays a role in the subjective psychological and physiological responses to pain, whereas a spinal cord- thalamic-somatosensory cortex pathway plays a role in pain sensation. A descending pathway involving the periaquaductal gray region modulates pain signals (pain modulation circuit). This system can augment or inhibit pain transmission at the level of the dorsal spinal cord. Endogenous opioids are particularly concentrated in this pathway. At the level of the spinal cord, serotonin and norepinephrine appear to play important roles.

Relaxation techniques as a group generally alter sympathetic activity as indicated by decreases in oxygen consumption, respiratory and heart rate, and blood pressure. Increased electroencephalographic slow wave activity has also been reported. Although the mechanism for the decrease in sympathetic activity is unclear, one may infer that decreased arousal (due to alterations in catecholamines or other neurochemical systems) plays a key role.

Hypnosis, in part because of its capacity for evoking intense relaxation, has been reported to reduce several types of pain (e.g., lower back and burn pain). Hypnosis does not appear to influence endorphin production, and its role in the production of catecholamines is not known.

Hypnosis has been hypothesized to block pain from entering consciousness by activating the frontal-limbic attention system to inhibit pain impulse transmission from thalamic to cortical structures. Similarly, other CBT may decrease transmission through this pathway. Moreover, the overlap in brain regions involved in pain modulation and anxiety suggests a possible role for CBT approaches affecting this area of function, although data are still evolving.

CBT also appears to exert a number of other effects that could alter pain intensity. Depression and anxiety increase subjective complaints of pain, and cognitive-behavioral approaches are well documented for decreasing these affective states. In addition, these types of techniques may alter expectation, which also plays a key role in subjective experiences of pain intensity. They also may augment analgesic responses through behavioral conditioning. Finally, these techniques help patients enhance their sense of self control over their illness enabling them to be less helpless and better able to deal with pain sensations.

Insomnia

A cognitive-behavioral model for insomnia elucidates the interaction of insomnia with emotional, cognitive, and physiologic arousal; dysfunctional conditions, such as worry over sleep; maladaptive habits (e.g., excessive time in bed and daytime napping); and the consequences of insomnia (e.g., fatigue and impairment in performance of activities).

In the treatment of insomnia, relaxation techniques have been used to reduce cognitive and physiological arousal and thus assist the induction of sleep as well as decrease awakenings during sleep.

Relaxation is also likely to influence decreased activity in the entire sympathetic system, permitting a more rapid and effective "deafferentation" at sleep onset at the level of the thalamus. Relaxation may also enhance parasympathetic activity, which in turn will further decrease autonomic tone. In addition, it has been suggested that alterations in cytokine activity (immune system) may play a role in insomnia or in response to treatment.

Cognitive approaches may decrease arousal and dysfunctional beliefs and thus improve sleep. Behavioral techniques including sleep restriction and stimulus control can be helpful in reducing physiologic arousal, reversing poor sleep habits, and shifting circadian rhythms. These effects appear to involve both cortical structures and deep nuclei (e.g., locus ceruleus and suprachiasmatic nucleus).

Knowing the mechanisms of action would reinforce and expand use of behavioral and relaxation techniques, but incorporation of these approaches into the treatment of chronic pain and insomnia can proceed on the basis of clinical efficacy, as has occurred with adoption of other practices and products before their mode of action was completely delineated.

Are There Barriers to the Appropriate Integration of These Approaches Into Health Care?

One barrier to the integration of behavioral and relaxation techniques in standard medical care has been the emphasis solely on the biomedical model as the basis of medical education. The biomedical model defines disease in anatomic and pathophysiologic terms. Expansion to a biopsychosocial model would increase emphasis on a patient's experience of disease and balance the anatomic/physiologic needs of patients with their psychosocial needs.

For example, of six factors identified to correlate with treatment failures of low back pain, all are psychosocial. Integration of behavioral and relaxation therapies with conventional medical procedures is necessary for the successful treatment of such conditions. Similarly, the importance of a comprehensive evaluation of a patient is emphasized in the field of insomnia where failure to identify a condition such as sleep apnea will result in inappropriate application of a behavioral therapy. Therapy should be matched to the illness and to the patient.

Integration of psychosocial issues with conventional medical approaches will necessitate the application of new methodologies to assess the success or failure of the interventions. Therefore, additional barriers to integration include lack of standardization of outcome measures, lack of standardization or agreement on what constitutes successful outcome, and lack of consensus on what constitutes appropriate followup. Methodologies appropriate for the evaluation of drugs

240

may not be adequate for the evaluation of some psychosocial interventions, especially those involving patient experience and quality of life. Psychosocial research studies must maintain the high quality of those methods that have been painstakingly developed over the last few decades. Agreement needs to be reached for standards governing the demonstration of efficacy for psychosocial interventions.

Psychosocial interventions are often time intensive, creating potential blocks to provider and patient acceptance and compliance. Participation in BF training typically includes up to 10-12 sessions of approximately 45 minutes to 1 hour each. In addition, home practice of these techniques is usually required. Thus, patient compliance and both patient and provider willingness to participate in these therapies will have to be addressed. Physicians will have to be educated on the efficacy of these techniques. They must also be willing to educate their patients about the importance and potential benefits of these interventions and to provide encouragement for the patient through the training processes.

Insurance companies provide either a financial incentive or barrier to access of care depending on their willingness to provide reimbursement. Insurance companies have traditionally been reluctant to reimburse for some psychosocial interventions and reimburse others at rates below those for standard medical care. Psychosocial interventions for pain and insomnia should be reimbursed as part of comprehensive medical services at rates comparable to those for other medical care, particularly in view of data supporting their effectiveness and data detailing the costs of failed medical and surgical interventions.

The evidence suggests that sleep disorders are significantly underdiagnosed. The prevalence and possible consequences of insomnia have begun to be documented. There are substantial disparities between patient reports of insomnia and the number of insomnia diagnoses, as well as between the number of prescriptions written for sleep medications and the number of recorded diagnoses of insomnia. Data indicate that insomnia is widespread, but the morbidity and mortality of this condition are not well understood. Without this information, it remains difficult for physicians to gauge how aggressive their intervention should be in the treatment of this disorder. In addition, the efficacy of the behavioral approaches for treating this condition has not been adequately disseminated to the medical community.

Finally, who should be administering these therapies? Problems with credentialing and training have yet to be completely addressed in the field. Although the initial studies have been done by qualified and highly trained practitioners, the question remains as to how this will best translate into delivery of care in the community. Decisions will have to be made about which practitioners are best qualified and most cost-effective to provide these psychosocial interventions.

What Are the Significant Issues for Future Research and Applications?

Research efforts on these therapies should include additional efficacy and effectiveness studies, cost-effectiveness studies, and efforts to replicate existing studies. Several specific issues should be addressed:

Outcomes

- Outcome measures should be reliable, valid, and standardized for behavioral and relaxation interventions research in each area (chronic pain, insomnia) so that studies can be compared and combined.

- Qualitative research is needed to help determine patients' experiences with both insomnia and chronic pain and the impact of treatments.

- Future research should include examination of consequences/outcomes of untreated chronic pain and insomnia; chronic pain and insomnia treated pharmacologically versus with behavioral and relaxation therapies; and combinations of pharmacologic and psychosocial treatments for chronic pain and insomnia.

Mechanism(s) of Action

- Advances in the neurobiological sciences and psychoneuroimmunology are providing an improved scientific base for understanding mechanisms of action of behavioral and relaxation techniques and need to be further investigated.

Covariates

- Chronic pain and insomnia, as well as behavioral and relaxation therapies, involve factors such as values, beliefs, expectations, and behaviors, all of which are strongly shaped by one's culture. Research is needed to assess cross-cultural applicability, efficacy, and modifications of psychosocial therapeutic modalities.

- Research studies that examine the effectiveness of behavioral and relaxation approaches to insomnia and chronic pain should consider the influence of age, race, gender, religious belief, and socioeconomic status on treatment effectiveness.

Health Services

- The most effective timing of the introduction of behavioral interventions into the course of treatment should be studied.

- Research is needed to optimize the match between specific behavioral and relaxation techniques and specific patient groups and treatment settings.

Integration Into Clinical Care and Medical Education

- New and innovative methods of introducing psychosocial treatments into health care curricula and practice should be implemented.

Conclusions

A number of well-defined behavioral and relaxation interventions are now available, some of which are commonly used to treat chronic pain and insomnia. Available data support the effectiveness of these interventions in relieving chronic pain and in achieving some reduction in insomnia. Data are currently insufficient to conclude with confidence that one technique is more effective than another for a given condition. For any given individual patient, however, one approach may indeed be more appropriate than another.

Behavioral and relaxation interventions clearly reduce arousal, and hypnosis reduces pain perception. However, the exact biological underpinnings of these effects require further study, as is often the case with medical therapies. The literature demonstrates treatment effectiveness, although the state of the art of the methodologies in this field indicates a need for thoughtful interpretation of the findings along with prompt translation into programs of health care delivery.

Although specific structural, bureaucratic, financial, and attitudinal barriers exist to the integration of these techniques, all are potentially surmountable with education and additional research, as patients shift from being passive participants in their treatment to becoming responsible, active partners in their rehabilitation.

Bibliography

Atkinson JH, Slater MA, Patterson TL, Grant I, Garfin SR. Prevalence, onset, and risk of psychiatric disorders in men with chronic low back pain: a controlled study. *Pain* 1991; 45: 111-21.

Berman BM, Singh BK, Lao L, Singh BB, Ferentz KS, Hartnoll SM. Physicians' attitudes toward complementary or alternative medicine: a regional survey. *JABP* 1995; 8 (5): 361-6.

Blanchard EB, Appelbaum KA, Guarnieri P, Morrill B, Dentinger MP. Five year prospective follow-up on the treatment of chronic headache with biofeedback and/or relaxation. *Headache* 1987; 27: 580-3.

Bonica JJ. General considerations of chronic pain in the management of pain (2nd ed.). *In:* Loeser JD, Chapman CR, Fordyce WE, eds. Philadelphia: Lea & Febiger, 1990. p. 180-2.

Carr DB, Jacox AK, Chapman RC, et al. Acute pain management. *Guideline Technical Report*, No. 1. Rockville, MD: US Department of Health and Human Services, Public Health Service, Agency for Health Care Policy and Research. AHCPR Publication No. 95-0034. February 1995. p. 107-59.

Crawford HJ. Brain dynamics and hypnosis: attentional and disattentional processes. *Int J Clin Exp Hypn* 1994; 42: 204-32.

Cutler RB, Fishbain DA, Rosomoff HL, Abdel-Moty E, Khalil TM, Steele-Rosomoff R. Does nonsurgical pain center treatment of chronic pain return patients to work? *Spine* 1994; 19 (6): 643-52.

Daan S, Beersma DGM, Borbely A. The timing of human sleep: recovery process gated by a circadian pacemaker. *Am J Physiol* 1984; 246: R161-78.

Eisenberg DM, Kessler RC, Foster C, Norlock FE, Calkins DR, Delbanco TL. Unconventional medicine in the United States. Prevalence, costs and patterns of use. *N Engl J Med* 1993.

Fields HL, Basbaum AI. Central nervous system mechanisms of pain modulation. In: Wall PD, Melzack R, eds. *Textbook of pain* (3rd ed.). London: Churchill-Livingstone, 1994. p. 243-57.

Fishbain DA, Rosomoff HL, Goldberg M, Cutler R, Abdel-Moty E, Khalil TM, Steele-Rosomoff R. The prediction of return to the workplace after multidisciplinary pain center treatment. *Clin J Pain* 1993; 9: 3-15.

Flor H, Birbaumeer N. Comparison of the efficacy of electromyographic biofeedback, cognitive-behavioral therapy, and conservative medical interventions in the treatment of chronic musculoskeletal pain. *J Consult Clin Psychol* 1993; 61: 653-8.

Gallagher RM, Woznicki M. Low back pain rehabilitation. In: Stoudemire A, Fogel BS, eds. Medical psychiatric practice (Vol. 2). APA Press, 1993. *Guideline for the clinical evaluation of analgesic drugs*. U.S. Department of Health and Human Services, Public Health Service (FDA) Docket No. 91D-0425, December 1992;1-26.

Hauri PJ, ed. *Case studies in insomnia*. York: Plenum Medical Books, 1991.

Hilgard ER, Hilgard JR. *Hypnosis in the relief of pain* (rev. ed.). New York: Brunner/Mazel, 1994.

Jacobs GD, Rosenberg PA, Friedman R, Matheson J, Peavy GM, Domar AD, Benson H. Multifactor behavioral treatment of chronic sleep-onset insomnia using stimulus control and the relaxation response. *Behav Modif* 1993; 17: 498-509.

Jacox AK, Carr DB, Payne R, et al. Management of cancer pain. *Clinical Practice Guideline*, No. 9. Rockville, MD: US Department of Health and Human Services, Public Health Service, Agency for Health Care Policy and Research. AHCPR Publication No. 94-00592. March 1994.

Jones BE. Basic mechanisms of sleep-wake states. In: Kryger MH, Roth T, Dement WC, eds. *Principles and practice of sleep medicine*. Philadelphia: WB Saunders, 1994. p. 145-62.

Kabat-Zinn J, Lipworth L, Burney R. The clinical use of mindfulness-meditation for the self- regulation of chronic pain. *J Behav Med* 1985; 8 (2): 163-90.

Kaplan RM. Behavior as the central outcome in health care. *Am Psychol* 1990; 45: 1211-20.

McCaffery M, Beebe A. *Pain: clinical manual for nursing practice*. St. Louis: CV Mosby, 1989.

McDonald-Haile J, Bradley LA, Bailey MA, Schan CA, Richter JE. Relaxation training reduces symptom reports and acid exposure in gastroesophageal reflux disease patients. *Gastroenterology* 1994; 107: 61-9.

Mendelson WB. *Human sleep: research and clinical care.* New York: Plenum Press, 1987. p. 1-436.

Morin CM, ed. *Insomnia.* New York: Guilford Press, 1993.

Morin CM, Culbert JP, Schwartz SM. Nonpharmacological interventions for insomnia: a meta- analysis of treatment efficacy. *Am J Psychiatry* 1994; 151 (8): 1172-80.

Morin CM, Galore B, Carry T, Kowatch RA. Patients' acceptance of psychological and pharmacological therapies for insomnia. *Sleep* 1992; 15: 302-5.

Murtagh DRR, Greenwood KM. Identifying effective psychological treatments for insomnia: a meta-analysis. *J Consult Clin Psychol* 1995; 63 (1): 79-89.

National Commission on Sleep Disorders Research. *Wake Up America: A National Sleep Alert, Vol. 1. Executive Summary and Executive Report*, Report of the National Commission on Sleep Disorders Research, January 1993. Washington DC: 1993, p. 1-76.

National Sleep Foundation. *Gallup poll survey: insomnia in America*, 1991.

Neher JO, Borkan JM. A clinical approach to alternative medicine (editorial). *Arch Fam Med* (United States) 1994; 3 (10): 859-61.

Prien R, Robinson D. Evaluation of hypnotic medications. *Clinical Evaluation of Psychotropic Drugs Principles and Guidelines* 1994; 22: 579-92.

Smith JC. *Cognitive-behavioral relaxation training.* New York: Springer, 1990.

Stepanski EJ. Behavioral therapy for insomnia. In: Kryger MH, Roth T, Dement WC, eds. *Principles and practice of sleep medicine.* Philadelphia: WB Saunders, 1994. p. 535-41.

Stoller MK. Economic effects of insomnia. *Clin Ther* 1994; 16(5).

Syrjala KL. Integrating medical and psychological treatments for cancer pain. *In*: Chapman CR, Foley KM, eds. Current and emerging issues in cancer pain: research and practice. New York: Raven Press, 1995.

Turk DC. Customizing treatment for chronic pain patients. Who, what, and why. *Clin J Pain* 1990; 6: 255-70.

Turk DC, Marcus DA. Assessment of chronic pain patients. *Sem Neurol* 1994; 14: 206-12.

Turk DC, Melzack R. *Handbook of pain assessment*. New York: Guilford Press, 1992.

Chapter 35

Sleepwalking

Until the early 1960s, sleepwalking (somnambulism) was thought to be a dissociative reaction that was related to dreaming. Now, however, sleepwalking is considered a disorder of arousal. [1] Polysomnographic studies have demonstrated that sleepwalking occurs during non-rapid-eye-movement (NREM) sleep (sleep stages 3 and 4), rather than during dreaming or rapid-eye-movement (REM) sleep. [2,3 Thus, the somnambulist remains deeply asleep despite motor arousal.

Somnambulism belongs to the group of parasomnias, which are disorders associated with sleep, sleep-stage transition or partial arousal. Included among the parasomnias are night terrors, nocturnal enuresis, nightmares, sleep-related bruxism, sleep-related head-banging, familial sleep paralysis and other medical conditions associated with sleep.

Epidemiology

Sleepwalking is much more common in children than in adults. Between 10 and 15 percent of children five to 12 years of age have at least one episode of somnambulism. [4] The prevalence of somnambulism is 1 to 6 percent in the general adult population, although a higher incidence has been reported in patients with schizophrenia, hysteria and anxiety neuroses. [5]

Sleepwalking is commonly associated with other parasomnias. Between 25 and 33 percent of somnambulists have nocturnal enuresis.

Reprinted with permission from *American Family Physician*, Feb 15, 1995 v5l n3 p649(6). © American Academy of Family Physicians.

[6] [In addition, some] children who are sleepwalkers, and 50 percent of adults who are sleepwalkers, have night terrors. Somnambulism affects both sexes equally The disorder is four to six times more common in patients with Tourette syndrome or migraine headaches. [8,9]

Clinical Features

As mentioned previously, sleepwalking typically occurs during stages 3 and 4 of NREM sleep. The episodes last 30 seconds to 30 minutes, but they can be longer in some instances. Rarely does more than one episode occur in one night. [10] Sleepwalking episodes occur earlier in the night in adults than in children. [6]

In children, sleepwalking is usually a benign, self-limited condition. [10] The first episode can occur as soon as a child is able to walk. However, sleepwalking is most prevalent in children four to eight years of age and usually disappears by adolescence. [11]

In adults, sleepwalking occurs almost three times more often per year and persists for a longer period of years than in children. In adults, the episodes are frequently associated with stress or major life events. [6] Onset of sleepwalking in old age is uncommon and is usually a manifestation of another disorder, such as delirium, drug toxicity or seizure disorder. [10]

During a typical episode, somnambulists sit up in bed. Most children do not actually walk, but they may make repetitive movements, such as rubbing their eyes or fumbling with their clothes. Some sleepwalkers get out of bed and walk about their bedroom, or even around the house; in rare instances, they leave the house. Children often walk to their parents' bedroom or to the toilet.

Somnambulists appear dazed. They have a blank, staring expression on their face, and they are relatively unresponsive to the communicative efforts of others. Their movements are clumsy. Researchers disagree about the dexterity and degree of motor performance possible during a sleepwalking episode, as well as its classification as an automatism (performance of a nonreflex act without conscious volition). [12,13]

On awakening from a sleepwalking episode, the person usually has no memory or only a vague awareness of what has happened. Immediately after awakening, however, the sleepwalker may experience a short period of confusion and disorientation. [10]

The potential danger of sleepwalking comes from the fact that somnambulists are not aware of what they do during an episode. Sleepwalking appears to be particularly dangerous in adults, for whom the risk of injury during an episode is twice as high as that in children. [10] In one study, [14] somnambulists represented 54 percent of 100 consecutive adults who came to a sleep disorders center complaining of repeated nocturnal injury. Sleepwalking can be accompanied by violent, often fatal injuries to others. [15] Somnambulists have been accused of sexual assault.

In children who sleepwalk, daytime functioning is usually normal, and psychologic tests demonstrate no consistent psychopathology in most patients. In one study [6] of sleepwalking, 72 percent of the adults were given a psychiatric diagnosis, compared with 33 percent of the children. The Minnesota Multiphasic Personality Inventory (MMPI) profiles of the adults in this study showed active, outwardly directed behavior patterns, which suggested that these adults had difficulty handling aggression. The profiles did not support an interpretation of sleepwalking as "hysterical dissociation."

Etiology

Genetic Causes

Genetic factors may play a role in sleep-walking. [16] Somnambulism has been found to occur six times more frequently in monozygotic twins than in dizygotic twins. The child of a parent with a history of sleepwalking is six times more likely to be a somnambulist than the child of parents who have never sleepwalked. First degree relatives of sleepwalkers are 10 times more likely to sleepwalk than persons in the general population. Second-and third-degree relatives of somnambulists also have a greater risk of sleepwalking. A multifactorial mode of inheritance has been suggested. [16]

Developmental Causes

The frequent onset of somnambulism in childhood and its termination by late adolescence strongly suggest that developmental factors, such as a delay in maturation, may have a role in this disorder. Also, the presence of sudden, rhythmic, high-voltage bursts of delta frequency during slow-wave sleep in somnambulists up to 17 years of age indicates that central nervous system (CNS) immaturity is a causative factor in childhood sleepwalking. [3]

Psychologic Causes

Psychologic factors are important in the etiology of sleepwalking in adults. Somnambulism was once thought to be a form of dissociative hysteria, but electroencephalographic (EEG) studies, MMPI profiles and psychiatric interviews do not support this view. However, a higher incidence of psychopathology has been found in adults who sleepwalk, and evidence shows that stress and major life events play a role in the disorder. [6]

Organic Causes

Fever may precipitate sleepwalking. In addition, some medications, including chlorpromazine (Thorazine), perphenazine (Trilafon), lithium, amitriptyline (Elavil, Endep) and beta blockers can precipitate sleepwalking episodes. [17,18]

Elevated temperature suppresses stages 3 and 4 of NREM sleep and is sometimes followed by a rebound phenomenon, a situation that can precipitate somnambulism. [19] Sleepwalking episodes associated with a fever are differentiated from delirium by their short duration, their occurrence early in the night and their persistence after the fever has abated.

Differential Diagnosis

Complex partial seizures occurring during sleep should be included in the differential diagnosis of sleepwalking. However, true somnambulism is rarely produced by seizures. Seizures last a short time, and they can occur any time during the day or night. Patients with seizures usually do not have a family history of sleepwalking or night terrors. [20] A sleep EEG can be helpful in distinguishing between seizure and somnambulism. Automatisms (e.g., chewing, swallowing and salivation) may occur in both seizures and sleepwalking.

In some cases, differentiating between sleepwalking and night terrors may be difficult. Like somnambulism, night terrors occur during NREM sleep. [11] However, sleep terrors are characterized by intense fear and panic, coupled with an initial scream.

REM behavior disorder is a relatively rare parasomnia that is characterized by punching, kicking, leaping and running from the bed during attempted dream enactment. [11,21] This disorder is most common in persons 70 to 90 years of age. The physical actions occur during REM sleep and are usually accompanied by vivid, violent, unpleasant dream content.

Occasionally, it may be difficult to distinguish sleepwalking from dissociative states such as amnesia, fugue states and multiple personalities. Unlike somnambulism, dissociative states may last for hours or days. In addition, patients in dissociative states are more alert than sleepwalkers, and they demonstrate complex and purposeful behavior. The amnesias are also examples of motivated non-recall in that patients are unable to retrieve an existing memory. In contrast, sleepwalkers have little memory trace. [6,15]

Malingering should be suspected when a patient demonstrates complicated goal directed activities during supposed episodes of sleepwalking. In malingering, the episodes usually last more than 15 minutes, and they may occur at any time during the night. The activities require considerable planning, but the next day the patient will claim amnesia for the episode. Larceny, sexual indiscretion and antisocial activities are among the motives for such behavior. [10]

Sleepwalking in the elderly is usually a sign of delirium or the adverse effect of a medication.

Assessment

The evaluation of a somnambulist should include a thorough medical, psychiatric and sleep history. The following information should be obtained: the patient's age at the onset of somnambulism; the frequency, duration and severity of the sleepwalking episodes; the time that the episodes occur after the onset of sleep; the presence or absence of a family history of sleep disorders; the degree of memory recall; the general daytime behavior, and the presence of triggering factors, such as alcohol, medications, stress and excessive fatigue. Much of this information must be obtained from the patient's parents, spouse or roommate.

Sleep laboratory evaluation is not usually required, except in patients with unusual clinical presentations, such as automatisms, postictal states, posturing or injury to self or others, or when the diagnosis cannot be otherwise established. [10]

Treatment

Since most children eventually outgrow sleepwalking, parents may simply be reassured and instructed about safety measures they can institute to protect their child. Insufficient sleep or irregular sleep schedules can precipitate episodes of sleepwalking, so parents should make certain that the child gets enough sleep and goes to bed at a set time. Because sleepwalking episodes can be dangerous, it is important that the somnambulist's environment be safe. For example, dangerous objects should be removed, and bolts should be placed on doors and windows. It may be necessary to have the somnambulist sleep on the ground floor. No attempt should be made to interrupt the sleepwalking episode, since such efforts may confuse or frighten the somnambulist. [6] Instead, the sleepwalker should be gently guided back to bed.

Studies and case reports indicate that benzodiazepines, particularly diazepam (Valium) and clonazepam (Klonopin), or the tricyclic antidepressant imipramine (Janimine, Tofranil) may be used to treat episodes of sleepwalking. [22]

A flexible psychotherapeutic approach is indicated in adult sleepwalkers who have evident psychopathology. It is important to help the patient identify stressors and deal with frustration in a healthy, nonaggressive manner. Other techniques, including hypnosis, have been used as alternative treatments in somnambulists, but the results have been inconsistent.

In elderly patients, treatment focuses on reversing the underlying causes of delirium or dementia. Withdrawal of a particular medication may be required. Low doses of a psychotropic medication, such as haloperidol (Haldol), 0.5 to 1.0 mg per day, may be more useful than benzodiazepines in treating nocturnal confusion.

References

1. Broughton RJ. Sleep disorders: disorders of arousal? Enuresis, somnambulism, and nightmares occur in confusional states of arousal, not in "dreaming sleep." *Science* 1968;159:1070-8.

2. Jacobson A, Kales A, Lehmann D, Zweizig JR. Somnambulism: All night electro-encephalographic studies. *Science* 1965;148:975-7.

3. Kales A, Paulson MJ, Jacobson A, Kales JD. Somnambulism: psychophysiological correlates. 11. Psychiatric interviews, psychological testing, and discussion. *Arch Gen Psychiatry* 1966;14:595-604.

4. Simonds JF, Parraga H. Prevalence of sleep disorders and sleep behaviors in children and adolescents. *J Am Acad Child Psychiatry* 1982;21:383-8.

5. Orme JE. The incidence of sleepwalking in various groups. *Acta Psychiatr Scand* 1967;43:279-81.

6. Kales A, Soldatos CF, Caldwell AB, Kales JD, Humphrey FJ 2d, Charney DS, et al. Somnambulism. Clinical characteristics and personality patterns. *Arch Gen Psychiatry* 1980;37:1406-10.

7. Vela-Bueno A, Soldatos CR. Episodic sleep disorders (parasomnias). *Semin Neurol* 1987;7:269-76.

8. Barabas G, Ferrari M, Matthews WS. Childhood migraine and somnambulism. *Neurology* 1983; 33:948-9.

9. Barabas G, Matthews WS. Homogeneous clinical subgroups in children with Tourette syndrome. *Pediatrics* 1985;75:73-5.

10. Berlin RM, Qayyum U. Sleepwalking: diagnosis and treatment through the life cycle. *Psychosomatics* 1986;27:755-60.

11. *The international classification of sleep disorders: diagnostic and coding manual.* Rochester, Minn.: American Sleep Disorders Association, 1990.

12. Crisp AH, Matthews BM, Oakey M, Crutchfield M. Sleepwalking, night terrors, and consciousness. *BMJ* 1990;300:360-2.

13. Mahowald MW, Bundlie SR, Hurwitz TD, Schenck CH. Sleep violence—forensic science implications: polygraphic and video documentation. *J Forensic Sci* 1990;35:413-32.

14. Schenck CH, Milner DM, Hurwitz TD, Bundlie SR, Mahowald MW. A polysomnographic and clinical report on sleep-related injury in 100 adult patients. *Am J Psychiatry* 1989;146:1166-73.

15. Oswald I., Evans J. On serious violence during sleep-walking. *Br J Psychiatry* 1985;147:688-91.

16. Kales A, Soldatos CR, Bixier EO, Ladda RL, Charney DS, Weber G, et al. Hereditary factors in sleepwalking and night terrors. *Br J Psychiatry* 1980;137:111-8.

17. Huapaya LV. Seven cases of somnambulism induced by drugs. *Am J Psychiatry* 1979;136:985-6.

18. Regestein QR. Reich P. Agitation observed during treatment with newer hypnotic drugs. *J Clin Psychiatry* 1985;46:280-3.

19. Karacan I., Wolff SM, Williams RL, Hursch CJ, Webb VY'B. The effects of fever on sleep and dream patterns. *Psychosomatics* 1968;9:331-9.

20. Tassinari CA, Dalia Bernardina B, Burea-Paillas M, Dravet C, Ambrosetto G, Roger J. Nocturnal epileptic seizures with exceptional clinical symptomatology (resembling pavor noctumus, terrific dreams, enuresis and sleepwalking). *Electroencephalogr Clin Neurophysiol* 1975;39:217.

21. Ishigooka J, Westendorp F, Oguchi T, Takahashi A, Sumiyoshi A, Inami M. Somnambulistic behavior associated with abnormal REM sleep in an elderly woman. *Biol Psychiatry* 1985; 20:1003-8.

22. Pesikoff RB, Davis PC. Treatment of pavor nocturnus and somnambulism in children. *Am J Psychiatry* 1971;128:778-81.

—*by Prakash Masand, M.D.,*
Anand P. Popli, M.D., and
Jeffrey B. Weilburg, M.D.

PRAKASH MASAND, M.D. is associate professor of psychiatry and director of the Psychiatric Consult Service at the State University of New York (SLNY) Health Science Center at Syracuse.

ANAND P. POPLI, M.D. is a fellow in psychopharmacology at McLean Hospital and Harvard Medical School, Boston.

JEFFREY B. WEILBURG, M.D. is assistant professor of psychiatry at Harvard Medical School, and director of the neuropsychiatry section of the clinical psychopharmacology unit at Massachusetts General Hospital, Boston, where he is also on the staff of the private consultation service of the Department of Psychiatry.

Chapter 36

Shiftwork:
Tactics to Ease the
Emotional and Physical Toll

Background Information

Defining Shiftwork

There are many work schedules that are called shiftwork. Shiftwork involves working outside the normal daylight hours. That is, outside the hours of around 7 a.m. to 6 p.m., the time period in which many people in our society work a 7-to 8-hour shift. Shift-workers might work in the evening, in the middle of the night, over-time or extra long workdays. They also might work regular days at one time or another. Many shiftworkers "rotate" around the clock, which involves changing work times from day to evening, or day to night. This might happen at different times of the week or at different times of the month. Police officers and firefighters, for example, often work rotating shifts. Other workers might have a "permanent" shift and only work at night or in the evenings. Waiters and wait-resses, for example, might work only the evening shift. Night watch-men, on the other hand, might work only the overnight or "graveyard" shift.

Society and Employer Reasons for Shiftwork

There are several reasons for shiftwork. A major reason is that modern technology has made it possible to do many activities at any

From *Plain Language About Shiftwork*, DHHS (NIOSH) Pub. No. 97-145.

257

time of the day or night. This "24-hour society" of ours requires that important services be provided at all times. Critical services include public safety, such as police and fire protection; military defense; health care; transportation; and public utilities, such as electrical power, water and telephone. Other industries must operate 24 hours per day because the production process is much longer than 8 hours and must be performed continuously. Many chemical products require such a process. Also, manufacturing industries often have expensive machinery that needs to be operated continuously in order to be profitable.

Because several occupations and industries operate around the clock, other services have expanded their hours to accommodate evening and nighttime workers. (They also have expanded access for all the rest of us who simply enjoy the convenience.) Some obvious examples are grocery stores, gas stations, and restaurants that are open 24 hours per day, seven days per week. The increase in these expanded-time services in the past decade or two has opened up the job market for new shiftworkers. This is ironic. Because there are so many shiftworkers, society now needs more shiftworkers.

Numbers of Shiftworkers

Estimates of the number of shiftworkers varies with the definition of shiftwork. The Bureau of Labor Statistics reports that about five percent of American adults work in the evening. Permanent night workers and workers with irregular schedules make up another four percent. Still another four percent are rotating shiftworkers. All together, this amounts to about 15.5 million people.

Almost any occupation or industry has some people doing shiftwork. A quick check of lists provided by the Bureau of Labor Statistics shows about 2 to 10 percent of almost any occupation working evening, night, or rotating shifts. These kinds of schedules happen quite often among police officers and firefighters. More than half of them work evenings and nights, and about a quarter of them rotate shifts. Many transportation and public utility workers—about one-fifth of them—also work shifts. Long-haul truckers often make their best time in the evening or at night.

Lately, many materials must be delivered "just in time," or just before they are used in manufacturing. For example, parts for making automobiles are delivered this way. This practice has forced more truckers to take trips at all hours and at the last minute to make their deliveries on time.

258

People Who Work Shifts

If we look only at full-time jobs, men work more night and rotating shifts, while women work more evening shifts and do more part-time work. However, full-time shiftworking women are not far behind in numbers. And more women are entering the workforce full time, so these numbers are changing quickly. Younger people are more likely to work shifts than older people. African-Americans do more shiftwork than Caucasian-Americans. Single people work more shifts than married people. If we look at married couples who each have paying jobs, about one-quarter to one-third of these couples have at least one partner who is a shiftworker. If we look at mothers with children at home, single mothers work shifts more often than married mothers.

Employee Reasons to Do Shiftwork

Some workers actually prefer non-day work, but most do not seek out shiftwork. Reasons for employees choosing shiftwork include better pay, more available time during the day for child care, more daylight hours for recreation, and more time to attend school. Some workers prefer the night shift because it is quieter and there are fewer supervisors. Usually, however, workers say they did not choose shiftwork. They do it either because it is required of the job, or no other job is available.

How to Examine Work Scheduling

Shiftwork experts often are asked what is the best or worst work schedule. There is no simple answer to this question because there is no ideal schedule that fits every situation. Both good and bad points can be found in most work schedules. In this section, we suggest ways to examine work schedules to identify their advantages and disadvantages.

Types of Work Schedules

There are hundreds of different shiftwork schedules. However, it is difficult to accurately count the many shiftwork schedules being used. No thorough records are kept by the federal government, trade organizations, or labor unions. Different schedules might be used by the same occupation, the same industry, or even the same workplace.

Table 36.1. Work Schedule Features

Feature	Particulars	Example
Time of Shift	Day, evening or night	
Shift Rotation		
Permanent	Fixed shift times (no rotation)	
Rotating Speed	Changing Shift times Number of workdays before shift change	Rapid: 2 days per shift Slow: 21 days per shift
Direction	Clockwise (forward) or counterclockwise (backward) change	Clockwise: day to evening to night Counter: day to night to evening

Work-Rest Ratios (or How Much Work Before a Rest)

Weekly	Number of workdays to number of restdays	5 workdays/2 restdays 7 workdays/3 restdays
	Overtime workdays	
Daily	Work hours to rest hours	8 h work/16h rest 12h work/12h rest
	Rest breaks within a day	Lunch, coffee break
	Overtime work hours	

How Regular or Predictable?

	Can affect any other part of the schedule	Emergency or "on-call" Unplanned overtime Demand-based scheduling or working off a "call board"

The most common shift schedule probably is five days on a single shift followed by two days off. If this is a rotating shift schedule, the worker will change to a new shift after the days off. Depending on the job, it is even possible to work 7, 10, or 14 days in a row. Offshore oil rig workers, for example, might work two weeks out on the rig followed by two weeks off at home.

Since so many different schedules exist, researchers have thought of ways to measure different features of the schedules. These features are used to study how work schedules might affect safety, health, or productivity. The features are listed in Table 36.1 with explanations below.

Work Schedule Features

We already have mentioned the time of the shift and whether shifts are permanent (fixed) or rotating. It also is important to consider:

- How long a shift might be.
- How many shifts are worked before a rest day.
- How many rest days are on weekends.
- Whether there is overtime.
- How much rest is taken between shifts.
- How much rest is taken during the shift.
- Whether the work schedule is regular and predictable.

As we will explain, all of these features can affect the amount of stress and fatigue a person feels because of the work schedule. If people experience too much stress and fatigue, then they might not do their jobs safely and efficiently. Or they might develop health problems. Here are some particulars about the different shift features.

Time of Shift: Twenty-four hour operations usually are divided into two or three shifts. Start-and end-times depend on the length of the shift. Day shift (also called morning or first shift) starts around 5 to 8 a.m. and ends around 2 to 6 p.m. Evening shift (also called afternoon or second shift) starts around 2 to 6 p.m. and ends around 10 p.m. to 2 a.m. Night shift (also called third, graveyard," or "mid" shift) starts around 10 p.m. to 2 a.m. and ends around 5 to 8 a.m.

Why is the time of shift important? Because people who work in the late night or early morning hours often feel sleepy and fatigued during their shift. This happens because their body rhythm (also called a circadian rhythm) tells them to be asleep at those times. Night workers also must sleep during the day, when their circadian rhythm tells them to be awake. Because of this, day sleep is short and feels "light" or unsatisfying. Often, night workers don't get enough sleep during the day to combat nighttime fatigue and sleepiness. Also, day workers sometimes must wake up very early to go to work. This might cause them to cut off their sleep, which makes them feel tired during the day.

Shift times also determine when a worker can see family and friends. Many social events take place in the evening, which means they might be missed by evening or night workers. Parents who work the evening shift might not see their children during the week because they are at work when the kids return from school. If this happens too often, it can be stressful.

Permanent versus Rotating Schedules: We might think that permanent night workers adapt or get used to their work times. Usually, the longer somebody does something, the easier it becomes. With experience, many night workers figure out tricks or personal methods to fight off some of the nighttime fatigue. However, research tells us that most permanent night workers never really get used to the schedule. That is, there are many nights when they still feel tired and sleepy. Fatigue occurs because most night workers go back to a day schedule on their days off. This is not surprising because family and friends are active during the day. Also, many errands and chores (like getting the car fixed) must be done during the day. Because most night workers often return to a day schedule, they never completely allow their sleep and body rhythms to adapt to being awake at night. They also sleep less during the day, so they don't recover from fatigue. This fatigue can carry over from day to day. over several days, fatigue can accumulate to unsafe levels.

People working rotating schedules face a similar situation. Because the shift times are always changing, they can never completely adapt to a set work schedule. Rotating schedules are often used because they are considered fairer to all workers. Everybody in the workforce takes their turn at both the popular and unpopular shifts. Rotating shift-workers are always trying to get used to changing work times. This is not easy, which is why rotating shiftworkers have more complaints than other workers about physical health and psychological stress. Research has shown that rotating shifts have special features that might affect a person's ability to get used to the schedule. These features are explained below.

Speed and Direction of Rotation: Adapting to rotating shifts can be affected by the speed of rotation and the direction of rotation. Speed of rotation means the number of consecutive day, evening, or night shifts before a shift change occurs. Direction of rotation means the order of shift change: A forward rotation is in the clockwise direction, from day to evening to night shift. A backward rotation is in the counterclockwise direction, from day to night to evening shift.

Different rotation speeds also affect a worker's ability to get used to change of shift times. We have already talked about the same situation under permanent versus rotating shifts. Longer rotations (for example, three to four weeks of working the same hours) are supposed to allow workers more time to get used to night shifts. However, workers usually return to a day schedule on their days off. A fast rotation (every two days, for example) allows no time to get used to night work. Some researchers prefer the fast rotation, because the worker quickly gets through the tough shifts and then has a couple of days off. Very fast rotations are used in Europe more than in America.

Direction of rotation can affect the ability of circadian (daily body) rhythms to adapt to the change in work times. Sleep, for example, is a circadian rhythm because each person sleeps for part of every day. Some researchers suggest that a forward, or clockwise, rotation is better for helping a worker adjust to new sleep times. This suggestion was made because it is easier to go to bed later and wake up later than earlier. Our body rhythms make us feel more awake and alert in the early evening. This makes it harder to fall asleep earlier. Backward rotations work against the body rhythm by forcing the worker to go to sleep earlier and earlier.

Although we don't have hard and fast numbers, it seems that backward rotation schedules are used frequently in the United States. It is not completely clear why. It is partly because of custom (We always did it this way) and partly because workers like the "long change." In the long change, workers pick up an extra day off when going to evening shifts after night shifts. This happens because evening shift starts late in the day, which leaves most of that day free for non-work activities.

Work-Rest Ratios (or How Much Work Before a Rest): The more a person works, the less time he or she will have for rest. People who work an 8-hour shift will have 16 hours left in a day to do everything else, and also to get some rest. People who work a 12-hour shift have only 12 hours to do everything else and to rest. In a situation like this, the extra work hours mean more tiredness and less time for rest. This is a two-edged sword. For example, many times a worker's home responsibilities, such as taking care of children, cannot change from day to day. So, if workers do overtime or a 12-hour shift, they still must take care of home duties. Since these duties take the same amount of time every day, workers may sacrifice rest and sleep after a long workday. This example shows us how important the length of shift can be in terms of stress and fatigue.

When looking at work versus rest, we also must consider how many breaks are taken during the shift and the length of breaks. Depending on the type of work and length of the day, several short breaks might be better than a few long breaks. Short breaks might be better particularly for jobs requiring heavy physical labor.

How tired a worker is also depends partly on how many days in a row he or she works. Fatigue builds up over several workdays, as well as over a single workday. This happens especially when a person gets less sleep between workdays than on rest days. As we mentioned earlier, a worker might not get enough sleep between long workdays because of home responsibilities. So, if a person works several days in a row, for example, six or seven, a good deal of sleep might be lost. Then the worker feels quite tired during the last one or two shifts.

How Regular or Predictable? Most jobs have a very regular, set schedule. A worker usually knows the schedule ahead of time. Even if the shift times change, a worker will know several days beforehand. This makes it easy to schedule other non-work activities, such as making sure somebody is at home when the children get there. Other jobs are not so regular or predictable. For example, health care workers might respond to emergencies that keep them on the job much longer than expected. Or, they might be on call for such emergencies. At a factory, a breakdown or a last-minute call for a product might keep workers at the plant working overtime. Railroad workers sometimes work off a "call board." This means they can be assigned to a train at the last minute to move a "just-in-time" order of goods.

If workers cannot predict their schedules, it is difficult to get adequate rest. Maybe they just get to sleep when they are called back to work, or maybe they have just worked a long shift when an emergency happens. So, they stay at work a few more hours. Maybe they are on call and never get deep, satisfying sleep because they are always listening for the phone. Some people call this "sleeping with one eye open."

Health and Safety Effects of Shiftwork

We have mentioned several positive points about shiftwork. Because of shiftworkers, our society is kept moving 24 hours a day. To the worker, shiftwork might mean extra pay or more free hours during the daytime. We also mentioned that shiftwork schedules are demanding and likely to produce stress and fatigue. Here we summarize ways that shiftwork might affect safety, health, or ability to do the job. Some of these things happen very soon after starting shiftwork. We talk about these under Immediate Effects. Health changes take a longer time to appear. We talk about health under Long-Term Health Effects.

Immediate Effects

Sleep

Soon after starting shiftwork, people notice changes in their sleep. Night workers usually get the least amount of sleep. Evening shiftworkers get the most sleep, and day shiftworkers get a medium amount of sleep. Night workers are forced to sleep during the day, when their circadian rhythm makes them feel more awake. Day sleep is usually shorter than night sleep,—sometimes two or three hours shorter. Day sleep also is lighter than night sleep. Day sleepers often say they don't sleep as deeply as they do at night. Because their sleep is lighter, they are easily awakened by sounds. This makes sleeping difficult. Since there is more activity during the day, there are more sounds to wake up the sleeping shiftworker. Both permanent night workers and rotating shiftworkers sleep worse when working nights. However, rotating shiftworkers sleep the least of all.

Sleep loss makes it much easier to fall asleep at inappropriate times. This affects a worker's ability to perform safely and efficiently. Sleepiness can affect performance both on and off the job. Driving to and from work is a major concern. Sleepiness affects our ability to concentrate or pay attention, and driving requires us to pay attention at all times. So, if a person is sleepy, it is easier to have an accident. Several jobs, such as operating dangerous machinery, also require us to pay attention at all times. So sleepiness can be risky in many different occupations. This risk is not simply a matter of falling completely asleep. After sleep loss, it is possible to have very brief periods of sleep that last only a few seconds. Most people may not even realize these short sleeps are happening. During those few seconds

265

of sleep, they are not paying attention at all. If something dangerous happens at those times, the worker or somebody else could get seriously hurt.

Circadian Rhythm, Performance, and Safety

The circadian rhythm is a major body rhythm with regular ups and downs in the 24-hour day. Many systems in the body are very active at certain times of day, and not active at all at other times of day. Usually the most activity happens in late afternoon or early evening. For example, the body's ability to produce energy from food (metabolism) is highest in the afternoon to evening. The least activity usually happens in the middle of the night when most people are asleep. This is one reason people feel most active and alert around 4 to 6 o'clock in the afternoon, and sleepiest at 4 to 6 o'clock in the morning.

There also are personal differences in circadian rhythms. Some people are morning types or "larks." Morning people feel most active and alert early in the day. They usually go to bed early in the evening. other people are evening types or "owls." Evening people feel most active in late afternoon or evening, and like to stay up late into the night. Fishermen who are out on the water before dawn usually are morning types. Musicians who perform in the evening usually are evening types. Most people, however, are somewhere in between the strict morning and evening types.

The internal circadian rhythm affects how alert people feel. This affects their ability to perform. People perform best when alertness and internal body activity is high, and worst when alertness and activity are low. In the normal day-work, night-sleep situation, people work when the circadian rhythm is high and sleep when it is low. On average, this schedule is best for performance, which means it also is best for safety. When workers perform poorly, they are more likely to make errors that could lead to accidents or injuries.

When working the night shift, a person is at work when his or her circadian rhythm is low and asleep when it is high. Such a schedule means that a person is trying to stay alert when the circadian rhythm is low. On average, this is not the best time of day for performance. This low-point affects physical activity and the ability to concentrate. If a worker also has lost sleep, fatigue could combine with the circadian low-point to double the effect on one's ability to perform. Poor performance could affect both productivity and safety. Studies of errors and accidents at different times of day show an increased risk at night when the circadian rhythm is low and sleep has been lost.

Interference with Social and Family Life

Most social and family events happen during the evening or on weekends. Because shiftworkers are on the job in the evening or on weekends, or because they sleep during the day, they often miss out on social or family activities. When shiftworkers are asked about problems with their work schedule, they usually say that the number one problem is missing family and friends. Most shiftworkers agree that sleep also is a problem, but sometimes they would rather lose a little sleep just to see other people, especially their spouse or children.

The amount of time shiftworkers spend with family and friends depends on their schedule. it also depends on their social and leisure activities and how flexible these activities are. Shiftwork interferes little with activities that are not on a strict time schedule. Gardening, woodworking, or fixing cars are these kinds of activities. Shiftwork does interfere with activities that are strictly scheduled, such as clubs or team sports. Shiftworkers often miss these activities because of work. Child care or visits to the children's school also can be a problem because of the work schedule.

A shiftwork schedule affects not only the worker but also the rest of the family. For example, children at play must be quiet during the day because the shiftworker is asleep.

Long-Term Health Effects

In the long run, it is possible for a demanding work schedule to affect a person's health. However, studying health problems in workers is difficult. If possible, workers will change jobs if they think the work is making them ill. A shiftworker might change to a day job for that reason. This is called the "healthy worker" or the "survivor" effect. Workers who stay on the job are those who can "take it." Because sick workers leave the job, it is much harder to show a relationship between job factors and poor health. Therefore, researchers have only fairly healthy shiftworkers to study.

With that in mind, it is not clear whether or not one's work schedule is the actual cause of health problems. But, workers who quit doing shiftwork often point to health problems as a major reason for quitting. Plus, a stressful schedule can combine with other factors to hurt a person's health. If a person has other major stresses in life, such as a bad marriage or a loved one with a chronic illness, a demanding work schedule certainly won't help the situation. If a worker has poor health habits, such as using too much alcohol or tobacco, it will be more difficult to resist the stress of the work schedule. A demanding schedule also might aggravate an existing health problem.

Digestive Problems: Some research has suggested that shift-workers have more upset stomachs, constipation, and stomach ulcers than day workers. Other research has not backed up this suggestion. But, there is always the problem of having only healthy workers to study. Digestive problems could be more common in shiftworkers because digestion follows a circadian rhythm. Usually people eat at regular times during the day. They also eliminate waste at regular times during the day. Shiftwork can interfere with regular eating and digestive patterns by changing work and sleep times frequently. So, it is not surprising that this could lead to nausea and other stomach problems. However, digestive problems also could be caused by lack of nutritious food. For example, sometimes on night shift only junk food from vending machines is available.

Heart Disease: Heart problems also have been noted more often among shiftworkers than day workers. For example, Swedish researchers studied paper mill workers in a small town for several years. This study is especially meaningful, because the paper mill was the only employer in town. This made it difficult for the employees to stop working shifts. Most of them had done shiftwork for most of their lives. Researchers found that the longer people worked shifts, the more likely they were to develop heart disease. However, the way in which the work schedule affects the heart is not at all clear. Work schedule stress might cause heart disease, but it is more likely a combination of stress, diet, smoking and drinking habits, other life stresses, and family history of heart disease.

It is difficult to say exactly how the work schedule fits in with all the other factors producing heart disease. Earlier we talked about several different work schedule features that could cause stress and fatigue. Right now we can only guess about which combination of those features has the most impact on a person's health. Constantly shifting from a day to a night schedule may be one of the stressful factors. But long work hours, high workloads, and irregular schedules also can play a role.

Improving Shiftwork Through the Organization

Work Schedule Design

There are few laws or regulations governing work hours or work scheduling in the United States. The federal government has placed a 10-hour limit on the length of time a long-haul trucker can drive each day. There also are federal regulations governing flight time and rest time for commercial airline pilots. Various state laws establish rules for overtime pay and child labor. Other than these regulations, the law does little to guide design of a work schedule to reduce stress or fatigue. Nevertheless, research has suggested that work schedules can be improved. Older, poorly designed work schedules might even be dangerous because new technologies can change both the physical and mental demands placed on a worker. A well-designed work schedule can improve health and safety, worker satisfaction, and productivity. Therefore, a good work schedule is an advantage for both the organization and the worker.

Changing a schedule is not easily done and must be handled carefully. Designing a work schedule has a large and immediate impact on all workers. All people on the job must abide by the work hours, or they will lose their jobs. Also, working hours affect how people arrange the rest of their lives. So any time a work schedule is changed, many aspects of job life and home life must be considered. It is recommended that any work schedule change should first be temporary and evaluated carefully. The benefits of the change must outweigh the possible negative aspects. If it really is a change for the better, then it can be established on a permanent basis. Because such a change is complex, it is a good idea to consult ergonomics, or human factors, specialists for help in work schedule design and evaluation.

Shown below are some possibilities that the organization could consider to improve a shiftwork schedule. Given the limited amount of knowledge and research at this time, these should be considered as suggestions and not as strict guidelines or regulations. Remember, all aspects of job and home life must be considered when changing a work schedule. Some suggestions may be useful in a particular work situation, and some may not.

Consider alternatives to permanent (fixed or non-rotating) night shift. Most workers never really get used to night shift because they go back to a daytime schedule on their days off. Also, some workers on fixed night shifts lose contact with management and the rest

269

of the workers in the organization. They may end up feeling too isolated or somehow "different" from the rest of the workers. This could make communication difficult. if possible, consider a rotating night shift schedule, but take measures to ease the burdens often experienced in the typical weekly shift rotation. Some suggestions for making rotation less taxing are given below. We realize, however, that permanent night shift sometimes is the only choice, such as in a nighttime security guard job.

Keep consecutive night shifts to a minimum. Some researchers suggest that only 2 to 4 nights in a row should be worked before a couple of days off. This keeps circadian rhythms from being overly disturbed and limits sleep loss.

Avoid quick shift changes: A break of only seven to ten hours should be avoided before rotating to a new shift, such as going from morning to night shift on the same day of the week. With so quick a change, it is difficult to get much rest before going back to work. On return to work after a quick change, most people are very tired and sleepy. At the end of a night shift, at least 24 hours are recommended before rotating to another shift. Some researchers even suggest that 48 hours should be the minimum between shifts.

Table 36.2. Improving Shiftwork Schedules

Avoid permanent (fixed or non-rotating night shift.)

Keep consecutive night shifts to a minimum.

Avoid quick shift changes.

Plan some free weekends.

Avoid several days of work followed by four-to seven-day "mini-vacations."

Keep long work shifts and overtime to a minimum.

Consider different lengths for shifts.

Examine start-end times.

Keep the schedule regular and predictable.

Examine rest breaks.

Plan some free weekends: If a seven-days-per-week schedule is required, allow one or two full weekends off each month. Loss of contact with friends and family is a major problem for shiftworkers. Weekends are the best time to meet family and friends who are on a day schedule.

Avoid several days of work followed by four-to seven-day "mini-vacations": Working several days in a row followed by several days off can be very fatiguing. For example, some schedules require 10 to 14 days of work followed by five to seven days off. Frequent "mini-vacations" are well liked by some workers, especially younger ones. However, older workers find it difficult to recover during the mini-vacations before they return to another long spell of work. Poor recovery from fatigue can produce accidents and damage health. A long work spell should be used only when there is no other choice, such as when long travel distances are required to do the work (e.g., mining or oil exploration).

Keep long work shifts and overtime to a minimum: Extra work hours add to fatigue. They also allow less rest time per day. If 12 hour shifts are used, two or three 12-hour shifts in a row should be the maximum. Two in a row is probably best for night shift. One or two days off should follow these night shifts.

Consider different lengths for shifts: Try adjusting shift length to the workload. Heavy physical or mental work or monotonous boring work is especially difficult at night. Maybe night shifts could be shorter. If possible, move heavy work to shorter shifts and lighter work to longer shifts.

Examine start-end times: Flexible start-end times, or "flextime," can be useful for those with child care needs or a long commute time. Consider moving shift start-end times away from rush hour. Morning shifts should not start too early (5 to 6 a.m.) because night sleep often is cut short before an early shift.

Keep the schedule regular and predictable: Workers should know their schedule well ahead of time, so they can plan their rest, child care, and contact with family and friends. Studies of train accidents showed that very irregular schedules contributed to the accidents by producing sleep loss and fatigue.

Examine rest breaks: Sometimes the standard lunch and coffee break are not enough to recover from fatigue. For example, card dealers in gambling casinos get a 10 to 15 minute break every hour because their jobs require so much concentration. If their concentration is low, it is easier for a player to cheat at cards, and the casino will lose money. In jobs requiring repetitive physical work, brief rest breaks each hour seem to be best for recovery from muscle fatigue.

Workload Distribution

In some jobs, it might be possible to schedule heavy or demanding work at times when workers are most alert or at peak performance. We mentioned that the afternoon and early evening hours are times of peak performance. If possible, avoid doing the heaviest or most dangerous work in the middle of the night or early morning hours. This is the time when circadian rhythms are low, and sleepiness is high. Especially avoid heavy or dangerous work if the worker is at the end of a 12-hour shift in the early morning hours. Extra fatigue from long work hours can combine with early morning sleepiness to increase accident risk.

Work Environment

Poor working conditions add to the strain of shiftwork. Adequate lighting, clean air, proper heat and air conditioning, and reduced noise will avoid adding to the shiftworker's burden. Shiftworkers also may be particularly sensitive to toxic substances because circadian rhythm changes make the body more sensitive to toxic exposure at certain times of day. Workers also should have access to hot and nutritious meals during evening and night shifts. If a cafeteria is not available, a microwave will allow workers to warm meals brought from home or bought from vending machines.

Electronic Monitoring

Modern computer technology makes it possible to check a worker's performance every minute of the day. Some people have suggested that a monitoring or test system could be used to check a worker for dangerous levels of fatigue. There are performance tests on the market that claim to test fatigue or determine whether the worker is using drugs. However, many of them have not been tested scientifically, so we cannot recommend them at this time.

Some computer systems actually measure worker output or productivity. For example, a computer might measure the number of times a worker taps a keyboard or how many phone calls are completed in an hour. If a worker slows down too much, it could be a sign of fatigue. It may be possible to use this system as a fatigue test. But this is tricky business. The feeling of being watched constantly can be very stressful to workers. ("Big Brother" is watching you.) It can make workers feel they have no control over their jobs. We suggest that computer monitoring be used only when the workers themselves choose it for safety purposes.

Access to Health Care and Counseling

Often, going to one's health clinic or to personal or marriage counseling is not possible in the evening or at night. Expanded access to these services will help improve shiftworkers' physical and mental health and boost morale. If services are not available within the organization, a directory of community health and counseling facilities with expanded hours could be provided.

Training/Awareness Programs

Meetings to make all workers aware of the ups and downs of shiftwork can be useful, especially for new shiftworkers. It is important to invite family members to these meetings, so they can know what to expect from the shiftworker. Use the meetings to share information on all issues mentioned in this document and in the recommended reading. Talking about personal experiences also is very valuable in these types of meetings. If people are having trouble adapting to shiftwork, it is important they know they are not alone. They might learn some tricks from other workers that could make their job life easier. The family will learn just how tough the work schedule can be. It will help to know when to go easy on the worker because of the schedule.

Social Programs

A little extra effort at organizing get-togethers, hobby clubs, or sports and game activities can lessen the feeling of isolation. There is no special reason for these activities to take place only in the day or evening. For example, nighttime or early morning bowling leagues are available in some places.

Coping Strategies for the Individual

Getting Enough Good Sleep

Take responsibility for getting enough sleep to feel rested and restored. For some people this happens without doing anything special. However, most shiftworkers need to become more aware of what to do to get satisfying sleep and when to do it.

When to Sleep after Night Shift: This depends on the individual. Try different times and see what works best for you. As you experiment with different sleep times, keep a written record of when you go to sleep, when you wake up, and how rested you feel. This will help you identify which sleep schedule works best for you.

Some workers like to sleep in one longer period, but many workers need two shorter sleep periods to get enough sleep after the night shift. It is a good idea to go to bed as early as possible after the night shift in order to maximize sleep. A second sleep also could be taken in the afternoon to get ready for night shift. Try taking advantage of the natural tendency to be sleepy in mid-afternoon. You might get your most satisfying sleep at that time.

Does Rest Equal Sleep? Just resting without sleep is not enough. The brain has to have sleep, or you will be sleepy later in the day or during night shift. However, rest without sleep still is valuable for body and muscle recovery. Schedule at least seven hours in bed, even if you don't sleep the whole time.

What Is the Minimum Amount of Sleep? The vast majority of workers need at least six hours of sleep but most need more than this. Most people do not feel refreshed and at their best with just six hours. Staying with your own preferred amount of sleep is best in the long run. You might find that you need less as you become more experienced with shiftwork.

Switching Back to Days: When switching back to days after the night shift, it is best to get most of your sleep the following night. Sleep just a couple of hours shortly after night shift to shake off sleepiness. Then stay awake all day and go to sleep at your regular' bedtime at night.

Napping. Shiftworkers frequently nap, especially when working night shift. Added to your regular sleep, a short afternoon or evening nap will help fight sleepiness during the night. However, napping is not long enough to replace regular sleep. If you nap, allow enough time for drowsiness to wear off before starting work. If you have time to nap at work during your break, don't make the nap too short. A nap of 15 minutes or less might actually make you more sleepy. Twenty to 30 minutes should be the minimum for a nap during a work break. Again, allow enough time for drowsiness to wear off before doing hazardous work. And don't use work-break naps to replace your sleep at home. Naps work best when they are extra sleep time. They don't work as well when you are trying to make up for lost sleep.

Protect Sleep

Block Out Noise: Switch off the phone and disconnect the door-bell. Use ear plugs. Ask the family to use headphones for the stereo or TV. Set strict times for noisy activity, such as vacuuming, clothes washing, or children playing. Don't allow these activities during your sleep times. Locate your bedroom in the quietest place. If possible, get away from outside noise and also away from the kitchen or bathroom. Soundproof the bedroom with insulation and heavy curtains. Put signs out to say you are sleeping. Tell friends and neighbors when not to call.

Keep a Regular Sleep Routine: Make the bedroom as dark as possible. Always sleep in the bedroom. Follow your regular bedtime routine every time you go to sleep. For example, wash up and brush your teeth so you feel comfortable. This can serve as a signal to your body that it is time to sleep. Don't use the bed for anything except what it is intended for. For example, don't read, eat, watch TV, write bills, or argue with your spouse in bed. Make sure you have a comfortable bed that won't disturb your sleep.

Avoid Heavy Foods and Alcohol Before Sleep: Heavy, greasy foods are anti-sleep because of stomach upsets. If you must eat, a light snack won't disturb your sleep. Alcohol might make you feel sleepy, but it will wake you up too quickly after falling asleep. Don't drink alcohol in the hour or two before sleep.

Exercise

In general, keeping physically fit helps resist stress and illness. Regular exercise also keeps a person from becoming tired too quickly.

A big question for the shiftworker is when to exercise. The timing of exercise is important, so that it does not make a person too tired to work. Exercise also should not interfere with sleep. If a worker does physical labor, too much exercise before work might make work too tiring. Twenty minutes of aerobic exercise before work (for example, a brisk walk, bike ride, jog, or swim) is enough to help any worker wake up and get going and also keep the heart in shape. Try to avoid exercise in the three hours before sleep. Exercise tends to activate the body or wake it up. This might make it difficult to fall asleep.

The timing of exercise also might help a person rotate from one shift to another. Since brisk exercising activates the body to produce energy, it also might help the body rhythm shift to the new work time. Try exercise before going on shift. Early morning exercise is good for day shift, afternoon exercise is good for evening shift, and early evening exercise is good for night shift. Don't overdo it or you will be too exhausted to work.

Relaxation Techniques

Being able to wind down and take it easy is just as important as being able to wake up and get going. Give yourself time to relax and get rid work-time stresses. This will make home life and sleep easier. Find out what is best for you personally to help you relax best. It could be just sitting down and closing your eyes for a while. Or it could be meditating, praying, reading, taking a bath, or watching TV.

The following simple exercise may help you start your quiet relaxation time. Try lying down on the carpet or bed, or sitting in an easy chair. One by one, slowly tense each muscle group in your body, then slowly let them relax. Do this for your arms, legs; stomach, neck, and face muscles. Breath deeply during this exercise and go slowly. Try to feel all the muscle tension draining away from your body. This is a simple way to let go of all the stresses of the day and to slow down.

Diet

TV and the newspapers have highlighted diets recommending certain foods to help people wake up and other foods to help them relax. Right now we cannot recommend either diet for the shiftworker. There have not been enough scientific tests to decide whether either diet really helps a person wake up or relax. In some cases the two diets recommend the same kinds of foods to do opposite things: one diet recommends eating protein to wake up, while the other diet recommends eating protein to relax or become sleepy. This conflict makes it even more difficult to decide whether either diet really works. There simply are not enough studies of people using these diets to be able to recommend them.

We can recommend sticking to a diet that, along with exercise, helps a person stay physically fit. This means avoiding fatty and sugary foods, which make a person gain too much weight. Heavy or fatty meals should be avoided especially in the middle of the night because they are the most difficult to digest at that time. Eating lighter meals in the middle of the night helps reduce stomach upsets.

Bright Light

Recent research tells us that bright light can affect our circadian rhythm. As we mentioned already, the circadian rhythm normally makes us feel most active and alert in the late afternoon, and most tired and sleepy in the middle of the night. Lately, we have learned that the high-point and the low-point of the circadian rhythm can be changed by exposure to bright light. By bright light we mean as much sunlight as on a bright summer day. Bright light affects melatonin, which is a chemical naturally produced by the brain. More melatonin makes us feel sleepier. Melatonin usually is produced during the early part of nighttime sleep. Bright light in the evening will reduce melatonin, or make it appear later in the night.

In laboratory research, people exposed to a few hours of bright light in the morning felt alert earlier in the day. They also felt sleepier earlier in the night. People exposed to bright light late in the afternoon felt most alert in late evening. Their low-point in alertness during the night also was delayed.

Some researchers have suggested that exposure to bright light could control the alertness of shiftworkers. The well-timed exposure of a worker to bright light could quickly increase alertness at night. After exposure to more bright light, they then could quickly switch back to being alert during the day. Right now, we see this as a promising idea that needs more work to be practical. Unlike use of drugs, it appears that there are no bad side effects from controlling bright light exposure. Still, workers have to be careful about using bright light, so that they will be alert at the right time. For bright light to work, a worker also must stay in low light or in darkness during some times of day. In other words, if you get too much bright light at the wrong time, this might change the circadian rhythm in the wrong direction. If this happens, you won't be alert at the times you really need to be.

To sum up, we think it is possible to use bright light to change peak alertness to different times of the day. But right now, it takes an expert to work out the right light-dark schedule to fit a particular work schedule. If workers are exposed to bright light and low light at the wrong times, they might end up moving their circadian rhythm in the wrong direction. Using this strategy requires a lot of careful effort from the worker. This might make it too impractical for some shiftworkers.

Caffeine, Alcohol, and Other Drugs

Just like many people in our society, some shiftworkers drink caffeinated beverages as a pick-me-up before or during work. They also might drink alcoholic beverages to relax or to be social. Other types of drugs, such as amphetamines and sleeping pills, also have been used to help people wake up or relax and go to sleep. Here we discuss these substances and whether we can recommend them at this time.

Caffeine: Caffeine is a mild stimulant that helps a person feel more alert and perhaps perform better. Caffeine is the most widely used drug in the world. It is a natural ingredient in coffee and tea (iced tea too!), and it is added to many soft drinks (for example, most colas, some root beers, Dr. Pepper, and Mountain Dew). Caffeinated beverages are a common part of our everyday diet and are easily available. Because of this, caffeine is used more than any other drug to maintain alertness and performance, or to help fight off sleepiness. Research backs up our everyday experience. There are many studies that show caffeine does help maintain alertness and performance. Research also tells us that caffeine is a fairly safe drug if used in small doses. By a small dose, we mean one to three cups of coffee or tea, or one to three soft drinks per day.

In small doses, caffeine is the only drug we can recommend as an aid for the shiftworker. If you drink caffeinated beverages, do so before the shift or early in the shift. Try to avoid caffeine late in the shift, especially late in the night shift. Too much caffeine, or caffeine late in the shift, makes it difficult to fall asleep after the shift. If you do get to sleep, caffeine makes sleep lighter and less satisfying. So don't drink too much and don't drink late in the shift.

If you now are drinking a lot of caffeine (say five to six cups of coffee every day), we recommend that you cut down. Cutting down may make relaxation easier and might improve sleep. Reduce caffeine use gradually over several days. Cut down only by one-half cup or one cup every couple of days. Cutting down too fast could produce headaches, nervousness, and bad moods or irritable feelings.

Amphetamines, Diet Pills, "Uppers": These types of drugs are very strong stimulants that increase alertness and can eliminate sleep all together. Unfortunately, they are too strong and cannot be recommended. Most of these drugs are either illegal or can be obtained only by prescription. It is too easy to become addicted to these drugs. A worker might end up using them every day just to get going. Also, over the long run a person has to take more and more of these drugs just to make them continue to work. This increases the possibility of becoming addicted. Frequent use produces extreme nervousness and mood changes, and performance actually becomes worse.

Alcohol: One or two alcoholic drinks per day, taken with food, is OK for relaxation and to be social. By one drink, we mean eight to twelve ounces of beer, four to six ounces of wine, or one ounce of hard liquor However, we recommend avoiding alcohol during work time, even during meal breaks. Also, we do not recommend using alcohol to help sleep. Alcohol can make a person sleepy, so falling asleep is easy. But, alcohol actually disturbs sleep. After drinking alcohol, a person wakes up more frequently and sleeps more lightly. Alcohol can also reduce sleep so a person doesn't sleep as long as they want or need to. Avoid alcohol for one to two hours before sleep, especially if you have to go to work after sleeping.

Sleeping Pills: These drugs can be divided into prescription and nonprescription (over-the-counter) types. Nonprescription sleeping pills usually contain the same drug used in allergy and sinus medicines. Nonprescription drugs sometimes make a person drowsy and help them fall asleep. However, most are fairly long acting, which means that the user can still feel drowsy after waking up. If used often (e.g, more than once or twice per week), nonprescription pills usually stop working and fail to make a person drowsy.

Prescription sleeping pills work pretty well to help a person fall asleep and stay asleep, even during the daytime. However, we cannot recommend regular use (e.g., more than once or twice per week) because there is no research on shiftworkers and long-term use of sleeping pills. It probably is not a good idea for shiftworkers to use sleeping pills every time they want to sleep during the day. For some people, it is too easy to become dependent on sleeping pills. They might end up using them every time they have to sleep. When this happens, they become nervous or irritable if they run out of pills. Also, some long-acting sleeping pills produce too much drowsiness after waking from sleep. This is less of a problem with the newer, short-acting sleeping pills. However, before considering prescription drugs, we recommend trying the other techniques for improving sleep. If all else fails and there still are problems with sleep, the worker should discuss taking prescription sleeping pills with his or her doctor.

Melatonin: As we mentioned already, melatonin is produced naturally by the brain at certain times of the day. The timing of the brain's melatonin production can be controlled by bright light. Melatonin also can be taken as a drug. Taken this way, melatonin makes a person feel sleepy. So it might help improve daytime sleep for the shiftworker.

Melatonin often is sold in health food stores and can be bought without a prescription. However, we cannot recommend melatonin for regular use by the shiftworker until more research is conducted. We need to find out how much melatonin should be taken. We need to learn the best time to take melatonin for a particular work shift. We also need to know if taking too much can damage your health. If taken too often, melatonin could create unknown problems. Also, the different brands of melatonin sold in stores might have different strengths or potency. So, we don't know whether taking one amount of one brand works as well as taking the same amount of another brand. Right now, we will have to take a wait-and-see attitude about melatonin until more research is done.

Recommended Reading

Authors: Corlett, E.N., Quiennec, Y., and Paoli, P.
Title: *Adapting Shiftwork Arrangements*
Publisher: European Foundation for the Improvement of Living and Working Conditions, Dublin, Ireland
Year Published: 1988

Authors: Folkard, S. and Monk, T.H. (editors)
Title: *Hours of Work: Temporal Factors in Work-Scheduling*
Publisher: John Wiley and Sons, New York
Year Published: 1985

Author: Lamberg, L.
Title: *Bodyrhythms: Chronobiology and Peak Performance*
Publisher: William Morrow and Company, New York
Year Published: 1994

Author: Monk, T.H.
Title: *How to Make Shift Work Safe and Productive*
Publisher: American Society of Safety Engineers, Des Plaines, Illinois
Year Published: 1988

Authors: Monk, T.H. and Folkard, S.
Title*: Making Shiftwork Tolerable*
Publisher: Taylor and Francis, London
Year Published: 1992

Author: Scott, Aj. (editor)
Title: *Shiftwork: Occupational Medicine State of the Art Reviews.* Volume 5, Number 2.
Publisher: Hanley and Belfus, Inc., Philadelphia
Year Published 1991

Author: U.S. Congress, Office of Technology Assessment
Title: *Biological Rhythms: Implications for the Worker (OTA-BA-463)*
Publisher: U.S. Government Printing Office, Washington, D.C.
Year Published: 1991

Author: Wedderburn, A.
Title *Guidelines for Shiftworkers*
Publisher: European Foundation for the Improvement of Living and Working Conditions, Dublin, Ireland
Year Published: 1991

Part Four

Sleep Medications

Chapter 37

How to Prescribe a Good Night's Sleep

Medication can go only so far in helping people with insomnia—and may not be appropriate for all. Patients need to be taught what they themselves can do to bring about lasting improvements.

Frequent or chronic insomnia affects more than 60 million Americans and is a severe problem for about half of these people. [1] Left unchecked, it can have significant psychosocial, occupational, health, and economic repercussions. Since recurring difficulties with sleep often lead to long-term insomnia, early detection and treatment are important.

Diagnosis

Healthy sleep is the quantity and quality of sleep required to maintain optimal alertness during desired waking hours. Insomnia results when the normal physiologic sleep pattern is disrupted, whether by external or internal causes. Asking the right questions helps to categorize the patient's insomnia most precisely. Determining the type of insomnia and its presenting characteristics, taking a good medical history, and, in the more chronic types of insomnia, performing a physical examination will generally provide the information you need to detect any underlying disorders and decide on treatment.

Reprinted with permission from *Patient Care*, Volume 31, Number 4, February 28, 1997. © 1997 Medical Economics Publishing

Types of Insomnia

The duration of the problem is the most basic diagnostic consideration in evaluating insomnia. In general, the longer the condition has persisted, the greater the chances that a significant underlying behavioral, medical, or psychiatric problem is involved. According to a recent review article, persistent insomnia is a risk factor for, as well as a herald of, mood disorders. [2] Successful treatment of the insomnia may prevent the development of major depression.

- Transient insomnia lasts no more than a few nights to a few weeks or occurs sporadically. It is a temporary condition resulting from a positive or negative stressor or a major change in routine. Sleep hygiene (the pattern of sleep and waking behaviors) should be evaluated whenever transient insomnia has no apparent or obvious cause, such as a recent life change, jet lag, a variable work shift, use of a new medication (including self-medication), a change in health, or the use or increased use of caffeine, alcohol, or illicit drugs. External sources of sleep disturbances may include environmental factors such as noise, light, temperature, and humidity—as well as exposure to substances in a new carpet at home or work. The most important question to ask is, "What has recently changed in your life?" The goal is to prevent an ongoing or escalating problem.

- Short-term insomnia persists for less than a month. Insomnia that lasts more than a few weeks is on the way to becoming habitual. Whether due to stress, a lifestyle change, environmental factors, or an underlying physical or psychological problem, a poor sleep pattern is developing, and potentially serious causes must be ruled out. After the history, a thorough physical examination is in order. Interviewing the patient's sleeping partner can provide clues to disorders such as sleep apnea, restless legs syndrome, or psychophysiologic insomnia, in which the patient sleeps better anywhere but in bed. The main question to ask is, Does this person just have poor sleep habits, or have the sleep habits changed because of new—and possibly health-related—circumstances?

- Long-term insomnia lasts from a few months to years. In these cases, an underlying behavioral, medical, or psychiatric problem or a primary sleep disorder is likely. As with short-term insomnia, the patient needs a thorough physical examination, and an interview with the sleeping partner is helpful. Ask the patient about symptoms of anxiety and depression. Many patients with chronic insomnia suffer from an underlying anxiety or mood disorder, particularly variants of depression. Carefully rule out alcohol abuse or overuse of sedatives or hypnotics as a cause of chronically restless and fragmented sleep. Substance-related insomnia may also result from the use of stimulants like caffeine, nicotine, cocaine, and amphetamines, as well as from withdrawal from sedative-hypnotics, alcohol, and other CNS depressants.

Chronic insomnia may develop because of a coexisting medical condition such as chronic headaches, respiratory problems, arthritis, fibromyalgia, anorexia nervosa, bulimia nervosa, or any disorder affecting the CNS. Sleep problems associated with obesity include sleep apnea and alveolar hypoventilation. Women who are perimenopausal or postmenopausal can experience serious sleep difficulties that may be ameliorated by hormone replacement therapy.

Patterns and Perceptions

The specific manifestations of insomnia may vary. Knowledge of the patient's sleep patterns, sleep quality, and daytime symptoms helps you pinpoint the problem and guide treatment. Initial insomnia—needing at least 30 minutes to fall asleep—generally indicates anxiety and stress, and terminal insomnia—awakening much earlier than desired—is often associated with depression. It is not unusual for a patient to be suffering from both types of insomnia at the same time. Maintenance insomnia—the inability to stay asleep—typically indicates a medical or psychiatric condition or a serious sleep disorder.

Occasionally, patients not suffering from true insomnia have misperceptions about sleep without objective findings; the American Sleep Disorders Association now classifies this as sleep state misperception. Affected persons typically perceive themselves as awake even though an EEG demonstrates that they're asleep.

Patients who have common misperceptions about their sleep needs include those with relatively low sleep requirements and good daytime functioning who believe they ought to sleep longer, or elderly patients complaining of the fragmented sleep that occurs naturally with aging. These patients may only need some facts about varying sleep requirements, sleep hygiene education, and reassurance (see "What are normal patterns of sleep?"). Older people need to know that experiencing less deep sleep and more light sleep with more arousals is normal. These physiologic changes may be exacerbated by remaining inactive during the day, taking naps, or going to bed too early in the evening.

Ruling Out Sleep Apnea

Patients who exhibit severe daytime symptoms and poor sleep quality may have sleep apnea or another underlying sleep disorder; consider referring them to a sleep study center. These patients have a proven higher incidence of motor vehicle accidents and are at significant risk of cardiac, CNS, and pulmonary mortality without treatment.

The classic manifestations of sleep apnea are heavy snoring, hypersomnolence, hypertension, and concomitant cardiovascular or pulmonary disease. Nuchal obesity—a neck size greater than 17 inches in men and greater than 16 inches in women—is also common. Sleep apnea must be ruled out before medications are prescribed.

Behavior Modification

Educating patients about sleep hygiene involves leading them to realize that they must take responsibility for improving the quantity and quality of their sleep. Any prescribed medication for insomnia will be a temporary measure, whereas good sleep hygiene can be practiced over a lifetime. All patients with insomnia, including those taking medication, will benefit from some of the following nondrug interventions.

Sleep Hygiene Basics

Maintaining a regular sleep schedule is the key to optimum daytime alertness and should lead to improved quality of sleep within 4-6 weeks. Going to bed and getting up at the same time each day is essential. If necessary, the bedtime may be varied, but the wake-up time must remain the same. The patient who is going to bed much too early needs to gradually stay up later each evening and continue to rise at the same hour until the sleep cycle is changed. Conversely, the late-to-bed patient must gradually retire earlier and continue to rise at the same hour each morning. Napping, unless very early in the day and for only about 20 minutes, is usually detrimental to about 80% of patients with insomnia.

A healthy diet is another important component of proper sleep hygiene. Patients should not go to bed either famished or too full from a heavy meal. Some people find it soothing to have a light snack or a warm, decaffeinated beverage—herbal tea, for example—before going to bed.

A daily walk or other exercise at least 5-6 hours before bedtime is generally beneficial, helping to reduce stress, lower blood pressure, and produce a feeling of well-being. These effects won't occur, however, if the exercise is considered just another stressful chore.

Relaxation Techniques

If patients tend to bring their problems to bed with them, suggest that they allot some "worry time" early in the evening for sitting quietly and reflecting on the day's events. After reviewing what's really bothered them that day, they should attempt to find one positive solution or make one decision that can be implemented soon. When the "worry period" is over, the rest of the evening is for relaxing. If stressful thoughts intrude, patients should plan to deal with them the next day and dispel them for the rest of the night.

People who have difficulty falling asleep may benefit from a regular presleep ritual to reduce anxiety. For some, it may be a lukewarm evening bath (hot baths are too stimulating) or a cup of warm milk. Relaxation can often be achieved simply by turning off the TV or enjoying some quiet time in the evening. Listening to soothing music or meditating may be helpful for some. Biofeedback techniques are beneficial for learning to control pain, lower blood pressure, and attain deeper levels of physiologic relaxation that lead to restful sleep. Many audiocassettes are available for learning guided imagery, self-hypnosis, deep-breathing techniques, and other forms of stress reduction.

Patients with psychophysiologic insomnia are prime candidates for relaxation and stimulus control techniques because they sleep better almost anywhere than in their bed, which is associated with worry and sleeplessness. Some of these insomniacs dread bedtime and become more anxious as they attempt to sleep. To divest the bed of negative or stressful connotations, activities in the bedroom must be restricted to sleep and sex (unless the patient has sexual dysfunction, in which case sexual activity may worsen insomnia).]

The Sleep Diary

An ongoing sleep diary or sleep log can help construct a correct pattern of sleep behavior. Elderly patients become aware of how often they nap and how naps affect their nighttime sleep. Patients who perceive an erratic pattern in their daily waking time can more easily formulate changes needed to enhance sleep quality. Some may notice that they feel rested only on nights when they get six, eight, or nine hours of sleep.

The diary must be kept daily, but the times can be approximate. The patient must make a commitment to keep the diary for several weeks to several months to track the changes. Besides making patients active, responsible participants in their own treatment, a sleep diary allows you to assess their sleep patterns and compliance.

Sleep Restriction Therapy

This approach is effective for those suffering from the vicious cycle of maintenance insomnia that causes daytime napping followed by more nighttime insomnia. Ask the patient to keep a sleep diary for two weeks. After reviewing this, you can estimate how much time a patient spends awake in bed each night (a total of all awake times). If, for example, the patient averages 90 minutes awake in bed, bedtime should be delayed by that amount. Do not change the wake-up time, and prohibit daytime napping.

Review the sleep diary weekly. If the patient is still having trouble, bedtime should be delayed for another 30 minutes. When improvement finally occurs, time in bed is gradually increased, in 15-minute increments, until the patient is well-rested in the morning and feels no need to nap. Encourage the patient to adhere strictly to this sleep schedule and to practice other sleep hygiene behaviors.

Psychotherapy

Psychotherapy may be useful in some patients, but it has not been proven effective in clinical trials and its cost can sometimes be prohibitive. With that in mind, candidates for psychotherapy may include patients with insomnia secondary to anxiety or mood disorders. Make sure you know the status of a patient's mental health and any medications the psychotherapist is prescribing. Other patients may benefit from counseling to learn to deal with underlying problems of anger, frustration, procrastination, or difficulty making important decisions. Psychotherapy may also be useful for psychophysiologic insomnia, especially if the patient is having serious problems with the sleeping partner.

Drug Therapy

Once you have confirmed the cause of insomnia, medications can provide temporary relief. Hypnotics are most helpful for managing severe insomnia or for short-term use to minimize sleep disruption during stressful periods. They should be used as an adjunct to the suggested behavioral techniques so that the patient is left with a daily strategy for keeping insomnia at bay when medication is discontinued.

Short-acting hypnotic agents such as triazolam and zolpidem tartrate cause minimal daytime sedation and are best used for sleep-onset insomnia, especially in cases of transient or psychophysiologic insomnia. Caution the patient about possible amnesiac episodes, especially with triazolam. The short-acting drugs allow patients to normalize their sleep pattern while practicing new sleep-related behaviors.

Zolpidem, a nonbenzodiazepine hypnotic of the imidazopyridine class, appears to cause less rebound and habituation and to have only minor antianxiety effects when compared to most benzodiazepines, although estazolam's pharmacodynamics are similar to zolpidem's. [2] Zolpidem might be a good first choice to use with behavioral techniques. It is also often prescribed with a selective serotonin reuptake inhibitor (SSRI) for patients whose insomnia is due to depression. In the weeks before the SSRI kicks in, zolpidem alleviates the insomnia. When the antidepressant starts to take effect, the zolpidem can be tapered and eventually withdrawn.

In patients with initial insomnia, a hypnotic agent with a half-life of less than 7-8 hours, such as triazolam or zolpidem, is a good choice. Patients whose initial insomnia is related to anxiety may benefit from the temporary use of clonazepam or alprazolam, combined with sleep hygiene techniques. Instruct the patient to use the anxiolytic on alternating nights and to begin all applicable sleep hygiene behaviors. As soon as the patient reports feeling calmer or able to get some sleep, the anxiolytic should be taken every third night, then every fourth night, and so on until the patient is relying solely on sleep hygiene.

Patients with early awakening, severe chronic insomnia, or insomnia from chronic anxiety or panic disorder may do better with an intermediate- or long-acting hypnotic. Long-acting drugs, such as flurazepam HC1 and quazepam, promote a full night's sleep but carry an increased risk of daytime drowsiness and drug accumulation, especially with chronic use. Advise patients to adopt an alternate-night regimen or to skip a nightly dose after one or two good nights of sleep.

Hypnotics should be prescribed at the lowest possible effective dose and frequency, and the patient should be monitored for adverse effects on normal sleep and daytime functioning. Benzodiazepines significantly change the natural pattern; slow-wave sleep and rapid eye movement (REM) sleep may be reduced, and REM sleep latency may be prolonged. These changes can affect dreaming, learning, memory, and adaptation to stress.

Hypnotic agents are not recommended for patients with a history of drug or alcohol abuse or dependence. Also avoid hypnotic agents if you suspect sleep apnea. Pregnancy is a contraindication to the use of many of these drugs, as is renal or hepatic insufficiency. Patients who must function well when awakened in an emergency, such as new mothers, physicians, caregivers, and firefighters, should be warned of possible impairment. Dosing of hypnotic drugs should receive especially careful consideration in people who are taking other CNS depressants, such as pain relievers or antidepressants, and the hypnotic should be tapered and discontinued as soon as possible.

The elderly are particularly sensitive to all hypnotic drugs. They may exhibit immediate side effects, such as confusion, amnesia, and dizziness, and the morning hangover effect of the medication may cause falls. Temazepam, an intermediate-acting benzodiazepine, is generally well tolerated. Blood levels of the long-acting drugs are more likely to accumulate to toxic levels in this population. Always start with the smallest possible dosage, and be sure you know every medication, including OTC drugs, that an elderly patient is taking before prescribing a hypnotic. Melatonin has been touted as a sleep aid in the elderly, but many experts remain skeptical of its effectiveness.

Withdrawing Medication

If taken nightly over an extended time, hypnotics lose their effectiveness. When use is abruptly discontinued, the rebound insomnia and withdrawal syndrome can be worse than the original condition. Symptoms of withdrawal from benzodiazepines include retrograde amnesia and daytime somnolence. Although withdrawal symptoms can occur with any benzodiazepine, they are most often associated with short-acting agents.

If the patient is taking a short-acting drug, you can very slowly taper the dosage, decrease the number of days a week it is taken, or both. Another approach is to switch to a longer-acting drug and then gradually reduce the dosage. Warn patients who are switched to longer-acting drugs that they may experience some daytime somnolence, amnesia, and confusion.

Continue to inquire whether the patient feels more rested and is sleeping better. If not, noncompliance with the sleep hygiene program or the drug regimen is one possibility; an unidentified underlying cause for the insomnia is another. Consider referral to a sleep laboratory for any patient with chronic insomnia that continues to affect waking function and does not respond to treatment.

Questions to Ask Patients with Insomnia

Sleep Pattern

- Do you feel sleepy during the day?
- Do you nap during the day?
- Do you have trouble concentrating during the day?
- Do you have trouble falling asleep when you first go to bed?
- Do you wake up during the night?
- How often?
- Do you wake up too early in the morning? Can you fall back asleep?
- How long have you had trouble sleeping? Can you connect this to any event or change in your life?
- What time do you usually go to bed? Get up in the morning?
- Describe the quality of your usual night's sleep.

Sleep Hygiene

- Do you keep a set sleep schedule during the week?
- How does this schedule vary on weekends and holidays?
- Do you sleep better or more easily on the couch or somewhere other than in the bed?
- Does anyone at home interrupt your sleep?
- Do you often get up during the night? How long do you stay awake?
- Do you regularly wake up because of pain, nasal congestion, or the need to urinate?

- Do you work rotating shifts at your job?

- Are you under great stress at home or at work?

- How much alcohol do you drink and how often?

- Do you use caffeine (coffee, tea, soda)? How many cups or drinks daily?

- Do you smoke or use chewing tobacco? How much daily?

- Do you use or have you ever used any over-the-counter (OTC) sleeping aids?

- Do you use any OTC aids to stay awake during the day?

- Do you use any other OTC medications regularly (nasal sprays, cough syrups, allergy medications)?

- Do you exercise? At what time of the day or night? For how long? How many days per week?

Medical History

- Do you have any medical problems?

- Have you ever taken a prescribed sleep medication? If so, which one(s)?

- Do you take any other prescription medications?

- Have you ever suffered from depression, anxiety, or similar problems?

- Do you snore? Do you ever wake up gasping for breath?

- Do you ever fall asleep at inappropriate times (for example, during meals, on the phone, while driving, at a social event, while watching TV)?

Questions for the Sleeping Partner

- Does your partner snore?

- Does your partner seem to stop breathing or gasp for breath at any time during the night?

- Does your partner jerk his (or her) legs or kick while sleeping?

- Does anything about your partner's sleeping habits keep you awake or wake you up?

- Does your partner ever fall asleep at inappropriate times?

What Are Normal Patterns of Sleep?

The pattern of normal sleep for a young person differs from that for an older one but is made up of the same components. The principal divisions of sleep are rapid eye movement (REM) and non-rapid eye movement (NREM) sleep. The sequence for most adults under normal sleep conditions is as follows:

- Stage 1, or light NREM sleep. It lasts just a few minutes and is a transitional sleep with dreamlike thoughts and a low-amplitude, fast-frequency EEG pattern.

- Stage 2, or relatively light NREM sleep. This lasts approximately 15-20 minutes and is characterized by fragmented thoughts and, on an EEG, sleep spindles and K complexes.

- Stages 3-4, or deep NREM sleep. These stages used to be considered separately but now are usually combined. Deep NREM sleep is also called slow-wave or delta sleep from the characteristic low-frequency, high-amplitude delta waves on the EEG. This stage begins 30-45 minutes after a person falls asleep and lasts approximately 40-70 minutes.

- REM sleep. After completing stages 1-4 of NREM sleep in about 90 minutes, the average adult enters REM sleep.

This pattern—beginning with light NREM followed by deep NREM sleep and then by REM sleep—is repeated during the night at intervals of 90-100 minutes, or about 4-6 times nightly. Toward the end of the night's sleep, REM periods lengthen and NREM periods shorten; a person may reach only stage 2 sleep before entering REM.

During REM sleep, body functions are less com trolled than during deep sleep. Pulse, respiration, blood pressure, and body temperature vary widely. Eyes move rapidly, penile erections occur, muscles twitch or become hypotonic, and laryngeal, head, and neck muscle tone decrease. in general, sleepers are later unaware of these changes but often recall the vivid dreams of REM sleep, This level of sleep probably has a role in learning and memory consolidation, perhaps through CNS protein synthesis or reorganization of CNS patterns scrambled during NREM sleep.

The Melatonin Controversy

The jury is still out on the safety of melatonin, but in the meantime consumers are already purchasing time-release melatonin tablets at their local pharmacy or health food store. According to a recent article, controlled-release melatonin improves sleep quality in the elderly by resetting their internal clock. [1] On the other hand, the National Sleep Foundation says that the long-term use of melatonin has not been adequately studied and that preliminary trials have been methodologically flawed. [2] Unresolved issues include identification of populations who can benefit from melatonin use, the types of sleep disorders in which melatonin may have a role, and optimal dosing.

The following Web sites offer information on melatonin:

1. http://www.aeiveos.com
   This Web site contains information and references on melatonin, including the MEDLINE Reviews.

2. http://pharminfo.com
   This URL brings you to the Pharmaceutical Information Network (sci.med.pharmacy) selected archives on melatonin.

References

1. Garfinkel D, Laudon M, Nor D, et al: Improvement of sleep quality in elderly people by controlled-release melatonin. *lancet* 1995;346:541-544.

2. Chronic melatonin use "cannot be justified for any sleep disorder." *F-D-C Reports, "The Tan Sheet*, "August 19, 1996, pp 13-14,

   —by Pagel, Zafralotfi, Zammit, Talarico

James F. Pagel, MD, is Director, Rocky Mountain Sleep Disorder Center, Colorado Springs; Director, Penrose-St. Francis Sleep Laboratory, Colorado Springs; and Director, Parkview Episcopal Sleep Laboratory, Pueblo, Colo. He is board-certified in family practice and sleep disorders medicine and a family practitioner at Pueblo Family Physicians Group.

Susan Zafralotfi, PhD, CSW, is Clinical Director, institute for Sleep-Wake Disorders, Hackensack University Medical Center, Hackensack, N.J.

Gary Zammit, PhD, is Director, Sleep Disorders Institute, St. Luke's-Roosevelt Hospital Center; and Assistant Professor of Clinical Psychology in Psychiatry, Columbia University College of Physicians and Surgeons, New York City. He is the author of *Good Nights: How to Stop Sleep Deprivation, Overcome Insomnia, & Get the Sleep You Need.*

Prepared by Lori D. Talarico, Senior associate editor

References

1. *Wake Up America: A National Sleep Alert: vol 1*, Executive Summary and Executive Report. Report of the National Commission on Sleep Disorders Research. Submitted to the United States Congress and to the Secretary, US Dept of Health and Human Services, January 1993, pp 36-37.

2. Kupfer DJ, Reynolds CF: Management of insomnia. *N Engl J Med* 1997; 336:341-346.

3. Johnson TA Jr, Deckert JJ: Sleep disorders, in Taylor RB (ed): *Family Medicine: Principles and Practices*, ed 4. New York, Springer-Verlag, 1994, pp 510-514.

Suggested Reading

Declerck AC: Is "poor sleep" too vague a concept for rational treatment? *J Int Med Res* 1994;22:1-16.

Farny RJ, Walker JM: Office management of common sleep-wake disorders. *Med Clin North Am* 1995;79:391-414.

Kryger MH, Roth T, Dement WC: *Principles and Practice of Sleep Medicine*, ed 2. Philadelphia, WB Saunders Co, 1994.

NIH Technology Assessment Panel on Integration of Behavioral and Relaxation Approaches into the Treatment of Chronic Pain and Insomnia: Integration of behavioral and relaxation approaches into the treatment of chronic pain and insomnia. *JAMA* 1996;276:313-318.

Mendelson WB, Jain B: An assessment of short-acting hypnotics. *Drug Saf* 1995;13:257-270.

Morin CM, Culbert JP, Schwartz SM: Nonpharmacological interventions for insomnia: A meta-analysis of treatment efficacy. *Am J Psychiatry* 1994; 151:1172-1180.

Pearse PAE: Use of the sleep diary in the management of patients with insomnia. *Aust Fam Phys* 1993;22:744-748.

Roth T, Roehers T, Vogel G: Zolpidem in the treatment of transient insomnia: A double-blind, randomized comparison with placebo. *Sleep* 1995;18:246-251.

Sloan EP, Hauri P, Bootzin R, el al: The nuts and bolts of behavioral therapy for insomnia. *J Psychosom Res* 1993;37(suppl 1):19-37.

Zammit G: *Good Nights: How to Stop Sleep Deprivation, Overcome Insomnia, & Get the Sleep You Need.* Kansas City, Mo, Andrews & McMeel, 1997.

Chapter 38

Over-the-Counter Medication for Insomnia

When your head hits the pillow but your body refuses to sleep, lying in the dark counting sheep just might induce tossing and turning instead of heavy eyelids.

Often, simple remedies can solve the problem of an occasional restless night. For some people, just a few minutes' reading or television gazing will lull the mind to sleep. Others coax slumber by taking a warm bath or light snack just before bedtime. Over-the-counter (OTC) nighttime sleep-aids, regulated by the Food and Drug Administration, are another option.

According to a 1993 report to Congress by the National Commission on Sleep Disorders Research, "frequent or chronic insomnia, estimated to affect more than 60 million Americans—about one of every three adults—is a severe problem for approximately half of those individuals."

Insomnia lasting just a few days—what the American Sleep Disorders Association (ASDA) calls "transient insomnia"—is a common aftermath of stress or excitement. It's not unusual to lose one or two days' sleep worrying about a spat with a spouse or a report due at work. Good things sometimes keep people awake, too, like an exciting sports event or anticipation of the start of a vacation.

"Short-term insomnia"—lasting two or three weeks—may result from ongoing stress. A job setback, illness, or death of a loved one can upset normal sleep habits for a while. If unresolved, "chronic insomnia"— defined by the ASDA as "poor sleep every night, most nights, or several nights a month"—may ensue.

FDA Consumer, September, 1994.

There are a lot of questions about sleep that scientists can't answer—why it's necessary, what its purpose is, how it's regulated, or what the brain does during sleep. But you don't have to be a scientist to recognize the effects of going without sleep. Anyone who has slept poorly for a few nights running knows that's the reason they are tired and irritable, and have trouble concentrating and staying alert.

Chronic insomnia can have more serious consequences. In a March 24, 1993, commentary in the *Journal of the American Medical Association*, sleep expert William C. Dement, M.D., Ph.D., notes that drowsiness is blamed for some 200,000 to 400,000 automobile accidents a year, accounting for almost half of all accident- related deaths in the United States.

The commission's report to Congress links sleep deprivation to increased psychosocial problems and illness and death, and to diminished productivity and performance. It names fatigue and drowsiness as contributors to accidents in hospitals, military operations, and the nuclear industry, and to major air, rail, road, and sea transportation disasters. The *Challenger* space shuttle explosion, the *Exxon Valdez* grounding, and the collision of two Conrail freight trains resulting in four deaths and $6 million dollars in damages are among several catastrophes cited.

So, while researchers want to learn more about sleep for many reasons, we plain folk who lie awake nights simply want to know how we can get more of it.

Professional or Self-Help?

People with chronic insomnia should see a doctor for treatment, which may include short-term use of prescription sleeping pills. Poor sleep for extended periods may be a symptom of an underlying disorder, such as depression, sleep apnea (repeated interruptions of breathing during sleep), pain from arthritis or other illness, or a neurological disease.

But if all that's needed is a little help to overcome a restless night or two, a do-it-yourself approach is sensible. Experts have come up with many useful tips to help people fall asleep and develop and maintain good sleeping habits (see "Tricks for the Tired").

Used appropriately, OTC and prescription sleep-aids also can help provide sounder sleep, the ASDA advises. The association cautions, however, that for some types of insomnia, such as that caused by breathing disorders, the products may be dangerous.

"Before taking any OTC drug product, you should read the label for directions on how and when to use it, and whether you should check with a doctor before taking it," says FDA regulatory review pharmacist Michael Benson. "Antihistamines are the ingredients in OTC nighttime sleep-aids that make you nod off, and some contain other ingredients, like an analgesic for pain," he says.

FDA allows three antihistamines—diphenhydramine hydrochloride (HCl), diphenhydramine citrate, and doxylamine succinate—to be used as the active ingredient in OTC nighttime sleep-aids.

In the early 1970s, FDA began a review of OTC drug products. Manufacturers were requested to submit data on the safety and effectiveness of the active ingredients for their intended uses. Expert panels on various classes of drug products were convened to review the data and make recommendations to the agency.

In 1978, FDA approved a new drug application providing for OTC marketing of doxylamine succinate for nighttime sleep-aid use. In 1982, the agency authorized the initial marketing of diphenhydramine HCl and diphenhydramine citrate for this use. These two drugs were the only ones included in the agency's final monograph on OTC nighttime sleep-aids, issued in 1989. After the monograph's publication, products containing active ingredients other than doxylamine succinate, diphenhydramine HCl, or diphenhydramine citrate had to be reformulated or taken off the market.

Read the Label

Consumers can find out what ingredients are in an OTC drug product by reading the label. Unisom contains doxylamine succinate, for example, while Nytol contains diphenhydramine HCl. Some products, such as Sominex Pain Relief Formula and Bufferin AF Nite Time contain an analgesic for pain relief as well as an antihistamine. You may find that one works better for you than another. Because of the different product ingredients, the label warnings and directions for use vary.

Most OTC sleep-aid product labels caution patients with certain conditions to check with a doctor before taking the product. Such conditions include shortness of breath, asthma, emphysema, chronic pulmonary disease, glaucoma, and difficulty urinating due to enlarged prostate gland. The labels also warn against taking the product along with alcohol or other central nervous system depressants, such as sedatives or tranquilizers, because they heighten the depressant effect.

(Recently approved revisions in wording will appear on all labels by April 11, 1995: The words "breathing problems" will be used to describe shortness of breath and difficulty breathing related to obstructive pulmonary disease; "chronic bronchitis" will replace "chronic pulmonary disease"; and the word "asthma" will be removed. These changes will help consumers recognize respiratory distress symptoms more readily.)

Sleep-aids that contain aspirin must carry a warning to consult a doctor about Reyes syndrome before giving the product to children and teenagers who have chickenpox or flu symptoms. Reyes syndrome is a rare but serious disease that has been associated with use of aspirin in children with these conditions. This warning may also appear on products containing other salicylates. These drugs should not be given to children under 12, and they should not be used for more than two weeks unless under a doctor's direction. Pregnant and nursing women should check with a doctor before taking these products.

OTC nighttime sleep-aids can provide welcome relief from a night of wide-eyed wakefulness. OTC status does not, however, guarantee the product is hazard-free. Just like prescription drugs, OTC drug products must be used with care.

"The bottom line for all OTC drug products," says FDA's Benson, "is to read the label and follow the instructions."

Tricks for the Tired

If you're having trouble sleeping, you may want to try modifying some behaviors that might be keeping you awake. The American Sleep Disorders Association suggests one or more of the following practices might help:

- Get up about the same time every day, regardless of when you go to bed.

- Go to bed only when sleepy.

- Establish relaxing pre-sleep rituals, such as a warm bath, light bedtime snack, reading, or watching television.

- Exercise regularly. Get vigorous exercise—such as jogging or squash—in the late afternoon, and mild exercise—such as simple stretching or walking—two or three hours before bedtime.

- Don't eat or drink caffeine-containing products within six hours of bedtime. It's better not to smoke at all, but if you do, avoid smoking at bedtime. Caffeine and nicotine are both stimulants. Even if they don't interfere with falling asleep, they may trigger awakenings later.

- Don't drink alcoholic beverages at bedtime. A nightcap may induce sleep, but it can interfere with sound sleep through the night.

- Don't nap, unless you find that naps don't interfere with sleep later on.

- If you often worry at bedtime, reserve another time of day for working on problems.

- If you can't sleep, get out of bed and go to another room to read or watch television.

You may want to try sleep restriction. This strategy is based on the finding that many insomniacs spend excessive time in bed, hoping to make up for lost sleep.

Go to bed later than usual, and get up at the same time each morning. Stay in bed only as long as you actually sleep, even if it's only a few hours. When you sleep at least 90 percent of your allotted time in bed for five days in a row, go to bed 15 minutes earlier. After a week or two you should be sleeping better and, after a few months, as long as you want.

While you can try this on a do-it-yourself basis, ASDA says, it is generally more easily done under the supervision of a sleep specialist.

—by Marian Segal

Marian Segal is a member of the FDA's public affairs staff.

Chapter 39

Melatonin

Melatonin, a hormone produced by the pineal gland, appears to help regulate the sleep-wake cycle. With further study and clinical experience, it may become an accepted therapy for insomnia. Although melatonin preparations are available without prescription in health food stores and pharmacies, their potency, purity, safety and effectiveness cannot be assured. Until large clinical trials provide further information about melatonin's efficacy, adverse effects, drug interactions and effects on various disease states, melatonin products should be used with the understanding that many questions about their safety remain unanswered.

Melatonin has been touted as a cure for everything from cancer to insomnia, and sales of melatonin now exceed those of vitamin C in the United States.[1] Since family physicians are likely to encounter patients taking melatonin, they need to be familiar with the possible benefits and dangers of this agent.

Melatonin and Sleep Disturbances

Insomnia

Melatonin is a hormone secreted at night by the pineal gland.[2] It is important in regulating sleep and, possibly, circadian rhythm.[1,2] Melatonin secretion decreases with age, and this decrease has been

Reprinted with permission from *American Family Physician*, Volume 56, Number 5, October 1, 1997. © 1997 American Academy of Family Physicians.

associated with sleep disturbances in the elderly.[2] Because melatonin's half-life is only 35 to 50 minutes, sustained-release formulations as well as immediate-release formulations have been studied in the treatment of insomnia in the geriatric population.[3]

One study[3] in elderly insomniacs with significantly lower melatonin levels than those in elderly patients without sleep disturbances showed that a sustained-release preparation improved sleep maintenance (sleep as a percentage of time in bed and activity during sleep), while an immediate-release preparation decreased sleep latency (time required to fall asleep).

In a double-blind, placebo-controlled, crossover study of 12 melatonin-deficient elderly subjects who complained of long-term insomnia, 2 mg of controlled-release melatonin, taken two hours before bedtime, improved sleep efficiency (sleep time as a percentage of time in bed) and decreased nocturnal awakenings. Melatonin was not found to decrease sleep latency or to increase total sleep time (time actually spent asleep).[4]

One unanswered question is whether only insomniacs with depressed melatonin peak concentrations are candidates for melatonin therapy. Identifying such patients is not practical, however, especially since the range of "normal" melatonin levels is very wide.[1] In addition, preliminary results of a five-year study[5] suggest that there is actually no relationship between melatonin levels and insomnia. In this study, being conducted at the University of California at San Diego, urine levels of melatonin metabolites did not correlate with nightly minutes of sleep in 42 insomniacs aged 60 to 79.

Melatonin's hypnotic effects have been studied in young patients without insomnia as well as in elderly patients with sleep disturbances. For example, in six healthy male volunteers free of sleep disorders, 0.3 mg of melatonin significantly decreased sleep latency as compared with placebo.[6] Polysomnography, the "gold standard" for objective measurement of hypnotic effectiveness,[7] was used to evaluate melatonin effectiveness in this double-blind study. The investigators found no difference in sleep latency between subjects receiving a 1-mg dose and those given a 0.3-mg dose. These findings were supported by a subsequent study by the same investigators.[8]

The authors of these two studies then compared melatonin in a dosage of 0.3 mg. with placebo in nine elderly patients who complained of insomnia.[9] Melatonin reportedly decreased sleep latency, reduced the number of nocturnal movements and awakenings, and improved subjective sleep quality, without increasing morning sleepiness. These parameters were assessed with a questionnaire and with monitoring of core body temperature and motor activity. The results of these studies[6,8,9] suggest that the therapeutic dose of melatonin is likely to be less than that found in many commercially available melatonin products.

Only two studies have examined the effects of melatonin in insomniacs under age 65.[7] One did not use polysomnographic sleep recordings, and the other failed to find any changes in sleep onset or duration in patients taking melatonin.

Comparison to Benzodiazepines

One study[10] compared the effects of triazolam (Halcion) and melatonin on cardiac autonomic function during sleep in six healthy male volunteers. Of the two drugs, triazolam was associated with a higher heart rate during sleep, presumably due to the benzodiazepine's reduction of parasympathetic tone via interaction at *-aminobutyric (GABA) receptors. Because melatonin does not interfere with autonomic activity, the authors suggested that it might be a more appropriate hypnotic in postmyocardial infarction patients. Melatonin, unlike benzodiazepines, does not appear to suppress rapid-eye-movement (REM) sleep.[6]

Jet Lag

Although several small studies involving airline passengers have shown some benefit in reducing jet lag symptoms, Canada's Committee to Advise on Tropical Medicine and Travel does not recommend the use of melatonin to treat or prevent jet lag.[11] Studies of melatonin in jet lag have yielded conflicting results, possibly because of differences in timing of the doses.[1,2,12] For example, in one study,[13] melatonin was found to relieve jet lag when taken before, during or after an eastward flight, but it was less effective for the return westward flight. In a later study of westward flight,[14] melatonin was reported to be effective when taken at bedtime for several nights after arrival in the new time zone, but not before.

Delayed Sleep Phase Syndrome

Melatonin has also been studied in patients with delayed sleep phase syndrome, a type of insomnia characterized by delayed sleep onset and inability to arise at a desirable hour.[15] In a 1991 study,[16] melatonin caused a statistically significant advance in time of awakening and sleep onset in eight men with this syndrome. The sleep symptoms had been present for at least one year and were not explained by medical or psychologic factors. However, three of the study participants reported suffering from depression, and seven reported social or occupational problems. Polysomnography revealed normal sleep architecture at baseline, except for delayed sleep onset.

The subjects were given 5 mg of melatonin or placebo, each for four weeks, with a one-week interval between treatments. The men were instructed to take the study medication at 10 p.m., which was five hours earlier than the mean sleep onset time recorded in the participants' sleep diaries before the study. Efficacy was based on the sleep diaries, not on polysomnography. Melatonin advanced sleep onset by a mean of 82 minutes and wake time by a mean of 117 minutes. Although total sleep time was reduced, alertness was not affected. Polysomnography would have been helpful in documenting more precisely the time of sleep onset and other sleep parameters during the study. Further investigation, with objective monitoring in larger numbers of patients, is needed to confirm melatonin's effectiveness in this disorder.

Use in Shift Workers

In a double-blind trial involving 27 shift workers, melatonin was found capable of "resetting" sleep patterns to match the change in schedule in approximately one half of the patients tested.[5] One investigator,[7] however, has stated that he "would not dream of giving melatonin to shift workers, except in experimental situations," presumably because administration of melatonin at the wrong time might impair job performance.

Melatonin shows promise as an alternative to the currently available hypnotics, which are far from ideal because of side effects, development of tolerance and rebound insomnia. Whether melatonin simply has hypnotic properties or actually causes a shift in the timing of the sleep-wake cycle is unclear.[7] The adverse effects and purity of current melatonin products are unknown.[2] Physicians should keep in mind the problems associated with over-the-counter preparations of l-tryptophan, another natural product that was popularly used as a sleep aid. Impurities in some preparations resulted in 36 deaths due to eosinophilia-myalgia syndrome, which led to l-tryptophan's removal from the market.[17]

Effects on Aging

Melatonin production decreases with age. Pineal gland transplants from young mice reportedly improved immune function and lengthened life span in old mice,18 but the strain of mice used in this study does not produce melatonin, which makes the results difficult to interpret.[17] In another experiment, the life span of mice given melatonin nightly was increased by 25 percent.[1] Even though effects on aging have not been demonstrated in humans, some persons have capitalized on this finding by touting melatonin as an "age-reversing, disease-fighting hormone."[18] No data are available, however, to support the claim that melatonin has any significant role in the human aging process.[17]

Effects on the Heart and Immune System

In a popular book entitled *The Melatonin Miracle*,[17] the authors claim that melatonin can lower cholesterol levels, reduce blood pressure, and prevent heart attacks and stroke. No human studies suggest these cardiovascular effects. The authors base their claim on the fact that a friend who took melatonin each evening became "stronger and healthier," and his cholesterol and blood glucose levels returned to normal within a few months. Because of this man's experience, the authors concluded that melatonin keeps the heart "strong and efficient."

Melatonin has been reported to have immunostimulant effects in animal models and in laboratory studies of T lymphocytes.[19,20] How this information can be applied to humans is unclear. Although melatonin has been touted as a cure for acquired immunodeficiency syndrome, no data support this claim.[17]

Use in Cancer

Melatonin has stimulatory effects on natural killer cells and antioxidant activity that might be responsible for its reported antineoplastic effects.[12] Other possible mechanisms include inhibition of stimulatory growth factors or decreasing expression or function of receptors (e.g., estrogen receptors) in cancer cells.[21] One study[22] suggested that melatonin is potentially active in conjunction with interleukin-2 in the treatment of metastatic endocrine tumors such as thyroid carcinoma, pancreatic tumors, and carcinoid lung tumors, although this study was of a very preliminary nature. Melatonin has also been used, with poor results, as monotherapy in the treatment of solid tumors resistant to standard regimens.[23]

The antitumor activity of interleukin-2 is thought to be augmented by melatonin, resulting in a decrease in the number of interleukin-2 doses needed to exert an anticancer response.[24] In a study of 50 patients with metastatic colorectal cancer refractory to chemotherapy with fluorouracil, the subjects were randomized to receive interleukin-2 plus melatonin and supportive therapy (analgesics, antidepressants and antianxiety drugs) or supportive therapy alone. One-year survival, tumor regression or stabilization, and well-being were greater in those patients who received interleukin-2 and melatonin. The combination therapy was well tolerated. Because of the study design, however, a placebo effect or investigator bias cannot be ruled out. A comparison group of patients receiving only interleukin-2 would have been optimal, especially since it is not a standard chemotherapeutic agent for colorectal cancer.

In vitro studies of melatonin have shown that it inhibits prolactin's stimulatory effects on breast cancer cells.[25] In addition, a statistical correlation between pineal gland calcification and breast cancer has also been noted, but considering that the risk of both conditions increases with age, a cause-and-effect relationship cannot be determined.[1]

Effects on Reproduction and Sexual Function

Administration of melatonin inhibits ovulation in humans by reducing luteinizing hormone concentrations. Thus, the melatonin can be viewed theoretically as a potential contraceptive.[26] Despite claims, no data support melatonin's use in prolonging sexual vitality in humans. In animal studies, gonadal shrinkage has been associated with melatonin administration.[1,17]

Use in Seasonal Affective Disorder

Some interest has been shown in using melatonin in seasonal affective disorder (SAD), because the disorder is believed to be caused by the release of melatonin at an inappropriate time.[1] However, melatonin has not been found effective in SAD, possibly because melatonin secretion increases in winter and might actually contribute to this disorder. Moreover, melatonin administration has been reported to cause or exacerbate depression.[1,2]

Other Clinical Considerations

Melatonin is available in health food stores and pharmacies in the United States, although it is now regulated as a medication in Canada and some European countries.[1] As mentioned previously, contaminated l-tryptophan was responsible for a series of deaths several years ago.[17] Melatonin is structurally similiar to tryptophan and is, in fact, synthesized from tryptophan in vivo.[2] Because melatonin is not regulated by any agency, contamination of melatonin products by harmful substances is a possibility. One investigator discovered several unidentified impurities in melatonin products tested.[2]

The proper melatonin dosage for insomnia is unknown, but too high a dose leads to daytime "hangover" and, possibly, to accidents.[18] Patients should be warned that melatonin causes drowsiness in 30 minutes, and its effects last for at least an hour.[12] Other adverse reactions associated with melatonin use include headache, the feeling of a "heavy head," stomach discomfort and depression. Humans have tolerated up to 6 g per night for up to one month with no apparent serious consequences,[12] while as little as 24 mg of oral melatonin has caused lethargy, disorientation and amnesia.[27] The variability in patient response to melatonin might be a reflection of interindividual variation in melatonin bioavailability.[28] Melatonin's drug interactions, long-term effects and effects on various disease states are unknown.[18]

Even though some melatonin supplement labels warn against the use of melatonin by persons with various diseases and persons taking certain medications, these warnings are not based on any studies or scientific knowledge. The National Sleep Foundation states that the long-term use of melatonin is not justified for any sleep disorder at this time.[29] Until more is known about this drug, it should be used cautiously, if at all.

References

1. Bonn D. Melatonin's multifarious marvels: miracle or myth? *Lancet* 1996;347:184.

2. Melatonin. *Med Lett Drugs Ther* 1995;37:111-2.

3. Haimov I, Lavie P, Laudon M, Herer P, Vigder C, Zisapel N. Melatonin replacement therapy of elderly insomniacs. *Sleep* 1995;18:598-603.

4. Garfinkel D, Laudon M, Nof D, Zisapel N. Improvement of sleep quality in elderly people by controlled-release melatonin. *Lancet* 1995;346:541-4.

5. Link between low melatonin and insomnia incidence absent in early study results. *The Tan Sheet*, 1996;4(34).

6. Zhdanova IV, Wurtman RJ, Lynch HJ, Ives JR, Dollins AB, et al. Sleep-inducing effects of low doses of melatonin ingested in the evening. *Clin Pharmacol Ther* 1995;57:552-8.

7. Lamberg L. Melatonin potentially useful but safety, efficacy remain uncertain [News]. *JAMA* 1996; 276:1011-4.

8. Zhdanova I, Wurtman RJ, Morabito C, Piotrovska VR, Lynch HJ. Effects of low oral doses of melatonin, given 2-4 hours before habitual bedtime, on sleep in normal young humans. *Sleep* 1996;19:423-31.

9. Wurtman RJ, Zhdanova I. Improvement of sleep quality by melatonin [Letter]. *Lancet* 1995;346:1491.

10. Ferini-Strambi L, Oldani A, Zucconi M, Stankov B, Castronovo C, Fraschini F, et al. Triazolam and melatonin effects on cardiac autonomic function during sleep. *Clin Neuropharmacol* 1995;18:405-9.

11. Paulson E. Travel statement on jet lag. *Can Med Assoc J* 1996;155:61-6.

12. Melatonin. *The Lawrence review of natural products*. St. Louis: Facts and Comparisons, January 1996.

13. Petrie K, Conaglen JV, Thompson L, Chamberlain K. Effect of melatonin on jet lag after long haul flights. *BMJ* 1989;298:705-7.

14. Petrie K, Dawson AG, Thompson L, Brook R. A double blind trial of melatonin as a treatment for jet lag in international cabin crew. *Biol Psychiatry* 1993;33:526-30.

15. Regestein QR, Pavlova M. Treatment of delayed sleep phase syndrome. *Gen Hosp Psychiatry* 1995;17:335-45.

16. Dahlitz M, Alvarez B, Vignan J. Delayed sleep phase syndrome response to melatonin. *Lancet* 1991;337:1121-4.

17. Turek FW. Melatonin hype hard to swallow. *Nature* 1996;379:295-6.

18. Butler RN. A wake-up call for caution. If insomnia is the patient's problem, is over-the-counter melatonin the cure? [Editorial] *Geriatrics* 1996;51:14,16.

19. Wichmann MW, Zellweger R, DeMaso CM, Ayala A, Chaudry IH. Melatonin administration attenuated depressed immune functions after trauma-hemorrhage. *J Surg Res* 1996;63:256-62.

20. Hofbauer LC, Heufelder AE. Endocrinology meets immunology: T lymphocytes as novel targets for melatonin. *Eur J Endocrinol* 1996;134:424-5.

21. Brzezinski A. Melatonin in humans. *N Engl J Med* 1997;336:186-95.

22. Lissoni P, Barni S, Tancini G, Mainini E, Piglia F, Maestroni GJ, et al. Immunoendocrine therapy with low-dose subcutaneous interleukin-2 plus melatonin of locally advanced or metastatic endocrine tumors. *Oncology* 1995;52:163-6.

23. Lissoni P, Barni S, Cattaneo G, Tancini G, Esposti G, Esposti D, et al. Clinical results with the pineal hormone melatonin in advanced cancer resistant to standard antitumor therapies. *Oncology* 1991;48:448-50.

24. Barni S, Lissoni P, Cazzaniga M, Ardizzoia A, Meregalli S, Fossati V, et al. A randomized study of low-dose subcutaneous interleukin-2 plus melatonin versus supportive care alone in metastatic colorectal cancer patients progressing under 5-fluorouracil and folates. *Oncology* 1995;52:243-5.

25. Lemus-Wilson A, Kelly PA, Blask DE. Melatonin blocks the stimulatory effects of prolactin on human breast cancer cell growth in culture. *Br J Cancer* 1995;72:1435-40.

26. Voordouw BC, Euser R, Verdonk RE, Alberda BT, de Jong FH, Drogendijk AC, et al. Melatonin and melatonin-progestin combinations alter pituitary-ovarian function in women and can inhibit ovulation. *J Clin Endocrinol Metab* 1992;74:108-17.

27. Holliman BJ, Chyka PA. Problems in assessment of acute melatonin overdose. *South Med J* 1997; 90:451-3.

28. Di WL, Kadva A, Johnston A, Silman R. Variable bioavailability of oral melatonin [Letter]. *N Engl J Med* 1997;336:1028-9.

29. Chronic melatonin use cannot be justified for any sleep disorder. *The Tan Sheet,* 1996;4(34).

—by Richard W. Sloan, M.D., R. PH.
and Melanie Johns Cupp, Pham. D.

Richard W. Sloan, M.D., R.PH., coordinator of this series, is chairman and residency program director of the Department of Family Medicine at York (Pa.) Hospital and clinical associate professor in family and community medicine at the Milton S. Hershey Medical Center, Pennsylvania State University, Hershey, Pa.

Melanie Johns Cupp, Pharm.D. is a clinical assistant professor at West Virginia University School of Pharmacy and a drug information specialist at West Virginia Drug Information Center, both in Morgantown. She earned her pharmacy degrees at West Virginia University School of Pharmacy and completed a hospital pharmacy practice residency at West Virginia University Hospitals. She is board-certified in pharmacotherapy.

Chapter 40

Benzodiazepine Use in Sleep Disorders

Physicians are often reluctant to prescribe benzodiazepines to patients with sleep disorders because of fears about dependence and tolerance. Schenck and Mahowald assessed the potential for medication abuse in patients receiving long-term benzodiazepine therapy.

The study included 170 patients who were evaluated and treated at a sleep disorder clinic over the course of 12 years. Patients underwent medical evaluation and completed questionnaires about their sleep cycles. Polysomnography also was performed for each patient. Each patient received at least a six-month course of benzodiazepines for the treatment of a sleep disorder.

Sixty-nine patients who were sleepwalkers or who had sleep terrors received 0.25 mg or 0.5 mg of clonazepam one to two hours before sleep. Fifty-two patients with rapid-eye-movement sleep behavior disorder received 0.25 to 0.5 mg of clonazepam immediately before sleep. Twenty-five patients with chronic psychophysiologic or idiopathic insomnia received either clonazepam or another benzodiazepine. Finally, 24 patients with restless leg syndrome/periodic limb movement disorder received the same dose of clonazepam on the same schedule as the group with sleep terrors. The dosage was increased every few days until control of the parasomnia was achieved or adverse

"Benzodiazepine Use in Sleep Disorders" (adapted from *American Journal of Medicine* 1996;100;333-7) (Tips from Other Journals); reprinted with permission from *American Family Physician*, Sept 1, 1996 Volume 54, Number 3. © American Academy of Family Physicians.

effects were noted. The outcomes measured were either control of the parasomnia or maintenance of satisfactory sleep.

Psychometric testing showed that the study patients were not more depressed or anxious than the general population. Most of the patients (86 percent) achieved control of their sleep disorder with the benzodiazepine treatment prescribed. Nearly three-quarters of the patients were taking the same dosage or a lower dosage of benzodiazepine at the most recent follow-up visit as the dosage that they received at the first-month follow-up visit. Drug discontinuation or substantial reduction in dosage did not cause withdrawal symptoms but did cause immediate reemergence of the symptoms of the sleep disorder.

Only 15.9 percent of patients experienced side effects of benzodiazepine treatment, and only 10 of these 27 patients had to stop taking the medication because of the adverse effect. A small percentage of patients (1.8 percent) were found to have taken the benzodiazepine in amounts exceeding what was prescribed. Of the 170 patients, 28 (16.4 percent) were known to have a past history of alcohol or substance abuse, but only 2.4 percent of the patients had a relapse of the substance abuse disorder.

The authors conclude that use of benzodiazepines for sleep disorders is not associated with dosage escalation, abuse of the medication or a high risk of adverse effects. However, the authors point out that good sleep hygiene and standard, nonpharmacologic methods for treating sleep disorders should always be the first-line treatment for sleep problems. (Schenck CH, Mahowald MW. Long-term, nightly benzodiazepine treatment of injurious parasomnias arid other disorders of disrupted nocturnal sleep in 170 adults. *Am J Med* 1996;100: 333-7.)

Part Five

Sleep and Other Disorders

Chapter 41

Sleep Disorders Associated with Physical and Mental Illness

Individuals suffering from a variety of medical illnesses frequently have trouble sleeping. For example, patients suffering from severe illnesses, such as cancer, may experience sleep disturbances as the result of factors associated with the primary illness, such as pain or depression. Often, medications used to treat serious illness have a disruptive effect on sleep. In turn, the sleep problem can be a significant barrier to recovery, potentially exacerbating the primary illness. The Commission investigated three areas of primary illness that are affected by sleep disorders: cardiopulmonary disorders, neurological disorders, and mental and addictive disorders. It is important to understand the interrelationship between sleep and other disorders to ensure appropriate treatment, particularly for older Americans, who tend to have a greater number of medical problems.

Sleep Disorders Associated with Neurological Disorders

Epilepsy, stroke, dementia, chronic pain, Parkinson's disease, Alzheimer's disease, and other central nervous system disorders can affect and be affected by sleep. For example, interaction between sleep and epileptic seizures may be key to understanding the process of

Excerpted from *Wake Up America: A National Sleep Alert*, Volume 1, Executive Summary and Executive Report, Report of the National Commission on Sleep Disorders Research, Submitted to the United States Congress and to the Secretary U.S. Department of Health and Human Services, January 1993.

abnormal neuronal excitability responsible for seizures. Certain stages of sleep inhibit the spread of abnormal neuronal discharges; other states facilitate this spread. We also know that sleep fragmentation, frequent awakenings, reduction in deep sleep, and deprivation of dream sleep can be a product of seizures. Seizures, thus, may lead to chronic sleep deprivation that, in turn, may exacerbate the incidence of seizures still further.

Thrombotic disease—the clotting of blood in the vessels—is more likely to occur during sleep or upon awakening, and has been implicated as a major cause of stroke and heart attack. Stroke occurs more often during sleep or upon awakening from sleep than at other times of day. Similarly, myocardial infarction has a peak incidence at 9 a.m. Moreover, blood flow to the brain varies with different stages of sleep. Sleep disturbances caused by stroke may lead to fatigue and depression, significantly complicating recovery.

> I have Parkinson's disease. (As a)side effect both of the medicines and the disease, I am plagued with sleepiness and lethargy. Outside of two to three good hours a day, the rest of the day is spent sleeping... at theaters, lectures, social gatherings, once even at a stop light...Stimulants from coffee to adrenaline... only exacerbate the Parkinson's and cause more problems than relief.
>
> —Witness, Commission Hearing, Chicago, IL

> It is estimated that about 60-90 percent of patients seeking medical treatment for Parkinson's disease have complaints of poor sleep yet sleep disturbances and subsequent daytime dysfunction are not even mentioned in neurology textbooks as a symptom of PD...Both the patient...and the caretaker...share chronic sleep deprivation and this inevitably results in poor daytime working performance and well-being of a caretaker, who is usually a breadwinner for the family as well.
>
> —Witness, Commission Hearing, Chicago, IL

Sleep disturbances are common in patients suffering from neurological disorders that cause dementia, and are a major contributing factor in the decision by caregivers to institutionalize such patients. Disordered sleep behavior, such as "sundowning," or unpredictable wandering and vocalization, is difficult to manage in the home and

often leads to institutionalization. These behaviors are equally difficult to manage in the nursing home, often leading to increased use of
physical and chemical restraints, with potentially serious cognitive,
psychological, physical, and economic sequelae. However, at present,
an ideal, broadly-effective drug therapy with minimal side effects does
not exist. The efficacy of the few drugs now available has not been
studied in this patient population; non-somatic approaches, such as
phototherapy, similarly, have been neglected.

The effect of chronic pain on sleep, and the effect of sleep loss on
chronic pain create a vicious cycle that compounds disability. Health
care needs, drug dependency, and need for social support services are
increased; productivity at home and in the workplace is compromised.
Scientific advances and treatments to alleviate sleep dysfunction in
these syndromes do exist. However, the inadequate translation of this
knowledge to practicing clinicians and to the public can lead to dismissal
of those afflicted as malingerers, hypochondriacs or depressives. Improved and increased public and professional education should help
dispel myths and prejudices about patients afflicted with chronic painful disorders that interfere with sleep.

Sleep Disorders Associated with Pulmonary and Cardiovascular Disease

A variety of pulmonary and cardiovascular disorders are affected
by and affect sleep disturbances. Asthma is a common respiratory
condition, frequently associated with worsening symptoms at night.
Evidence suggests that, in a substantial number of patients, asthma
attacks may worsen during sleep. In a recent study of asthmatics, 39
percent of individuals reported respiratory symptoms every night; 64
percent had symptoms at least three times a week. Mortality rates
for asthma continue to climb. Despite improvements in treatment, 70
percent of deaths occur during normal sleeping hours. Nocturnal
symptoms of asthma are believed to be related to the narrowing of
the airway during sleep. However, information about the pathogenesis, etiology, and treatment of nocturnal asthma is limited. Circadian changes in hormones and other neurologically active agents have
been implicated in the pathogenesis of nocturnal asthma Careful attention must be paid to the phasing of the medications to achieve
nighttime relief. Asthma is especially common in children; disturbances of sleep may well be the link between childhood asthma and
learning disabilities.

Chronic obstructive pulmonary disease (chronic bronchitis and emphysema) and interstitial lung disease also impede sleep. In both cases, oxygen desaturation can occur, compromising the ability to sleep. In addition, the decrease of respiratory drive associated with sleep exacerbates the diminution of oxygen in the blood, setting up a vicious cycle.

A significant proportion of death and illness attributed to cardiovascular disorders actually may be a result of obstructive sleep apnea (OSA). The prevalence of hypertension among OSA patients is so high that OSA syndrome itself becomes a possible risk factor for hypertension. Additionally, both myocardial infarction and cardiac arhythmias have been found to be more common in patients suffering from OSA. Sleep apnea patients have twice the prevalence of hypertension, three times as much heart disease, and four times as much cerebrovascular disease than is found in the normal population.

Sleep Disorders Associated with Mental and Addictive Disorders

Within any six-month period, one in five Americans suffers from a mental or addictive disorder. Commonly, sleep disturbances are associated with these disorders and may influence their development, course, and treatment. Prevalent in nearly all mental illnesses, sleep disturbances differ among specific mental and substance abuse disorders, although particular clusters of sleep problems may characterize a variety of mental disorders. These alterations in sleep function change across the lifespan and also may vary with gender. Sleep disturbances of specific kinds may provide markers of biological processes contributing to the development of certain mental illnesses. The treatment of sleep abnormalities may improve the management of mental illnesses and substance abuse disorders; conversely, the treatment of the mental illness may significantly improve the sleep disturbance. Individuals reporting abnormal sleep patterns frequently are found to be suffering from a primary psychiatric disorder such as schizophrenia, Alzheimer's disease, depression, or adjustment disorder.

An NIMH study of sleep disturbances and psychiatric disorders found that nearly half of those with insomnia or hypersomnia suffered from a mental disorder. In contrast, those with no sleep complaint infrequently had a mental disorder. The combination of sleep problems, and mental and addictive disorders costs millions of dollars in lost productivity, medical costs, accidents, lost educational opportunities among the young, and long-term care expenses among the elderly.

Depression, anxiety, alcoholism, and drug abuse affect more than one-third of the population. In addition stress related disorders are at least as common. Each of these conditions adversely affects sleep. One of the cardinal features of depression is insomnia. While this association has been known for over 100 years, it has recently been shown sleep loss itself can produce depression. It is common for the overworked person who obtains insufficient sleep to feel irritable the next day, but if the sleep loss persists, chronic depression can occur.

—Witness, Commission Hearing, Pittsburgh, PA

Twelve million Americans suffer from depression, with annual costs to our society of $10 billion per year. Sleep plays an important role in the onset, course, and treatment of this very prevalent and painful illness. Sleep disturbances may herald the onset of mood disorders; the majority of these patients suffer from early morning awakening, difficulty falling asleep, and, for some, excessive sleepiness. Patients may engage in self-medication of their sleep disturbances, using alcohol or sedative-hypnotic drugs, leading to further disruption in the sleep-wake cycle and deepening depression. Recent research strongly suggests that persistent insomnia is a risk factor for the subsequent development of depression; the treatment of sleep disturbances in mood disorder patients may itself be an opportunity for preventive mental health care.

Disturbed sleep is a prominent feature of manic-depressive illness—bipolar disorder—that affects one million Americans. Sleep manipulation may alter the course of this disorder. For example, sleep loss may trigger symptoms in certain patients in remission, and temporarily may alleviate depression and even induce mania in those who are depressed.

About three percent of the population suffer from chronic low-grade depression called dysthyrnia, a disorder characterized by periods of too much sleep or, less commonly, insomnia. Even when clinical symptoms of acute depression largely are absent, the sleep abnormalities persist; this continued aberrant sleep may represent a physiological "vulnerability" to new severe depressive episodes. Seasonal affective disorder, a depressive illness in which patients suffer from diminished energy, hypersomnia, overeating and other depressive symptoms, appears to be alleviated by treatment with phototherapy—bright light treatment.

323

Most people have little awareness of the importance of sleep in maintaining mental health. It is commonly assumed that productive people sleep less, and if one can get by on less sleep that is laudatory....These are incorrect assumptions.

—Witness, Commission Hearing, Portland, OR

Insomnia and sleep disruption are common features of the psychoses, including schizophrenia, a disorder that alone affects over two million Americans over the course of their lifetimes and represents the diagnosis of 40 percent of all hospitalized psychiatric patients in the United States. Reduced sleep efficiency actually may precede psychotic episodes, and some aspects of sleep may remain abnormal, even when the disease is in remission. Medication may help to regulate the sleep-wake cycle and increase sleep efficiency in people suffering from psychotic disorders.

Sixteen million Americans suffer from anxiety disorders, the most prevalent mental health problem in the United States. Insomnia is a common complaint. Moreover, depression and substance abuse often coexist in patients suffering from these disorders, further complicating accurate diagnosis and treatment. One type of anxiety disorder, panic disorder, afflicts two percent of Americans and is characterized by discrete periods of intense fear or discomfort, accompanied by unpleasant physical symptoms—including chest pain, rapid and pounding heartbeats, and sweating—that occur unexpectedly and for which there is no associated medical explanation. While the secondary complications in response to daytime-wake panic attacks have been recognized for many years, only within the past several years have we learned that many panic disorder patients also suffer from nocturnal panic attacks, characterized by sudden awakening and the onset of typical symptoms coupled with difficulty returning to sleep.

Sleep disturbances, particularly recurrent dream anxiety episodes, may be the hallmark of post-traumatic stress disorder, an anxiety disorder that affects as many as 20 percent of wounded Vietnam veterans and also affects people suffering other traumatic experiences, such as sexual abuse or a natural disaster.

Addictive disorders take a tremendous toll on our society and involve over 20 million people. Alcohol use is particularly pernicious. Although alcohol initially promotes sleep, it later may disrupt and fragment sleep. In alcoholism, sleep abnormalities appear not only during bouts of drinking, but also during the acute, subacute, and chronic abstinence syndrome. Insomnia, hypersomnia, circadian disturbances, and parasomnias all may occur. Ironically, many substance abusers relate that concern about sleep provided part of the motivation for initial substance use, patterns of continued use, and fears about cessation of use.

Unfortunately, no well-established treatment is now available for sleep disturbances in the chronically abstinent alcoholic. Addictive disorders also affect the sleep of others. The newborns of drug addicted mothers and infants suffering from fetal alcohol syndrome suffer from aberrant sleep patterns themselves.

Increased understanding of sleep and disturbances of sleep that are associated with mental and addictive disorders has considerable potential to advance both our understanding of mental illness and the clinician's ability to diagnose, treat, and prevent these disabling disorders that afflict over 40 million Americans.

Chapter 42

Sleep Cycles and Mood Disorders

The cycle of waking and sleeping, one of the fundamental biological rhythms of our lives, is also one of the most telling indicators of disturbed behavioral regulation. Studying sleep patterns helps to define and explain normal sleep, sleep disorders, and the sleep disturbances seen in some mental disorders. It also shows that sleep is part of broader rhythms that involve a person's body chemistry, mental outlook, behavior, and emotion all interacting with changes in the physical and social environment.

The need for sleep is powerfully motivating, as any sleepy person will testify, and it is a prime example of rhythmic factors that determine behavior. Although sleep can be temporarily postponed, it cannot be delayed for long. Behavioral research has shown that when rats are totally deprived of sleep, they die within 2 to 3 weeks almost as rapidly as they would if deprived of food.

Pioneering research using physiological monitoring in sleep laboratories during the past few decades has uncovered the normal stages of sleep, identified a variety of sleep pathologies, and developed many treatments to address those sleep disorders. We now know that sleep is not simply a state of unconsciousness punctuated by dreams; rather, it a regular procession of rhythmic cycles and stages.

Five major sleep stages have been identified in humans, each with a different pattern of muscle tone and electrical activity in the cortex. Dreaming usually occurs in the fifth stage (dubbed "rapid-eye-movement (REM)" sleep because during it, the eyes quickly move back

Excerpted from NIH Pub. No. 96-3682, 1995.

327

and forth under closed lids). Although sleepers are immobile during REM sleep (except for isolated finger or facial twitches), their heart rate and respiration both become irregular, and their brains become very active.

In mood disorders such as manic-depressive illness or clinical depression, the normal patterns of sleep and its stages are often altered. People with clinical depression often wake up involuntarily in the early hours of the morning and cannot return to sleep. Even when they do sleep, the structure of sleep is often abnormal; they tend to enter the REM sleep stage much sooner after falling asleep than do other people.

Among people with manic-depressive illness, the pattern of sleep disturbance varies with the phase of their disorder. In episodes of depression, they are typically very tired and sleep excessively; in episodes of mania, they are dynamos of activity and barely sleep. These dramatic changes have led many researchers to view this illness as a disorder of the multiple biological clocks or "pacemakers" that regulate brain and body rhythms especially the sleep-wake cycle.

Recent research findings suggest that the circadian pacemaker, which regulates cycles that recur daily, is indeed unstable; it is constantly resetting itself to a slightly different time in patients with manic-depressive illness. The pacemaker also seems to be readily disrupted in patients with clinical depression. Levels of the hormone melatonin, which is normally secreted in response to messages from the body's major timekeeper, are lower in their brains than in the brains of other people.

Whether the sleep disturbances are causes or symptoms of these disorders remains to be seen. However, several kinds of sleep treatment have been shown to improve the mood of depressed patients, at least temporarily. These treatments include total or partial sleep deprivation and shifting the sleep period (such as moving an 11 PM-7 AM sleep period to 5 PM-1 AM). Research has shown that the timing of sleep may be more important for these patients than the total time spent sleeping. Other studies confirm that treatment with bright light, which is presumed to stabilize the circadian pacemaker, offers another therapeutic option for some patients whose mood disorders, such as seasonal affective disorder or "winter depression," appear to be linked to seasonal variations in daylight.

Chapter 43

Sleep Research: Mental and Addictive Disorders

Overview

Mental illnesses are among the most widespread, destructive and costly public health problems in the United States. Nineteen percent of the adult US population suffers from a diagnosable mental or substance use disorder within any six-month period (Robins and Regier 1991). The direct and indirect costs to our society from these illnesses is estimated at $273 billion a year (Rice et al. 1990).

Sleep disturbances—deviations from normal sleep patterns—accompany many mental illnesses and may influence their development and course. Poor sleep is widely prevalent in our society and has been reported in as many as 25-30 percent of the population (Ford and 1989). Sleep disturbances affect performance, cognitive capacity, and other significant aspects of daily life. Researchers have found that women, widowed and divorced persons, unemployed individuals and those of lower economic status report higher rates of disturbed sleep than others in the general population (Ford and Kamerow 1989). Life stresses—around family issues, age, work or economic condition—may precipitate sleep disturbances that, if not treated, may become exacerbated and, in some instances, may trigger a more serious mental disorder. The closely intertwined relationship between sleep disturbances

From *Wake Up America: A National Sleep Alert*, Volume 1, Executive Summary and Executive Report, Report of the National Commission on Sleep Disorders Research, Submitted to the United States Congress and to the Secretary U.S. Department of Health and Human Services, January 1993.

and mental disorders knows no age, socioeconomic, race or ethnic distinction. The combination of mental and addictive disorders and sleep disturbances cost millions of dollars in lost productivity, medical costs, accidents, lost educational opportunities among the young, and long-term care expenses for the elderly.

Sleep disturbances differ among psychiatric diagnoses, although particular clusters of specific sleep problems may characterize a variety of mental disorders. Furthermore, the sleep disturbances associated with mental illnesses are often subject to a developmental progression and, thus, may differ across the lifespan. Gender, too, may account for significant differences in these sleep findings. For example, the menstrual cycle has been found to affect circadian rhythms and sleep. Additionally, sleep disturbances of specific kinds may provide markers of biological processes contributing to the development of mental illnesses and substance abuse disorders; conversely, in certain disorders, the sleep disturbances themselves may cause or contribute to the psychiatric manifestations. The treatment of sleep disturbances may aid in, or improve the management of, mental illnesses and substance abuse disorders. Finally, primary sleep disorders may have significant psychiatric comorbidity that needs to be evaluated. Therefore, sleep has an important role in at least four areas relevant to mental illness: etiology, diagnosis, treatment and prevention.

If most psychiatric and substance abuse disorders are accompanied by sleep disturbances, the converse also can be true. Individuals reporting abnormal sleep patterns are frequently found to be suffering from a primary psychiatric disorder, such as schizophrenia, Alzheimer's disease, adjustment disorders, or depressive illness. The National Institute of Mental Health Epidemiologic Catchment Area (ECA) study of sleep disturbances and psychiatric disorders (Ford and Kamerow 1989) found that 40.4 percent of those with insomnia (too little sleep) and 46.5 percent of those with hypersomia (too much sleep) suffered from a mental disorder. In contrast, only 16.4 percent of those with no sleep complaint had a psychiatric problem. Kamerow and Ford found that study respondents who had insomnia at both the baseline interview and a follow-up interview a year later were far more likely to develop a new major depressive episode than were those whose sleep disturbance had been resolved by the second interview. This study and other recent research suggest that abnormal alterations in sleep may be predictive of the onset of certain mental disorders.

Thus, an understanding of sleep and disturbances of sleep that arise concomitant with mental and addictive disorders has considerable potential to advance both our understanding of mental illness and our ability to diagnose, treat and, ultimately, prevent these disorders. Unfortunately, the study of sleep disturbances among those with mental illness and substance abuse disorders is seriously underfunded, understaffed, and, consequently, underexplored. This chapter provides an overview of the state-of-the-art research into the relationship between sleep and mental and addictive disorders, highlighting the progress to date; it concludes with suggestions about promising prospects for future study, underscoring the urgent need for public policy that will facilitate research in this field to the end of the 20th century and beyond.

Sleep and Specific Mental and Addictive Disorders

Schizophrenia and Other Psychotic Disorders

Psychoses, including schizophrenia (one of the most severe and intractable of psychiatric disorders) are a large group of illnesses that involve disturbances of thought, language and communication, perception, affect and behavior. Reality may be misinterpreted; delusions and hallucinations are common. Behavior may be withdrawn, regressive and bizarre, and social and work functioning are severely impaired. Schizophrenia affects over two million Americans over the course of their lifetimes; approximately 40 percent of all hospitalized psychiatric patients in the U.S. suffer from diagnosed schizophrenia (National Advisory Mental Health Council 1988). Indeed, schizophrenia results in a greater loss of total years of expected life than any other psychiatric disorder. Treatment costs for schizophrenia exceed $7 billion annually, and indirect costs account for at least twice that figure (National Advisory Mental Health Council 1988). Ten to 15 percent of all schizophrenics end their lives by suicide (Blumenthal 1988). Insomnia and excessive sleepiness are common features of the psychoses and add to the considerable suffering and human misery imparted by schizophrenia and other severe psychotic disorders.

Dreaming has some similarities to psychosis. Dream sleep is a state in which hallucinations, perceptual distortions, bizarre thinking and temporary delusions are intimately mixed with more normal thought and perceptual processes. This similarity led to the speculation some twenty-five years ago that schizophrenia is an intrusion of the dream state into wakefulness. Indeed, the NIMH's first area of involvement in sleep and mental disorders centered around this potential relationship between dreaming during sleep and hallucinations in schizophrenia. The hope engendered by the early discovery of the association between dreaming and REM sleep was that schizophrenia was an intrusion into wakefulness or at least that REM sleep was abnormal in schizophrenics (Dement 1955). Intense study has suggested that there are no unique or specific disturbances of REM sleep variables in the baseline sleep of schizophrenics. Furthermore, the related hypothesis that REM or sleep deprivation might precipitate schizophrenia has not been supported; the majority of the literature suggests that such deprivation often activates sleep within a normal baseline and might precipitate hypomania or mania in those predisposed to bipolar disorder (Vogel et al. 1980).

However, a recent meta-analysis of a large number of studies comparing sleep variables in schizophrenic and mood disorder patients suggest that both groups have low REM latency (Benca et al. 1992). Studies of severe depressive disorder based on these findings have suggested a potential genetic relationship between depression and this particular form of sleep dysfunction (see discussion below). These studies require further replication. Unfortunately, similar genetic studies have not been undertaken with regard to schizophrenia.

Acute psychosis and chronic schizophrenia are often associated with significant sleep disruption, generally characterized by severe difficulty in initiating sleep. Because of major disruptions of sleep-wake timing, there may be other rhythm disturbances, e.g., meals may be taken at odd times. The patient may suffer from hyperactivity resulting from anxiety and preoccupation with delusions and hallucinations. Patients so agitated may remain awake until exhaustion overtakes them; for some, day and nighttime patterns become inverted. Even in remission, some aspects of sleep may remain abnormal, such as reduction in slow wave sleep.

Reduced sleep efficiency may actually precede psychotic episodes and may accompany the acute exacerbation of psychotic symptoms. Among those suffering from schizophrenia, sleep efficiency may be more compromised during periods of exacerbation (van Kammen et al. 1986). For some patients, adequate antipsychotic medications may regulate the sleep-wake cycle and increase sleep efficiency.

A panoply of research opportunities that may shed light on the potential relationship between sleep and schizophrenia exist. Much work needs to be done to determine whether or not the sleep dysfunction identified in schizophrenia represents a marker for a trait that may predispose to this illness. The ability to identify those at risk of this highly disruptive, highly disabling disorder may help prevent suffering and potentially move the research field one step closer to identifying better clinical methods to treat, control, and, ultimately, eliminate this devastating disorder.

In order to pursue these goals, a useful general strategy may be the longitudinal study of sleep in adolescents genetically at risk for schizophrenia. The central question is whether adolescents at risk for schizophrenia develop abnormalities of sleep architecture, particularly slow wave sleep, before the explicit onset of the first episode. Slow wave sleep deficits may be markers for an abnormal brain development process. To investigate this relationship requires the longitudinal study of sleep and brain imaging (CT or MRI) during the second decade of life. Such an approach exemplifies the investigation of sleep as a marker of vulnerability to mental disorders and, as such, cuts across several diagnostic boundaries. If these studies show that trait dominates state, then some permanent underlying mechanism is implied. With that mechanism in hand, science may be advanced markedly in its understanding of these most serious of mental disorders.

The Affective Disorders

Thirteen million Americans suffer from depression. The annual financial burden of depression and other affective disorders is estimated to be more than $ 10 billion. Another $4.2 billion in potential earning power lost (not to mention the toll in human suffering) due to premature death from suicide (Rice and Miller 1991) because 15 percent of people with severe depression commit suicide (Blumenthal 1988). A recent study examining six major medical conditions— including hypertension, diabetes, lung diseases and arthritis—found only severe heart disease to be associated with more disabling interruption of daily functioning than depression (Wells et al. 1989).

The affective disorders are characterized by a prominent and persistent disturbance of mood (depression or mania) and a full syndrome of associated symptoms, including changes in appetite, weight, sleep, libido, self-esteem, interest in daily activities and cognitive functions. These disorders are usually episodic; recent research has suggested they arise from a low-grade chronic depressive base (Akiskal 1983). Depressive disorders represent a spectrum of illnesses. They are not the everyday "blues" that we all experience after a loss or disappointment, but are disabling illnesses that interfere with how one perceives the world and performance. Mood disorders include bipolar disorder, major depressive disorder, cyclothymia and dysthymia. Bipolar disorders are characterized by cycling between periods of depression and elation, often showing a seasonal pattern. Major depression—sometimes known as "unipolar' disorder—manifests with a persistent sad mood and clusters of symptoms that may recur. Dysthymia and cyclothymia are more chronic, less severe forms of affective disorder, but appear to manifest the same types of sleep disturbances associated with more severe mood disorders.

As noted elsewhere in this article, ECA data have suggested that sleep disturbances may represent risk factors that herald the onset of affective disorders (Ford and Kamerow 1989). Two separate sleep disturbance patterns appear to occur in patients with mood disorders. Typically, individuals with major depression suffer from difficulty falling asleep, trouble maintaining sleep, and problems with premature awakening. They often complain of nocturnal restlessness and tired feelings. Patients in the manic phase of bipolar disorder, however, suffer from sleep onset insomnia and short sleep duration. Interestingly, they often do not complain about the lack of sleep. Affective disorder patients may engage in self-medication of their sleep disturbances by using alcohol or sedative-hypnotic drugs. This may lead to further disruptions in the sleep-wake cycle.

A recent meta-analysis evaluating the scientific literature on mental illness and sleep disorders lends further credence to the finding that sleep, in fact, may be an indicator of major depression, the most prevalent of the affective disorders (Knowles and MacLean 1990; Benca et al. 1992). The sleep abnormalities occur in inpatients as well as outpatient populations of depressives (Hudson et al. 1982). To date, the vast majority of research has focused on the pathophysiology concurrent with or underlying acute clinical signs and symptoms. If a linkage between depression and sleep dysfunction is to be validated scientifically, it is important to evaluate issues of sleep dysfunction both during, before and after a depressive episode. Further research may disclose whether it is possible to determine the likelihood of either a past history of affective disorder or predict the development of such a disorder based upon sleep-related data.

Unipolar Depression

Recent family studies of sleep and depression are beginning to shed light on the role REM latency may have in the development and course of unipolar depression (Giles et al. 1988; Giles et al. 1989). REM latency, the interval from sleep onset to the first period of rapid eye movement sleep (the so-called dream state) has been found to be shortened not only in patients suffering from unipolar depression, but in first-degree relatives of those patients as well. Indeed, "the relative risk for unipolar depression among relatives with reduced REM latency was almost three times greater than for relatives with non-reduced REM latency" (Giles et al. 1988; Giles et al. 1989). However, the question arises whether the same sleep dysfunctions occur in other mental disorders. If so, the power of the findings regarding affective disorder is diminished. In contrast, if REM latency reduction is restricted to those with current or past affective disorder, then these findings regarding first-degree relatives suggests that reduced REM latency may be a vulnerability marker specific to affective disorders. To examine this hypothesis further, family history should be evaluated in any future studies in the field.

REM sleep disturbance is but one of a constellation of findings that characterize the sleep of depressive patients during the acute stages of their illness. As mentioned earlier, the majority of such patients suffer from wakefulness or difficulty falling asleep. While younger depressive patients often report difficulty falling asleep, middle-aged and older depressive patients are more likely to complain of difficulty maintaining sleep, including early morning awakenings. This range of complaints suggests an age-dependent continuum in affective disorder. Indeed, the sleep changes that characterize depression may also occur, to a lesser extent, during the course of normal aging as well. Studies of both the young and the old lend further support to the concept of an interaction between aging and disease in determining the sleep abnormalities of depression. However, for more careful delineation of differences in the manifestation of sleep dysfunction in depressed patients across the lifespan, it is necessary to undertake further research into the sleep patterns in the normal population across the life cycle.

Since one of the biologic changes in and frequently experienced symptoms of depression is alteration in sleep patterns, this set of measures should continue to represent a major focus of both basic and clinical investigation. It has been suggested that EEG sleep analyses offer a unique quantitative opportunity to uncover a CNS 'signature' of depressive disorders (Kupfer and Ehlers 1989). With that "signature," it may be possible to determine who may be of heightened vulnerability to affective disorders in general and to depression, in particular. Additionally, recent research shows persistent abnormalities in the sleep of remitted depressed patients (Kupfer et al. 1988).

Most antidepressant medications have similar effects on the sleep disturbance in depression: they facilitate falling asleep and enhance sleep continuity; they acutely suppress REM sleep and prolong REM latency; and they increase early slow wave activity during the first NREM sleep period (Kupfer et al. 1989). Many subtypes of depression appear to be associated with nocturnal hyperarousal, as evidenced by decreased sleep continuity, decreased slow wave or deep sleep (particularly early in the night), and increased REM sleep. Thus, many antidepressant medications appear to decrease these symptoms, suggesting that the efficacy of many antidepressant therapies may depend upon decreasing arousal in a way that permits restitution of slow wave sleep, particularly early in the night, and that suppresses REM sleep.

Further research into the effects of nonpharmacologic therapies for depression on sleep and sleep-wake rhythms is necessary. For example, nonpharmacologic treatment approaches that stabilize sleep-wake rhythms may have particular value in the long-term management of patients. Additionally, studies have suggested that sleep deprivation has an antidepressant effect in some patients.

Bipolar Disorder

Bipolar disorder (also known as manic-depressive illness) is characterized by alternating periods of mania (highs) and depression (lows). During manic episodes, patients display euphoric or irritable mood, hyperactivity, grandiosity, paranoia, other delusions, and poor judgment. During depressive episodes, they exhibit sadness and loss of interest, often complaining of decreased energy, poor concentration and feelings of worthlessness. Depressive episodes in bipolar disordered patients tend to be similar to those experienced by individuals with major depression (with the possible exception that the slowing of motor activity (known as psychomotor retardation) and excessive sleep (hypersomnia) are more commonly observed in younger bipolar depressives (Detre 1972).

Bipolar disorder affects one percent of Americans, occurs equally in men and women, and usually has its onset between the ages of 15 and 40 (Goodwin and Jamieson 1990). As in unipolar depression, disturbed sleep is a prominent feature of both manic and depressive episodes. With the "highs" and "lows" of bipolar disorder, both insomnia and hypersomia, respectively, are common. It has been found that sleep manipulation may alter the course of bipolar disorder. For example, sleep loss may trigger symptoms of mania or hypomania in certain bipolar patients who are in remission, and may alleviate depression and even induce mania in bipolar patients who are depressed (Wehr 1989).

However, in contrast to the large number of studies of sleep in major depression, the field has undertaken little systematic study of sleep in bipolar disorders, particularly during the manic state. The limited data available (Hudson et al. 1992) suggest that mania (and its milder variant, hypomania) may be associated with the same disturbed sleep continuity and REM measures found by those studying patients suffering from unipolar depression. Studies focusing on sleep disturbances among patients with bipolar depression, however, have yielded inconsistent findings. It remains unclear to what extent the sleep disturbances in bipolar depression may be similar to those encountered in unipolar depression. Virtually no research has evaluated the potential relationship between sleep changes in bipolar disorder and other mental disorders. For example, since patients with bipolar disorder commonly exhibit psychotic symptoms—most often hallucinations and delusions—comparison of the sleep disturbances in bipolar disorder and psychotic disorders such as schizophrenia, might yield fruitful findings.

Further exploration of the relationship between sleep disturbances and affective disorders should include an increased effort devoted to bipolar illness. If, as suggested in depressive disorders, sleep disturbances may be predictive of new bipolar illness episodes, the treatment or even preventive options could be expanded considerably; the toll in human suffering might be reduced significantly.

Dysthymic Disorders and Other Related Disorders

As many as 3.3 percent of the population suffer from low-grade chronic affective disorders (i.e., dysthymic and related disorders) (Regier et al. 1988). These disorders account for at least half of all those with affective disorders at any point in time or one-third of the affectively ill over a lifetime. Lacking the acute exacerbations typical in "classical" affective disorders, individuals with these subtypes of depressive disorders nevertheless frequent the medical care system (Weissman et al. 1988) and suffer disability comparable in severity to chronic physical conditions (Wells et al. 1989).

Dysthymia itself typically begins in childhood or adolescence and then continues a lifelong course of low-grade chronicity. Presenting complaints include chronic fatigue, "being depressed all the time," periods of hypersomnia (too much sleep), poor concentration, and, less commonly, insomnia (Akiskal 1983). The sleep EEG findings in theses patients generally parallel those of major affective disorders, thereby supporting the link between chronic and major forms of affective illness. However much research needs to be conducted on how to distinguish dysthymia from personality disturbances.

Sleep disorders also arise in patients recovering from major depressive episodes. Recovery does not always occur within a few months. In fact, depressive symptoms may linger for many months, even years, in one out of every three patients (Akiskal 1983). This is particularly true for those who have experienced a single depressive episode after age 40. Another group of such "recovering" patients may actually suffer from ongoing depressive episodes; the residuum of such successive episodes may eventually coalesce into chronic low-grade depression. Sleep research on patients with such residual depression have shown that while relevant clinical symptoms of acute depression are largely absent, the sleep abnormalities persist. It is possible that this continued aberrant sleep may serve as a physiological "vulnerability" to new severe depressive episodes. However, as is the case with sleep disturbances in severe depressive illness, substantial research will be necessary to confirm this potential link between sleep and residual depression.

At the clinical level, sleep clinicians and mental health professionals who serve as consultants to primary care settings should pay particular attention to the issue of chronic insomnia of adult onset; such a sleep disorder may actually reflect the presence of chronic depression. Unless expertly questioned, patients may not provide the health professional with a history of a major depressive episode. Alcohol abuse or overuse of sedatives may further mask the affective origins of the insomnia (Akiskal 1982).

Cyclothymia, a milder form of bipolar disorder, manifests in an alternating pattern of short depressive and hypomanic periods. To date, no formal sleep studies have been undertaken on this disorder. Nonetheless, clinical studies (Akiskal et al. 1977; Akiskal 1979) have shown a similar changing pattern of periods of hypersomnia and decreased sleep need. These sleep disturbances, in turn, are associated with substance abuse, alternating between the use of "uppers" and "downers." Because of the diagnostic overlap between cyclothymia and borderline conditions, coupled with the fact that borderline sleep is similar to that of depressives (Akiskal et al. 1985), it has been suggested that the sleep of cyclothymics probably parallels that of persons suffering from bipolar disorders. Hence, the provocative possibility arises that treatments found effective in bipolar disorder might prove equally effective for cyclothymia and its attendant sleep and substance abuse problems. Indeed, recent studies (Steinberg 1989; Mirin et al. 1991) have shown high rates of dysthymia and cy-

clothymia in polysubstance abusers. Given its public health significance, this lead should be followed up in more systematic study.

Because different mechanisms seem to underlie the sleep abnormalities found in the heterogeneous group of the chronic affective
disorders, the sleep disturbances may aid in differential diagnosis as
well as provide new insights into the pathophysiology of these disorders. Sleep research in this area must vigorously continue, since a
better understanding of the disturbed circadian patterns of these conditions may lead to promising treatment strategies.

Further epidemiologic and treatment research addressing the overlap of chronic insomnia and chronic depression is needed. The NIMH
ECA studies have suggested that persistent insomnia is a risk factor
for the subsequent development of depression, and the treatment of
sleep disturbance may itself be an opportunity for preventive mental
health care (Ford and Kamerow 1989). The value of non-pharmacologic approaches to chronic insomnia, such as sleep restriction therapy
and strengthened stability of sleep-wake rhythms, needs to be evaluated as a primary or adjunctive therapy in patients with dysthymia
and other mood disorders.

Seasonal Affective Disorder

Seasonal affective disorder (SAD) is a mood disorder occurring in
the winter months, characterized by diminished energy, hypersomnia, overeating, and other depressive symptoms. It is now generally
accepted that bright light administered at the onset or the end of sleep
exerts an antidepressant effect on patients with winter seasonal affective disorder (Rosenthal et al. 1984). Studies are needed to explore
the mechanisms by which this effect is exerted. Because of the difficulty in designing an adequate placebo control, it has been difficult
to rule out a placebo effect. Renewed efforts to develop an appropriate environmental placebo control should be a high priority in this
area of research. Studies also need to focus on the effects of bright
light on general levels of alertness and on the underlying circadian
rhythms of temperature and sleep in order to determine if these effects on biology are critical to antidepressant efficacy. Such research
embodies the increased focus on the mechanisms of action of antidepressant interventions, to test the general hypothesis that effects on
sleep and sleep-wake rhythms are crucial to the antidepressant effect.

As a whole, sleep research in affective illness has produced exciting leads
over the past decade. Progress in conceptual and methodologic areas has
yielded new insight into the abnormalities of sleep in depression, new

information about the potential use of sleep disturbances as a predictor of vulnerability to affective disorder, and new data about some of the specific "internal clock' related disturbances of depression. One of the major challenges for the field in the next decade will be to integrate biologic and psychologic concepts of the etiology of depression. Another area of fruitful investigation is to advance the understanding of the specific changes in the brain related to depression and antidepressant response through the use of new brain imaging techniques that allow quantification and identification of changes in brain metabolism during illness and recovery (e.g., PET, etc.). Such an integration of structural and functional studies may help elucidate the specific role sleep may play in mediating the course or even the manifestation of the affective disorders.

Anxiety Disorders

According to recent epidemiological studies, the anxiety disorders—including panic disorder, post-traumatic stress disorder, generalized anxiety disorder, and phobias—represent the most prevalent mental health problem in the United States. Approximately 16 million Americans suffer from one or more anxiety disorders, a significant proportion of whom experience severe distress resulting in work and social disability (Regier et al. 1988). Many of these disorders may be precipitated in childhood and an increasing body of research suggests that early forerunners of adult anxiety syndromes may develop in childhood. Comorbid conditions such as depression, avoidance behavior (social withdrawal), and alcohol or drug abuse are commonly associated with the anxiety disorders. Post-traumatic stress disorder (PTSD), too, has been established as a chronic disorder that can originate in childhood, since children are not immune from the trauma of natural disaster, victimization or other devastating events. Most, but not all, anxiety disorders appear to be associated with disturbances in sleep.

Insomnia is a common complaint of patients with primary anxiety disorders. Frequent awakenings occur either with or without anxiety dreams. Acute anxiety attacks or ruminative thinking may occur during periods of wakefulness while lying in bed, not only at sleep onset but also during awakening. Patients may express intense anxiety during the daytime about the inevitability of a poor night's sleep. Those in this category display chronic anxiety, with features that include trembling, muscle tension, restlessness, easy fatigability, shortness of breath, palpitations, tremor, sweating, dry mouth, dizziness, keyed up feelings, an exaggerated startle response, and difficulty in concentration. It is also a widely held notion among general medical practitioners that patients who have "problems falling asleep" are worried, anxious or undergoing stressful life events. Despite the almost universal assumption that anxiety and sleep disturbances are tightly linked in a causal manner, few studies have investigated sleep disorders systematically in patients with primary anxiety disorders.

Panic Disorder

Panic disorder is a mental illness afflicting one to two percent of Americans (Regier et al. 1988). It is characterized by discrete periods of intense fear or discomfort accompanied by several somatic symptoms that occur unexpectedly and for which there is no medical cause. The disorder is more common in women, usually beginning in young adulthood and has a chronic course. Typical symptoms of panic attacks include light-headedness, shortness of breath or choking sensations, numbness and tingling, hot or cold flashes, rapid and pounding heart, chest pain, sweating, changes in the intensity of light or sound, floating sensations, feelings of being unreal, and a fear of dying. The symptoms are so pronounced that it is not uncommon for these patients to be admitted to hospitals to rule out heart attacks or other life-threatening medical illnesses. If panic attacks continue to occur, many patients develop secondary avoidance behaviors and phobias. Up to 60 percent of panic disorder patients develop major depression.

While the secondary complications in response to daytime-wake panic attacks have been recognized for many years, it has only been within the past several years that we have learned that a similar pattern of impairment occurs in panic disorder patients who suffer from nocturnal-sleep panic attacks (Mellman and Uhde 1989a; Mellman and Uhde 1989b; Mellman and Uhde 1990; Uhde, in press). Episodes that occur during sleep are associated with a sudden awakening and the onset of typical symptoms (Hauri et al. 1989). The patient becomes agitated and has difficulty falling back to sleep. Patients with panic disorder may have marginally increased sleep latency and decreased sleep efficiency. Panic episodes tend to occur in NREM sleep, particularly at the transition from stage 2 to slow wave sleep. More rarely, the panic attack occurs at sleep onset. Despite frequent subjective complaints of insomnia by patients with panic disorder, only a small number of studies have evaluated the phenomenology and polysomnography of sleep in patients with this disabling condition.

341

Generalized Anxiety Disorder

Generalized anxiety disorder is diagnosed in patients who have persistent, pervasive, unrealistic or excessive anxiety, given the circumstances, and who have been worried about two or more life circumstances for at least six months. Patients with generalized anxiety disorder have many somatic complaints: sweating, irritability, feeling agitated or on edge, restlessness and fatigue. The majority of these patients also complain of insomnia; 30 percent of the time, the insomnia is of moderate to severe intensity (Uhde and Nemiah 1989). Additional research is required to delineate the prevalence, character and treatment of insomnia found in these patients. Additional research activity is required to determine whether electrophysiological or neuroendocrine correlates of poor sleep can be identified in these and other, patients with anxiety disorders.

Post-Traumatic Stress Disorder

One of the most perplexing of the anxiety disorders is post-traumatic stress disorder (PTSD), first brought to light in the wake of the Vietnam war. The Epidemiologic Catchment Area survey of the prevalence of a range of mental disorders in representative U.S. communities found that 20 percent of wounded Vietnam veterans had a history of post traumatic stress disorder (PTSD). The National Vietnam Veterans Readjustment Study found that the lifetime prevalence of PTSD is 30.6 percent among male Vietnam theater veterans (Kulka et al. 1990). PTSD also occurs after other traumatic experiences, such as sexual abuse or natural disaster. In marked contrast to the magnitude of the public health problems raised by PTSD is the dearth of information about the pathophysiology of the disorder. In general, PTSD is characterized by the re-experiencing of a traumatic event in the form of repetitive dreams, recurrent, intrusive daytime recollections, and dissociative flashback episodes. Some have suggested that the sleep disturbance associated with PTSD, including the recurrent dream anxiety episode, may be a "hallmark" of the disorder. This hypothesis follows from the observation that the particular sleep problems that are highly prevalent in PTSD are not typically seen in other mental disorders.

Yet, despite the likely importance of an understanding of disordered sleep in PTSD to disclosing the overall pathophysiology of the illness, few studies using polysomnography, the current best method for analyzing human sleep, have been conducted. Equally, few studies have investigated in detail the range of somatic and nonsomatic treatments for the disorder, notwithstanding its significantly high prevalence and high rates of excess disability and comorbidity.

Thus, some anxiety disorders have special sleep related symptoms, such as the abrupt and frightening arousals from sleep experienced by patients with panic and post-traumatic stress disorders. Methodological advances and innovative approaches to the study of these sleep-related phenomena are required to develop new treatments for these disabling conditions.

Currently, we have a poor understanding of the causes and treatments of the other types of sleep disturbances found in the anxiety disorders. It is unknown whether identical treatments are effective in waking and sleeping phenomena characteristic of an anxiety syndrome. It has been speculated that effective treatments during the wake state may actually worsen the same symptom during sleep. Clinical and epidemiological research is needed to address this notion and related questions in greater depth.

Although sleep panickers often become fearful of sleep and, as a consequence of the resultant sleep deprivation, experience a worsening of their clinical symptomatology, the role of acute or chronic sleep deprivation in the etiology or maintenance of the anxiety disorders is unknown. Clinical and basic science approaches to the study of sleep and sleep deprivation would be useful in identifying neurobiological systems that mediate the important biological functions of alarm and arousal. With etiological information of this nature in hand, development of appropriate interventions becomes more likely. An improved ability to diagnose and effectively treat abnormal anxiety states is pivotal for prevention, especially given that most anxiety conditions are thought to have their onset in late adolescence or early adulthood. It is possible that some sleep disturbances common in childhood might represent early expressions of the adult anxiety disorders. Research is required to answer this question. The prevention or early detection and treatment of the anxiety disorders will lead to marked improvement m the long-term quality of life and productivity of millions of Americans.

Eating Disorders

Anorexia nervosa and bulimia nervosa afflict 0.5-2 percent of the population having profound psychological and biological consequences (Halmi 1989). Ninety percent of cases occur in women; approximately 10 percent occur in males. Anorexia results in some of the highest mortality of any of the mental disorders. Anorexia nervosa is a mental disorder associated with dieting and abnormal preoccupation with food and body image. Bulimia nervosa is a disorder associated with binge eating and purging behavior.

Since the 1960s, the influences on sleep of nutritional status, nutrient intake and psychopathology associated with eating disorders such as anorexia nervosa and bulimia nervosa have been examined from several perspectives. Relatively little work has been published on nutrient intake and sleep; the majority of the work has focused on the effects of starvation and eating disorders on sleep behavior. To date, studies of otherwise healthy individuals whose diets have been severely restricted or regimented (Phillips et al. 1975; Lacey et al. 1978) have not determined whether dietary manipulations can change sleep parameters, and whether these changes are slight or of clinical significance. Research has not examined the potential effect of such dietary restriction on mental disorders that have been related to specific sleep dysregulation (e.g., depression may be associated with nutritionally imposed reduced REM latency). Little of the research on healthy populations has been undertaken with women subjects, a problem that should be rectified.

Several well-designed studies have examined sleep patterns of patients with anorexia nervosa (Walsh et al. 1985; Levy et al. 1988; Lauer et al. 1988). These studies suggest that there is not a strong relationship between anorexia nervosa and mood disorders, based on findings regarding reduced REM latency, now becoming a hallmark of depressive illness, as described elsewhere in this paper. However, to determine whether sleep dysfunction among anorexics alters with recovery, longitudinal studies over the course of treatment into remission would be helpful.

Similarly, a substantial number of excellent studies have been undertaken of patients with bulimia nervosa (Walsh et al. 1985; Hudson et al. 1987; Byrne et al. 1990) Taken together, these studies suggest that the sleep of bulimics does not differ substantially from that found in agematched normal controls. While comorbidity for symptoms of major depression is high, the sleep patterns of bulimics appear closer to normal than they are to those of patients with major depression (Hudson et al. 1987). An interesting subpopulation of patients with binge eating exhibit this behavior apparently only when sleep-walking. The comorbidity of this nocturnal binge eating with other mental and substance abuse disorders may be high, a finding requiring further study (Whyte et al. 1988; Schenck et al. 1989a). Moreover, the sleep patterns of this subgroup have not been adequately studied; such research must be undertaken if we are to characterize and understand this disorder fully.

At present, relatively little data are available on the influence of nutrient intake and subsequent sleep. The effects of normal metabolism as well as the effects of metabolic disturbances resulting from diseases like anorexia nervosa need to be better understood. It would be informative to study the sleep of these patients over time as their symptoms remit. The need for this type of clinical study is underscored by animal research into the metabolic effects of prolonged sleep deprivation. Prolonged sleep deprivation, particularly REM sleep deprivation in rats, is associated with the development of a hypercatabolic state in which the animal loses weight progressively, despite increasing food intake and may be fatal (Rechtshaffen 1989). Anorexia nervosa also offers an excellent opportunity to study sleep/energy relationships in the human.

Somatoform Disorders

As many as 11.6 percent of the population seek medical care for unexplained physical symptoms. Those with numerous somatic symptoms experience poor health and often are severely impaired in their day-to-day activities. They frequently experience anxiety and depressive symptoms (Walsh and Sugarman 1989) and often complain of sleep difficulties that are attributed to their mysterious ailments (Katon et al. 1991; Moldofsky 1989).

Somatoform disorders embrace a group of disturbances that are characterized by physical symptoms for which there is no acknowledged objective evidence of disease or physiologic disorder. Psychologic factors are presumed significant for the disorder (APA 1987). The mysterious complaints are grouped into a number of different categories for the purposes of nosology. They include disorders in which the patient is preoccupied with an imagined physical defect in which a particular physical function is lost or impaired, in which the patient is preoccupied with the fear or belief that he or she suffers from a serious disease, in which pain of no known etiology exists, and in which unexplained recurrent somatic complaints arise.

Of all unexplained physical symptoms, diffuse muscular pain, chronic fatigue and unrefreshing sleep have perplexed patients and physicians for a long time. For more than 85 years, rheumatologists have considered such people to have "fibrositis" because, initially, physicians believed that the disability was the result of an infection that affected the fibrous tissue of muscle. Eighty percent of those affected are young women in the prime of their lives (average age, approximately 40 years). The reason for this sex predilection is unknown. Twenty to 50 percent describe the onset of their symptoms following a nonphysically injurious industrial or automobile accident (Bennett 1989). Today, the diagnostic label now widely preferred in the U.S. is "fibromyalgia," a descriptive term that emphasizes the ubiquitous pain of fibrous tissue and muscle. Another newly-described condition closely related to fibromyalgia is "chronic fatigue syndrome," a disorder that has recently attracted considerable public and media attention.

In both disorders, patients usually complain of muscular chronic pain, profound physical fatigue and light, unrefreshing sleep. Such sleep disorders have been reported in between 76 and 95 percent of fibromyalgia and chronic fatigue syndrome patients (Moldofsky 1989; Goldenberg 1989). Both disorders take an untold cost on both the individual and the economy. Data suggest that 30 percent of fibromyalgia patients change jobs and 17 percent cease work altogether as the result of disability (Wolfe et al. 1988). Chronic fatigue syndrome also places an extraordinary burden on the health care system in costly diagnostic procedures, uncertain remedies, and disability payments. Losses to the workforce have not been estimated in the US, but are projected to be of major economic and social consequence.

Knowledge of the basic biologic mechanisms that affect sleep-wake behavior is fundamental to determining the causes of fibromyalgia and chronic fatigue syndrome. Better understanding of and potential intervention into the sleep dysfunctions in these and other somatoform disorders may help identify their prevalence, unravel their etiology and disclose potential treatments. In the meantime, it is critical that the medical profession, other health professionals and the public be educated to understand somatoform disorders in order to dispel the myths and prejudice associated with fibromyalgia and chronic fatigue syndrome. Because of ignorance about recent scientific advances about these syndromes and the contribution of sleepwake brain dysfunction to these disorders, those afflicted have been dismissed as malingerers or hypochondriacs. Additionally, clinicians must be trained to the importance of differential diagnosis, particularly in identifying the presence of underlying mental disorders, including depression, in order to ensure proper patient treatment.

Adjustment Disorders

Although most people adjust to upsetting events in their lives without developing psychiatric symptoms, others have a period of poorer functioning, whether at work or in their interactions with others. These responses are referred to as adjustment disorders. People who suffer from these disorders are likely to have a transient period of poor sleep as well. Persons who respond to stressful events with these disturbed waking and sleep reactions usually recover once the consequences of the precipitating event are resolved or corrected. Others, however, may develop a more serious mental disorder.

Adjustment disorders commonly are associated with a mood disturbance. During waking time, those with depressed mood may show tearfulness and express hopelessness. Their energy is lowered; they do not concentrate well. Those with anxious mood exhibit nervousness, worries and hyperalertness, changes that are known to be counterproductive to good sleep.

The nature of the sleep disturbance in adjustment sleep disorders is popularly known as insomnia, though in a small proportion of cases, stress can be followed by the opposite effect, a period of oversleeping. Most frequently the sleep is of poorer quality and of shorter duration than is typical for that individual, often including a delay in the onset of sleep, or an early morning awakening after which the patient is unable to return to sleep.

Little research has been conducted directly on this disorder, consequently, prevalence data is either anecdotal or deduced from information gathered for other study purposes. For example, in a study of 5,713 people, (Lugaresi et al. 1983) one question asked was "How often do you sleep well without using sleeping pills?" Those who responded "rarely" or "never" were rated as poor sleepers. A greater number of women (23.1 percent) than men (14.7 percent) fell into this group. The percentage of women who were poor sleepers increased dramatically with age, with 40 percent of those surveyed meeting this criterion at age 45 and up. Men, on the other hand, did not show an age-related increase in sleep difficulty until after the age of 60. When asked the reason for their poor sleep, the most common response was "worries." Among poor sleepers, family or work difficulties were identified in over 60 percent of the cases. Because the study did not evaluate whether the sleep difficulties emanated from a precipitating event, it is of limited value in evaluating the prevalence of adjustment disorders of sleep. We know only that sleep disturbances arise among those with ongoing worries about family and work, and that women appear more vulnerable to this sleep dysfunction than do men. The Epidemiologic Catchment Area survey provides somewhat more precise data (Ford and Kairnerow 1989). As described earlier in this paper, the study found that poor sleep that extended over the one year

347

penod between study initiation and follow-up might be an early warning sign of more serious psychiatric disorders than an adjustment disorder of sleep.

Two ongoing longitudinal laboratory studies are attempting to evaluate the impressions of previous work that detail the nature of both the sleep disturbance in adjustment disorders and the consequences these problems have on waking behavior (Reynolds et al. 1992; Cartwright and Wood 1991). Even if adjustment disorders of sleep are found to be highly transitory and self-limiting, they remain worthy of further research investigation; as sleep suffers, so does the capacity to function well the next day. As fatigue accumulates from poor sleep, it has been found that work performance is compromised. In such cases, the temptation is to induce sleep using a hypnotic medication, alcohol, or an over-the-counter preparation that may have some untoward health effects. Because each of these may become habitual, a psychological, if not physiological addiction may follow.

While the long-term effects associated with today's short-acting sleeping medications and over-the-counter sleep aids are not known, too often their use leads to long-term dependency. Thus, non-pharmacologic approaches to improving sleep depth and continuity should be tested for their efficacy in helping those suffering from this disorder. It is also important to specify the selection criteria for these interventions, since patients respond differently to various approaches. Students in all of the mental health disciplines should be taught sensitivity to these issues and to the alternatives to medications for those complaining of poor sleep.

In addition to treatment research, basic research is needed to distinguish individuals who will suffer adjustment disorders of sleep in the face of stress and who will develop more serious disorders such as anxiety or mood disorders. Little is known about who is at risk for this development. Longitudinal studies of persons undergoing specific stressful life events may help elucidate the issue.

Dissociative Disorders

Dissociative disorders, as defined in the Diagnostic and Statistical Manual of Psychiatry IIIR, include four psychiatric conditions closely associated with traumatic antecedents (Putnam 1989). Psychogenetic amnesia and psychogenetic fugue usually are acute responses to an immediate traumatic experience. Multiple personality disorder (MPD) and dissociative disorder not otherwise specified (DDNOS) are chronic conditions, typically related to prior childhood trauma. Few data have been compiled on the incidence or prevalence of these conditions. However, recent research on both general population samples and sequential admissions to an inpatient unit suggest that MPD occurs in one percent of the general population and four to six percent of psychiatric inpatients (Ross et al. 1989; Ross et al. 1991). Clinical experience suggests that DDNOS is more common than MPD, but no comparison data are available.

A number of sleep disturbances have been reported in patients with multiple personality disorder or DDNOS; however only a few small-scale studies have examined these questions (Fleming 1987; Salley 1988; Schenck et al. 1989b). Clinically, sleep problems in patients with dissociative disorders closely resemble those seen in posttraumatic stress disorder and include traumatic nightmares, decreased sleep efficiency, difficulty initiating sleep, and fear of returning to sleep after being awakened. In addition, MPD patients often experience somnambulism (sleep walking). A polysomnographic study of 150 patients presenting with sleep-related injury found that 5.3 percent experienced a dissociative disorder (Schenck et al. 1989b). In every case, these patients presented with apparent sonambulism. However, sleep EEG studies revealed that sleepwalking episodes in dissociative disorder patients occurred during wakeful EEG sleep, not during non-REM sleep, the period during which somnambulism is most likely in other patients. Sleepwalking among dissociative disorder patients often involves complex or bizarre activities. For example, one patient "turned into" a large jungle cat, walked consistently on four legs, left bite marks on the furniture, and lifted very heavy objects—including a marble table—with his mouth. In contrast, classic nonREM somnambulism involves a limited repertoire of "automatic" behaviors.

Current treatment for the dissociative disorders relies primarily on psychotherapy, often augmented with hypnosis (Putnam 1989). Antidepressants and anti-anxiety medications are useful adjunctive treatments for many patients. In open clinical trials, clonazepam has been reported to be of benefit, particularly for sleep disturbances occurring with these disorders (Loewenstein et al. 1988).

Addictive Disorders

Substance abuse takes a tremendous toll on our society, increasing morbidity and mortality. An estimated 18 million people over the age of 18 are alcoholics or problem drinkers. One alcohol-related traffic death occurs every 22 minutes, and 16-24 year olds are involved in 42 percent of all fatal alcohol-related crashes (Rice et al. 1989). The incidence of Fetal Alcohol Syndrome, one of the leading causes of mental retardation, is estimated at 0.1-0.5 percent of all live births (Rice et al. 1990). At least seven million Americans regularly use stimulants, sedatives, tranquilizers, or analgesics for non-medical purposes; five million use cocaine. Substance abuse is certainly involved in many aspects of sleep disorders, but we are only beginning to grasp the magnitude of the problem. Nevertheless, there is little current research on substance abuse in sleep disorders treatment and the impact of substance abuse on sleep disorders in psychiatric and other medical illnesses, whether at the basic, clinical or epidemiological levels. These gaps represent a missed opportunity, because the convergence of the neuropharmacology of alcohol and benzodiazepines, implicating common binding sites, might reveal important knowledge about the mechanisms involved in both sleep and substance abuse.

Although morphine was named for Morpheus, the Greek god thought to produce human figures in dreams, research has recently found that acute administration of morphine and heroin cause arousal and actually reduce REM sleep. With chronic administration, tolerance develops and, during withdrawal, the "nods" and insomnia are well known. Stimulants such as amphetamine and cocaine inhibit sleep and reduce REM time. Tolerance may develop. Withdrawal in stimulant abusers is associated with depression, hypersomnia, hyperphagia, and anhedonia. For the first seven to ten days, total sleep time and REM percentage are elevated, while REM latency is shortened. Preliminary evidence suggests that the changes in REM sleep are not correlated with the severity of depressive symptoms.

The use of alcohol in self-medication of sleep disorders is better known and understood than the use of other drugs of abuse. Although alcohol initially promotes sleep in low to moderate amounts, it often disrupts and fragments sleep as a result of falling blood alcohol levels over the night, somatic discomfort, tolerance, or withdrawal upon discontinuation. Interestingly, sleep researchers have recently suggested that the sedative effects of alcohol may reflect the "unmasking" of a prior sleep "debt" rather than inherent sleep-inducing properties. That is, alcohol-induced sleep affects individuals based on the amount of prior sleep deprivation; it may have less effect on fully rested individuals.

It is also known that alcohol exacerbates sleep-related breathing disorders, apparently by potentiating sleep-related atonia in the upper airways and thereby increasing sleep apnea (Issa and Sullivan 1982; Krol et al. 1984; Scrima et al. 1982). In the case of alcoholism, sleep abnormalities appear not only during bouts of drinking, but also during the acute, subacute, and chronic abstinence syndrome. These disturbances may take the form of insomnia, hypersomnia, circadian disturbances or parasomnia (Allen et al. 1971; Gillin et al. 1990; Gross and Hastey 1976; Lester et al. 1975; Skoloda et al. 1979; Snyder and Karacan 1985; Zarcone 1979b).

Insomnia is very common. During periods of heavy drinking, alcoholics have difficulty initiating and maintaining sleep. During acute withdrawal, sleep is short, fragmented, and shallow, with a particular loss of delta sleep and inconsistent changes in REM sleep. With delirium tremens (DTs), very little sleep may occur for days at a time. During prolonged abstinence, recovered alcoholics may complain of insomnia and fatigue; during this time, alcohol may improve sleep and may, therefore, predispose to renewed drinking. Patients with poor subjective sleep may be more inclined to drink again than those who sleep relatively well. Unfortunately, no well established treatment is now available for sleep disturbances in the chronically abstinent alcoholic.

Hypersomnia in alcoholics also occurs and may result from (a) direct hypnotic effects in sleep deprived individuals, (b) an intermittent hypersomnia during brief periods of abstinence, sometimes seen in the midst of recurring cycles of heavy alcohol intake, and (c) terminal sleep, a prolonged, often restful deep sleep, that occurs during withdrawal.

In recent years, it has been recognized that a significant number of patients with primary alcoholism develop secondary depression during and shortly after drinking episodes. In many ways, these patients show most of the symptoms and signs of major depressive disorder, except that the condition occurs in the context of drinking and is self-limited over a period of a month or less. Research has found that alcoholic patients with secondary depression have shortened REM latency, while primary alcoholics without depression did not. Thus, short REM latency is associated with the depressive syndrome not only in primary but secondary depression.

Addictive disorders also affect the sleep of unintended others. The newborns of drug addicted mothers, including, but not limited to "crack babies" and infants suffering from fetal alcohol syndrome, suffer from aberrant sleep patterns themselves. Otherwise "normal" infants born to addicted mothers may develop altered sleep patterns as the result of the addicted parent's abnormal day-night patterns and attendant lack of regulation of feeding and bed routines for the child.

Substance abuse also coexists in many individuals with major psychiatric disorders, including mood disorders, schizophrenia, and anxiety disorders, among others. At this time, scant information exists to determine whether patients with a single diagnosis differ from those with dual diagnoses in terms of clinical presentation, natural history, optimal treatments, or psychobiology.

These issues are particularly relevant to the relationship between substance abuse and sleep disorders. At present, it is generally recognized that substance abuse, particularly the use of alcohol, is an important consideration in the differential diagnosis of sleep disorders. About 10-15 percent of patients with chronic insomnia, for example, have underlying substance abuse (Gillin and Byerley 1990). Indeed, many drug abusers relate that concerns about sleep provide part of the motivation for initial substance use, patterns of continued use and fears about cessation of use. Both complaints of sleep problems and documented sleep disorders are clearly associated with intoxication and withdrawal states related to central nervous system depressants and stimulants; sleep disorders may well be involved in other parts of the addiction cycle, such as vulnerability to relapse.

We need more research on the etiology and epidemiology of substance abuse in sleep disorders, the impact of alcohol and other drugs on sleep disorders in psychiatric and other medical patients, the neurobiology of sleep disturbances associated with substance abuse, the natural history of these sleep disturbances, and the treatment for such sleep difficulties. Other problems worthy of additional research include alcohol-related exacerbation of sleep-related breathing disorders and disturbances of circadian sleep-wake patterns in the midst of drinking episodes and withdrawal.

REM Behavior Disorders

Rapid eye movement (REM) sleep behavior disorder is a fascinating condition relevant to neurology, psychiatry and sleep disorders medicine (Moore-Ede and Richardson 1985; Wehr and Rosenthal 1989; Tamarkin et al. 1985). Simply put, patients with this disorder enact their dreams. While most people are essentially paralyzed during REM sleep (the dreaming phase of sleep), the patient with REM sleep behavior disorder has abnormally "normal" muscle tone during REM sleep and can carry out purposeful, sometimes dangerous, behaviors consistent with the context of the dream itself. Thus, the mechanisms that produce muscle paralysis during normal REM sleep do not operate properly.

The most typical case is that of an elderly male with no previous psychiatric history who describes increasing disturbance at night. As the disorder develops, complex behaviors begin to appear in association with dreaming. When a dream-enactment episode occurs the patient will usually remember a vivid, action-oriented dream. Often, the dream involves a confrontation or a chase; there is vigorous physical activity. The dreams need not necessarily be frightening; sometimes they are pleasant. The patient may jump out of bed, believing he is diving into a swimming pool. The enactment behavior is usually quite brief; the patient is awakened by bumping into an object or person or by falling out of bed. If violent episodes are directed toward a bed partner, the patients are remorseful and frightened by a behavior that is completely out of character. Often, a precipitating event—a fall or an injury to the bed partner—brings the patient to medical attention.

REM sleep behavior disorder is a good example of how basic research on sleep mechanisms has helped understand particular pathologies. Even before the disorder was found to exist in humans, animal models were identified that demonstrated abnormal muscle tone during REM sleep as the result of tiny lesions in the brain stem near the centers for REM sleep (Gordon et al. 1986). Apparently, muscle paralysis is one component of REM-sleep that can be isolated from other components. Prior to this understanding, most patients with this disorder were considered to have deep-seated psychiatric disease, nocturnal seizures or personality disturbances. Ineffective treatments were pursued, or patients were told that no treatment was available for this "problem."

Today, diagnosis and treatment are relatively uncomplicated. The medical history, if taken carefully, is quite suggestive of the disorder, though it could also suggest nocturnal seizures, night terrors, post-traumatic stress disorder, psychogenic dissociative states, and nocturnal panic attacks. Sudden, vigorous activity during sleep in an older male that makes sense given the circumstances perceived by the dreamer, is highly suggestive of REM behavior disorder. A polysomnographic evaluation is usually pathognomonic for rapid eye movement sleep behavior disorders, although the interpretation must be undertaken by someone familiar with the disorder since the episodes of REM sleep may be mistaken for wakefulness. A striking increase in muscle tone is observed in all of the limbs.

Rapid eye movement sleep behavior disorder is readily diagnosable and readily treatable with medication. Although high rates of treatment success using clonazapam have been reported, controlled clinical trials have not yet been carried out (Schenck et al. 1989c). In some refractory cases, other medications may need to be tried.

Rapid eye movement sleep behavior disorders are but one of a series of disorders known as 'parasomnias,' disorders that occur during sleep, including teeth grinding, enuresis, night terrors and others. While some of these events are quite benign, others such as REM sleep behavior disorders and certain cases of sleep walking can be quite dangerous. Very little is known of the true incidence of these problems, since patients are frequently embarrassed to bring them to medical attention. Fortunately, many of these conditions probably have an organic basis and, even with current limited knowledge of the etiology of the disorders, treatment is quite good.

Nonetheless, these disorders deserve further investigation. These conditions underscore the importance of continuing research on the basic neurobiology of sleep. Increased effort should be devoted to this languishing scientific focus. Further, efforts should be directed toward a better appreciation of the epidemiology of these conditions, which may help develop better hypotheses regarding their etiology (Wehr 1990). Equally important is the need for better education of both the public and the medical profession to ensure that patients come forward with their problems and that physicians accurately diagnose and appropriately treat these disorders. Given the optimistic outlook for both diagnosis and treatment, broader recognition of these disorders will ultimately benefit the patient, the family and our society.

Issues in Differential Diagnosis: Evaluating Insomnia

Insomnia is highly prevalent, ranging from 30-35 percent of the adult US population and 45-57 percent of those over 65 years of age. Some form of sleep disruption affects over half of the 29 million Americans over age 65 (Coroni-Huntley et al. 1986; Hunt et al. 198 1). Women suffer from insomnia more often than men; their problems are serious enough to require them to use sleeping medication more often than men. Although widespread, insomnia is often considered to be more of a nuisance than a threat to health and well-being. However, amassing research evidence suggests that insomnia, in fact, may be predictive of serious health problems. As noted in many of the previous sections of this paper, insomnia is a frequent symptom of mental and addictive disorders.

The cornerstone of the treatment of insomnia is accurate diagnosis. A thorough diagnostic psychiatric and medical evaluation should be conducted to determine whether the insomnia is a symptom of another underlying illness. The most widespread cause of serious insomnia appears to be the affective disorders, especially unipolar depression.

It is vital that this cause of insomnia be promptly recognized and treated. Nevertheless, insomnia may be the depressed patient's major complaint. The treating physician must decide whether treatment should be limited to antidepressant methods, awaiting resolution of the insomnia as a collateral effect of the treatment of depression, or whether treatment should aggressively pursue both the depression and the accompanying insomnia.

Anxiety disorders, also discussed earlier in this paper, may exist alone or in combination with depression. A promising area of investigation has been posed with the realization that panic attacks can occur during sleep as well as during wakefulness. Sleep also appears to be disturbed in patients with panic attacks even on nights when no such attacks occur. While the relationship between insomnia and anxiety associated with specific life events is well established, it is less clear that chronic anxiety can be regarded as a "cause" of insomnia. The efficacy of long-term use of anti-anxiety medications for the management of insomnia is controversial, and in need of substantially greater study.

In addition to the need for further research into the relationship between mental disorders and insomnia, it is critical that clinicians more carefully evaluate the potential causes of patient complaints of insomnia before prescribing hypnotic-sedatives. Such somatic treatments may actual exacerbate the underlying cause(s) of the sleep dysfunction, actually resulting in greater sleep disturbance at the same time. Patients and physicians must be educated in techniques of sleep hygiene. Better education of health care professionals to the relationship between sleep dysfunction and mental disorders is urgently needed.

Further, mental health professionals need to be aware of the importance of primary insomnia, that is the chronic inability to sleep (extending beyond one month) that is not associated with an underlying psychiatric or other medical disorder, but which is probably due to negative conditioning factors such as overanxious concern about not sleeping. As conceptualized in both drafts of DSM-IV and in the International Classification of Sleep Disorders (ICSD, where it is called "psychophysiologic insomnia"), primary insomnia is seen in about 15 percent of patients referred to university-based sleep-disorder centers. Its complications include sedative-hypnotic dependency and alcohol abuse. It may also be a precursor to such psychiatric disorders as major depression. Hence, its early recognition and treatment actually may be a fon of preventive psychiatry. Non-pharmacologic approaches such as sleep restriction therapy are showing much promise for the treatment of primary insomnia. However, implementation of additional controlled clinical trials is necessary for this important public health problem.

Sleep and Mental Disorders Across the Lifespan

Child and Adolescent Mental Disorders

Although the basic function of sleep remains a mystery, research evidence suggests that sleep is particularly important during periods of growth and development, with the implication that children and adolescents may be particularly vulnerable to the effects of sleep loss. Age is the most significant factor influencing the amount and architecture of sleep. Symptoms of disturbed sleep are a common manifestation of many child and adolescent mental disorders. Indeed they may serve as a biological marker for a risk factor among adolescents for the development of subsequent mental disorders.

However, symptoms of inadequate sleep (or disrupted sleep/wake cycles), such as irritability, decreased concentration, mood swings (emotional lability), and decreased impulse control, may be mistaken by the inadequately trained clinician as aspects of common childhood disorders such as attention deficit disorder or depression. Moreover, the rates of psychopathology in children and adolescents appear to be increasing with evidence for an earlier age of onset of depression and suicidality (Dahl 1990; Blumenthal 1990; Shaffer and Fisher 1981). Over the same time, increasing evidence points to the fact that children and adolescents are getting less sleep. This set of parallel developments poses provocative questions about the growing numbers of young people obtaining inadequate amounts of sleep.

Sleep loss occurs in wide variety of childhood and adolescent psychiatric and behavioral disorders and can exacerbate symptoms and complicate management. In many cases—particularly in populations with severe disorders, mental retardation or multiple handicaps—nighttime and sleep-related problems tilt the balance, resulting in institutional care. Thus, sleep disturbances in the presence of child or adolescent physical or mental disorders may claim a toll on the individual, the family and the economy.

Recent studies of severe affective disorders in adults (Gillin et al. 1981) posit a relationship between sleep disturbances and major depressive disorder. However, studies in the child and adolescent age group have not found the same consistent pattern of sleep changes with severe affective disorders. A recent meta-analysis of studies

356

across age groups (Knowles and MacLean 1990) as well as other studies (Giles and Roffwarg 1990) suggest that age and depression interact in producing some of the psychobiological changes associated with depression. These findings focus attention on the early end of the age spectrum, noting that insufficient data are available in the child and adolescent age range to address the key questions as to when and how these sleep-related changes in depression begin.

The apparent infrequency of sleep changes in depression in the very young as measured in studies utilizing EEG and sleep laboratory evaluation stands in contrast to measures of subjective sleep complaints that occur very frequently in child and adolescent depression (Ryan et al. 1987). Seventy-five percent of depressed adolescents suffer from insomnia; twenty percent suffer with hypersomnia (Ryan et al. 1987). Among adolescents, depression and sleep/schedule problems seem to overlap; depressed adolescents frequently have problems with erratic schedules, delayed sleep onset, and difficulty awakening for school. A complex set of interrelationships among sleep, mood and motivation may account for some of these subjective complaints of sleep disturbances, an interrelationship that may be difficult, but important to disentangle (Ferber 1983; Carskadon and Marrcuso 1988). Adolescence represents a crucial interval with respect to both depression and sleep regulation, during which time the rates of depression increase, the depression sex ratio changes, bipolarity of the disorder increases, and suicidality increases (Blumenthal 1990; Shaffer and Fisher 1981). During the same period, profound changes in sleepiness and the response to sleep deprivation occur. How and why depression arises in this and younger age cohorts and how and if sleep may hold a clue to the etiology, treatment and course of early life depressive disorder remains the province of future research.

Disruptive disorders of childhood and adolescence, such as attention deficit disorder, present a paradigm similar to that of depression in this population, in which there are numerous subjective complaints of sleep disturbance, but little EEG or other sleep study evidence of disturbed sleep (Greenhill et al. 1983; Busby et al. 1981; Kaplan et al. 1987). While the evidence linking sleep and ADD is little more than circumstantial, clinicians working in this area are not surprised to find that children with inadequate or disrupted sleep appear irritable, have decreased attention spans, are oppositional, and can often appear hyperactive in structured settings. The fact that stimulants improve some of these symptoms following sleep deprivation is also consistent with current understanding of arousal control. However,

357

unless carefully utilized in controlled settings in combination with sleep deprivation, stimulant medication used to treat ADD can produce even greater sleep disturbances that create the possibility of vicious cycles in some cases.

Both in depression and in disruptive behavior disorders, a wide range of critical questions with respect to sleep and mental disorders arise, spanning the psychobiologic to the pragmatic issues of clinical management. Regrettably, the data to address these questions are inadequate. We have yet to understand fully the relationship of inadequate sleep to disturbed behavior patterns; equally we do not know the long-term consequences of inadequate sleep during childhood. The embryonic state of our current understanding produces a number of current priorities. The first priority is the clear necessity for better basic knowledge of child and adolescent sleep. Basic knowledge of sleep and development, methodologic issues addressing the measurement of sleep in this age group, naturalistic studies looking at sleep and sleep schedules, and basic relationships among sleep, mood and arousal in children and adolescents are central questions. Moreover, better coordination and focus among the fragments of work being done in the field needs to be achieved. Specifically, the wide range of disciplines engaged in research into sleep and child and adolescent mental disorders makes communication and coordination of efforts difficult. A focused effort in this area to pull together and build upon these fragments and to address some of the key questions outlined above is a critical step with respect toward progress in the psychobiology of child and adolescent mental disorders.

Sleep and Mental Disorders in Geriatric Populations

Approximately 10 percent of the elderly population have clinically significant cognitive defects—dementia—resulting in problems with memory, reasoning, speech, normal self-care or other functions of daily living. Over half of these individuals, some three million today, are now recognized to suffer from Alzheimer's disease, a progressive degeneration of critical cortical brain tissue that remains of unknown cause (Terry and Katzman 1983). The annual cost of nursing home care alone for these patients now exceeds $12 billion; the toll on their families is incalculable. The remaining cases generally involve other disorders, such as Parkinson's disease, alcohol-related dementia, and cerebrovascular disorders such as multi-infarct dementia, although other rare disorders may also contribute to the toll of dementia on the Nation's elderly.

Impaired sleep is commonly associated with abnormalities of brain function, such as Alzheimer's disease (AD). Persons with AD or other forms of dementia often experience excessive sleepiness in the daytime, disrupted sleep at night, or both. These changes become more severe as the course of the illness progresses. Several studies have documented nocturnal sleep disruption in patients with Alzheimer's disease and other dementing disorders. Most studies have shown that the amount of movement and wake time in the night is increased in those patients compared to nondemented elderly normals. Over the course of a night, orderly sleep cycles are disrupted, with less deep sleep and less REM (dreaming) sleep. Daytime napping is increased as a form of compensation. These changes are more severe in the more severely demented.

In addition to this common pattern, a variety of specific primary sleep disorders, such as sleep apnea, nocturnal myoclonus, and REM behavior disorder appear to be more prevalent in certain subgroups, and interact with cognitive changes to exacerbate poor nocturnal sleep and daytime neurocognitive dysfunction. Exacerbation of the sleep problem may result in evening and nighttime agitation, confusion, and disruptive behavior, a disorder known as "nocturnal delirium" or "sundowning' " occurring in an estimated 12-20 percent of demented patients. Typical patterns include wandering outside of the home, turning on kitchen appliances, accidentally breaking household items, and shouting inappropriately. Whether occurring in the home or in an institutional facility, sundowning is frightening for the patient and burdensome to the patient's caregivers.

Causes of sleep disruption in dementia may well be attributable to many of the same changes that result in mental dysfunction in the dementing disorders. Brain mechanisms producing and maintaining sleep are widespread and interactive; optimal sleep-wake functioning depends on the integrity of many neuronal systems and networks. Degeneration and alternation of brain neurochemical, neurovascular and neuroanatomic systems seem to underlie both the mental dysfunction and the sleep disruption. Regrettably, the underlying causes of the neurodegenerative conditions such as Alzheimer's disease remain unknown.

Additional and contributing factors to the sleep disturbances found in dementia include alterations in circadian rhythms (daily cycles of wake-sleep, seasonal changes, etc.), in part caused by immobility and confinement to bed with resulting loss of regulating factors such as social interaction and exposure to sunlight. Pain and secondary medical illnesses can decrease cerebral function, further contributing to sleep disruption. Moreover, specific primary sleep disorders such as sleep apnea often co-exist and worsen nighttime sleep and daytime alertness in the elderly (Ancoh-Israel et al. 199 1). Depression and anxiety are often present and may further heighten sleep problems.

While research progresses, unfortunately there are still no adequate treatments available today for Alzheimer's disease. Sometimes, concomitant physical or mental illnesses or specific sleep disorders can be treated, relieving the problem somewhat. The treatment of sundowning remains difficult. Tranquilizers, the most common form of treatment, are not well tolerated by the elderly in general and by those suffering from Alzheimer's disease in particular. Recent suggestions regarding manipulation of the wake-sleep cycle, the use of bright light and chronotherapy, and alterations in ambient temperature hold some promise, but require further study.

Sadly, until the basic causes of Alzheimer's disease and other dementing disorders are elucidated through research, only the complications of the disorders, such as the serious loss of quality sleep, can be managed. Nonetheless, the proper application of resources can produce both an understanding of the causes of these sleep problems as well as better treatment. Epidemiologic and clinical research is needed to determine the effect of medical illnesses and primary sleep disorders on sleep quality and daytime functioning in demented patients. Pharmacologic research into specific deficits in sleep-promoting pathways could provide valuable insight into the treatment of dementia-related insomnia. Circadian rhythm physiology in the elderly must be further characterized, especially as it applies to Alzheimer's disease. Markers of circadian rhythms include the temperature cycle, hormone levels and their cycles, and, obviously, the sleep-wake cycle. Such information may improve treatment opportunities not only for the dementia related insomnias but also the difficult problem of sundowning.

While research may help reduce some of the excess disability caused by sleep dysfunction that accompanies the dementing disorders, public and medical education programs are also needed. The elderly, their families and their physicians should be educated to the importance of good sleep habits and the effect of external factors on internal body rhythms. They should learn about the dangers of multiple medications, the sleep disruptive effects of common drugs, and the potential interaction of sleep disorders, medical illness, medicines and cognitive dysfunction.

Chapter 44

Sleep Disturbances Occur with Some Antidepressants

The most commonly prescribed antidepressant drug can help overcome a mood disorder, but often that pharmaceutical help comes at a price, according to a recent study sponsored by Bristol-Myers Squibb, manufacturer of nefazodone (Serzone).

Researchers say that selective serotonin reuptake inhibitors (SSRIs), which include the drug fluoxetine (Prozac), can interrupt sleep patterns, make consumers feel as if they haven't had a good night's sleep and cause them to feel sleepy and drowsy during the day.

But newer, third-generation antidepressants that act on specific neurotransmitters don't seem to have the same sleep-interrupting side effects.

Eduardo Estivill, PhD, head of the Sleep Disturbance Unit at the Dexeus Clinic in Barcelona, Spain, compared electronic sleep patterns of people on fluoxetine to those on nefazodone. He found that patients on fluoxetine had on average eight more awakenings during the night than did patients taking nefazodone for depression. About 120 patients took part in three separate studies.

Estivill said that during normal sleep, people have a number of brief, unnoticed awakenings. But depressed patients have considerably more disturbed sleep, often leaving them feeling tired all day. SSRIs further damage sleep patterns, he said.

Norman Sussman, MD, clinical associate professor of medicine at New York University School of Medicine, said the sleep studies are

Reprinted with permission from *Behavioral Health Treatment*, November 1997, Volume 2, Number 11, pp.3(1). © 1997 Manisses Communications Group.

important because side effects have an impact on compliance. Side effects such as sexual dysfunction, sleep disturbance, sweating and other problems associated with SSRIs—complications that will make a person quit taking antidepressant medication—are not found in newer medications, he said.

However, Sussman said nefazodone has its own set of side effects that include dizziness, dry mouth, constipation and some visual symptoms. He said that patients generally tolerate these problems more easily than they do the problems associated with SSRIs.

Presented at the October meeting of the European College of Neuropsychopharmacology, Vienna, Austria. Drs. Estivill and Sussman can be reached through Bristol-Myers Squibb. Contact Ami Knoefler at (609) 252-4533.

Chapter 45

Alcohol and Sleep

The average adult sleeps 7.5 to 8 hours every night. Although the function of sleep is unknown, abundant evidence demonstrates that lack of sleep can have serious consequences, including increased risk of depressive disorders, impaired breathing, and heart disease. In addition, excessive daytime sleepiness resulting from sleep disturbance is associated with memory deficits, impaired social and occupational function, and car crashes (1,2). Alcohol consumption can induce sleep disorders by disrupting the sequence and duration of sleep states and by altering total sleep time as well as the time required to fall asleep (i.e., sleep latency). This *Alcohol Alert* explores the effects of alcohol consumption on sleep patterns, the potential health consequences of alcohol consumption combined with disturbed sleep, and the risk for relapse in those with alcoholism who fail to recover normal sleep patterns.

Sleep Structure, Onset, and Arousal

Before discussing alcohol's effects on sleep, it is helpful to summarize some basic features of normal sleep. A person goes through two alternating states of sleep, characterized in part by different types of brain electrical activity (i.e., brain waves). These states are called slow wave sleep (SWS), because in this type of sleep the brain waves are

National Institute on Alcohol Abuse and Alcoholism, *Alcohol Alert*, No.41, July 1998.

very slow, and rapid eye movement (REM) sleep, in which the eyes undergo rapid movements although the person remains asleep.

Most sleep is the deep, restful SWS. REM sleep occurs periodically, occupying about 25 percent of sleep time in the young adult. Episodes of REM normally recur about every 90 minutes and last 5 to 30 minutes. REM sleep is less restful than SWS and is usually associated with dreaming. Although its function is unknown, REM appears to be essential to health. In rats, deprivation of REM sleep can lead to death within a few weeks (3). In addition, a transitional stage of light sleep occurs at intervals throughout the sleep period (4).

Sleep was formerly attributed to decreased activity of brain systems that maintain wakefulness. More recent data indicate that sleep, like consciousness, is an active process. Sleep is controlled largely by nerve centers in the lower brain stem, where the base of the brain joins the spinal cord. Some of these nerve cells produce serotonin, a chemical messenger associated with sleep onset (5) and with the regulation of SWS. Certain other nerve cells produce norepinephrine, which helps regulate REM sleep and facilitates arousal (6). The exact roles and interactions of these and other chemical messengers in orchestrating sleep patterns are not known (6). Significantly, however, alcohol consumption affects the function of these and other chemical messengers that appear to influence sleep.

Alcohol and Sleep in Those Without Alcoholism

Alcohol consumed at bedtime, after an initial stimulating effect, may decrease the time required to fall asleep. Because of alcohol's sedating effect, many people with insomnia consume alcohol to promote sleep. However, alcohol consumed within an hour of bedtime appears to disrupt the second half of the sleep period (7). The subject may sleep fitfully during the second half of sleep, awakening from dreams and returning to sleep with difficulty. With continued consumption just before bedtime, alcohol's sleep-inducing effect may decrease, while its disruptive effects continue or increase (8). This sleep disruption may lead to daytime fatigue and sleepiness. The elderly are at particular risk, because they achieve higher levels of alcohol in the blood and brain than do younger persons after consuming an equivalent dose. Bedtime alcohol consumption among older persons may lead to unsteadiness if walking is attempted during the night, with increased risk of falls and injuries (3).

Alcoholic beverages are often consumed in the late afternoon (e.g., at "happy hour" or with dinner) without further consumption before bedtime. Studies show that a moderate dose of alcohol consumed as much as 6 hours before bedtime can increase wakefulness during the second half of sleep. By the time this effect occurs, the dose of alcohol consumed earlier has already been eliminated from the body, suggesting a relatively long-lasting change in the body's mechanisms of sleep regulation (7,8).

The adverse effects of sleep deprivation are increased following alcohol consumption. Subjects administered low doses of alcohol following a night of reduced sleep perform poorly in a driving simulator, even with no alcohol left in the body (9,10). Reduced alertness may potentially increase alcohol's sedating effect in situations such as rotating sleep-wake schedules (e.g., shift work) and rapid travel across multiple time zones (i.e., jet lag) (9). A person may not recognize the extent of sleep disturbance that occurs under these circumstances, increasing the danger that sleepiness and alcohol consumption will co-occur.

Alcohol and Breathing Disorders

Approximately 2 to 4 percent of Americans suffer from obstructive sleep apnea (OSA), a disorder in which the upper air passage (i.e., the pharynx, located at the back of the mouth) narrows or closes during sleep (11). The resulting episode of interrupted breathing (i.e., apnea) wakens the person, who then resumes breathing and returns to sleep. Recurring episodes of apnea followed by arousal can occur hundreds of times each night, significantly reducing sleep time and resulting in daytime sleepiness. Those with alcoholism appear to be at increased risk for sleep apnea, especially if they snore (12). In addition, moderate to high doses of alcohol consumed in the evening can lead to narrowing of the air passage (13,14), causing episodes of apnea even in persons who do not otherwise exhibit symptoms of OSA. Alcohol's general depressant effects can increase the duration of periods of apnea, worsening any preexisting OSA (14).

OSA is associated with impaired performance on a driving simulator as well as with an increased rate of motor vehicle crashes in the absence of alcohol consumption (9,10). Among patients with severe OSA, alcohol consumption at a rate of two or more drinks per day is associated with a fivefold increased risk for fatigue-related traffic crashes compared with OSA patients who consume little or no alcohol (15). In addition, the combination of alcohol, OSA, and snoring increases a person's risk for heart attack, arrhythmia, stroke, and sudden death (16).

Age-Related Effects and the Impact of Drinking

Little research has been conducted on the specific effects of alcohol on sleep states among different age groups. Scher (17) investigated the effects of prenatal alcohol exposure on sleep patterns in infants. Measurements of brain electrical activity demonstrated that infants of mothers who consumed at least one drink per day during the first trimester of pregnancy exhibited sleep disruptions and increased arousal compared with infants of nondrinking women. Additional studies revealed that infants exposed to alcohol in mothers' milk fell asleep sooner but slept less overall than those who were not exposed to alcohol (18). The exact significance of these findings is unclear.

Normal aging is accompanied by a gradual decrease in SWS and an increase in nighttime wakefulness. People over 65 often awaken 20 times or more during the night, leading to sleep that is less restful and restorative (3). Age-related sleep deficiencies may encourage the use of alcohol to promote sleep, while increasing an older person's susceptibility to alcohol-related sleep disturbances (3,19). Potential sources of inconsistency among study results include different doses of alcohol employed and failure to screen out subjects with preexisting sleep disorders (3).

Effects of Alcohol on Sleep in Those With Alcoholism

Active Drinking and Withdrawal. Sleep disturbances associated with alcoholism include increased time required to fall asleep, frequent awakenings, and a decrease in subjective sleep quality associated with daytime fatigue (3). Abrupt reduction of heavy drinking can trigger alcohol withdrawal syndrome, accompanied by pronounced insomnia with marked sleep fragmentation. Decreased SWS during withdrawal may reduce the amount of restful sleep. It has been suggested that increased REM may be related to the hallucinations that sometimes occur during withdrawal. In patients with severe withdrawal, sleep may consist almost entirely of brief periods of REM interrupted by numerous awakenings (3,20).

Recovery and Relapse. Despite some improvement after withdrawal subsides, sleep patterns may never return to normal in those with alcoholism, even after years of abstinence (3,21). Abstinent alcoholics tend to sleep poorly, with decreased amounts of SWS and increased nighttime wakefulness that could make sleep less restorative and contribute to daytime fatigue (22). Resumption of heavy drinking leads to increased SWS and decreased wakefulness. This apparent improvement in sleep continuity may promote relapse by contributing to the mistaken impression that alcohol consumption improves sleep (23-25). Nevertheless, as drinking continues, sleep patterns again become disrupted (3).

Researchers have attempted to predict relapse potential using measures of sleep disruption. Gillin and colleagues (26) measured REM sleep in patients admitted to a 1-month alcoholism treatment program. Higher levels of REM predicted those who relapsed within 3 months after hospital discharge in 80 percent of the patients. A review of additional research (3) concluded that those who eventually relapsed exhibited a higher proportion of REM and a lower proportion of SWS at the beginning of treatment, compared with those who remained abstinent. Although additional research is needed, these findings may facilitate early identification of patients at risk for relapse and allow clinicians to tailor their treatment programs accordingly.

Alcohol and Sleep: A Commentary by NIAAA Director Enoch Gordis, M.D.

According to recent news reports, Americans are at risk for a variety of sleep-related health problems. Alcohol use affects sleep in a number of ways and can exacerbate these problems. Because alcohol use is widespread, it is important to understand how this use affects sleep to increase risk for illness. For example, it is popularly believed that a drink before bedtime can aid falling asleep. However, it also can disrupt normal sleep patterns, resulting in increased fatigue and physical stress to the body. Alcohol use can aggravate sleeping disorders, such as sleep apnea; those with such disorders should be cautious about alcohol use. Many nursing mothers are still regularly advised by their physicians to have a drink to promote lactation (so-called let-down reflex). Babies who receive alcohol in breast milk are known to have disrupted sleeping patterns. Because researchers do not yet know what effect this disruption has on nursing infants, physicians should reconsider this advice.

Alcoholism treatment also can be complicated by sleep problems during withdrawal and during subsequent behavioral treatment, where sleeping problems experienced by many recovering alcoholics may increase their risk for relapse. Because it is likely that alcohol may act on the same neurotransmitters involved in sleep, increased knowledge of alcohol's effects on the brain will help to promote new therapeutic techniques for alcohol-related sleep disorders and, perhaps, improve the chance for long-term sobriety.

References

1. Roehrs, T., and Roth, T. Alcohol-induced sleepiness and memory function. *Alcohol Health Res World* 19(2):130-135, 1995.

2. Kupfer, D.J., and Reynolds, C.F. Management of insomnia. *N Engl J Med* 336(5):341-346, 1997.

3. Aldrich, M.S. Effects of alcohol on sleep. In: Lisansky Gomberg, E.S., et al., eds. Alcohol Problems and Aging. *NIAAA Research Monograph No. 33.* NIH Pub. No. 98-4163. Bethesda, MD: NIAAA, in press.

4. Guyton, A.C. *Human Physiology and Mechanisms of Disease.* 5th ed. Philadelphia: W.B. Saunders, 1992.

5. Zajicek, K., et al. Rhesus macaques with high CSF 5-HIAA concentrations exhibit early sleep onset. *Neuropsychopharmacology*, in press.

6. Shepherd, G.M. *Neurobiology.* 3d ed. New York: Oxford University Press, 1994.

7. Landolt, H.-P., et al. Late-afternoon ethanol intake affects nocturnal sleep and the sleep EEG in middle-aged men. *J Clin Psychopharmacol* 16(6):428-436, 1996.

8. Vitiello, M.V. Sleep, alcohol and alcohol abuse. *Addict Biol* (2):151-158, 1997.

9. Roehrs, T., et al. Sleepiness and ethanol effects on simulated driving. *Alcohol Clin Exp Res* 18(1):154-158, 1994.

10. Krull, K.R., et al. Simple reaction time event-related potentials: Effects of alcohol and sleep deprivation. *Alcohol Clin Exp Res* 17(4):771-777, 1993.

11. Strollo, P.J., and Rogers, R.M. Obstructive sleep apnea. *N Engl J Med* 334(2):99-104, 1996.

12. Aldrich, M.S., et al. Sleep-disordered breathing in alcoholics: Association with age. *Alcohol Clin Exp Res* 17(6):1179-1183, 1993.

13. Mitler, M.M., et al. Bedtime ethanol increases resistance of upper airways and produces sleep apneas in asymptomatic snorers. *Alcohol Clin Exp Res* 12(6):801-805, 1988.

14. Dawson, A., et al. Effect of bedtime ethanol on total inspiratory resistance and respiratory drive in normal nonsnoring men. *Alcohol Clin Exp Res* 17(2):256-262, 1993.

15. Aldrich, M.S., and Chervin, R.D. Alcohol use, obstructive sleep apnea, and sleep-related motor vehicle accidents. *Sleep Res*, in press.

16. Bassetti, C., and Aldrich, M.S. Alcohol consumption and sleep apnea in patients with TIA and ischemic stroke. *Sleep Res* 25:400, 1996.

17. Scher, M., et al. The effects of prenatal alcohol and marijuana exposure: Disturbances in neonatal sleep cycling and arousal. *Pediatr Res* 24(1):101-105, 1988.

18. Mennella, J.A., and Gerrish, C.J. Effects of exposure to alcohol in mothers' milk on the infants' sleep and activity levels. *Pediatrics*, in press.

19. Block, A.J., et al. Effect of alcohol ingestion on breathing and oxygenation during sleep. *Am J Med* 80(4):595-600, 1986.

20. Allen, R.P., et al. Electroencephalographic (EEG) sleep recovery following prolonged alcohol intoxication in alcoholics. *J Ner and Ment Dis* 153(6):424-433, 1971.

21. Williams, H.L., and Rundell, Jr., O.H. Altered sleep physiology in chronic alcoholics: Reversal with abstinence. *Alcohol Clin Exp Res* 5(2):318-325, 1981.

22. Gillin, J.C., et al. EEG sleep studies in "pure" primary alcoholism during subacute withdrawal: Relationships to normal controls, age, and other clinical variables. *Bio Psychiatry* 27:477-488, 1990.

23. Lester, B.K., et al. Chronic alcoholism, alcohol and sleep. In: Gross, M.M., ed. Advances in Experimental Medicine and Biology: Volume 35. *Alcohol Intoxication and Withdrawal*: Experimental Studies. New York: Plenum Press, 1973. pp. 261-279.

24. Skoloda, T.E., et al. Sleep quality reported by drinking and non-drinking alcoholics. In: Gottheil, E.L., et al., eds. *Addiction Research and Treatments: Converging Trends*. New York: Pergamon Press, 1979. pp. 102-112.

25. Zarcone, V., et al. Alcohol, sleep and cerebrospinal fluid changes in alcoholics: Cyclic AMP and biogenic amine metabolites in CSF. In: Gross, M.M., ed. *Advances in Experimental Medicine and Biology: Volume 85A. Alcohol Intoxication and Withdrawal—IIIa: Biological Aspects of Ethanol.* New York: Plenum Press, 1977. pp. 593-599.

26. Gillin, J.C., et al. Increased pressure for rapid eye movement sleep at time of hospital admission predicts relapse in non-depressed patients with primary alcoholism at 3-month follow-up. *Arch Gen Psychiatry* 51:189-197, 1994.

[1]A standard drink is generally considered to be 12 ounces of beer, 5 ounces of wine, or 1.5 ounces of distilled spirits, each drink containing approximately 0.5 ounce of alcohol. In addition, terms such as light, moderate, or heavy drinking are not used consistently by alcoholism researchers. Therefore, in each case, the terms used in this text are those of the author or authors cited.

Copies of the *Alcohol Alert* are available free of charge from the National Institute on Alcohol Abuse and Alcoholism Publications Distribution Center, P.O. Box 10686, Rockville, MD 20849-0686.

Chapter 46

Caffeine in Medications Induces Sleep Problems in Elders

Medications that contain caffeine can exacerbate sleep problems in older adults, according to an article published in a recent issue of the *Journal of the American Geriatrics Society*.

In fact, say researchers from the National Institutes on Aging, regular use of over-the-counter pain medications unknowingly can provide a daily dose of caffeine equivalent to that found in four cups of coffee—and can cause similar difficulties in falling asleep.

The researchers based their conclusions on a study of 2,885 participants in the Iowa 65+ Rural Health Study, a longitudinal study of the health status of elderly men and women (age range 67-105). Participants completed an in-person survey that included questions on sleep problems. The subjects also were asked about any prescription and over-the-counter medications they had taken in the past two weeks, as well as chronic or painful health problems that might interfere with sleep.

The investigators found that 155 (5.4%) of subjects reported taking medications that contained caffeine. Most of these drugs were analgesics that contained either aspirin or acetaminophen along with caffeine 85.2%); others were prescription analgesics 10.3%), cold remedies 3.8%), and miscellaneous (0.6%).

"Caffeine in Medications Induces Sleep Problems in Elders." (over-the-counter)(adapted from the *Journal of the American Geriatrics Society*, 43:860-864, 1995); reprinted with permission from *The Brown University Long-Term Care Quality Letter*, December 11, 1995, Volume 7, Number 23. © 1995 Manisses Communications Group Inc.

Subjects who were taking medications that contained caffeine were significantly more likely to report trouble falling asleep most of the time; 20.7% reported this problem, compared with only 12.9% of subjects who were not taking caffeinated medications. Use of caffeinated drugs was not associated with waking in the night, waking too early, or daytime sleepiness.

The investigators also found that subjects who took many medications [excluding those containing caffeine) were likely to have sleep problems, as were subjects suffering from hip fracture. Depression and the perception of poor health also were associated with trouble sleeping. The authors say that it is important to distinguish among the possible sources of sleeplessness.

The researchers acknowledge that their study was limited by the data set in that they don't know whether the sleep problems reported were current or in the past. Nor do the data indicate how much and what time of day the caffeinated medications were taken.

Nevertheless, taking medications containing caffeine was associated with "a 60% greater risk for having trouble falling asleep." The authors suggest that although older people who have trouble sleeping may try to avoid beverages with caffeine, "the presence of caffeine in medications may be unknown to older consumers of these drugs so that they do not have the opportunity to avoid them even if they know that they may be sensitive to the effects of caffeine."

Therefore, the authors say, "healthcare providers should be aware of the potential problems with over-the-counter medications that contain caffeine and counsel patients about the potential of sleep problems."

—by S. Lori Brown, Marcel E. Salive, et al

Chapter 47

Chronic Headaches and Sleep Disorders

Headache is a common complaint in Western societies as is the complaint of poor sleep. Both complaints are addressed first to the general practitioner.[1-4] Different types of relationships can be postulated by the physician: (1) the sleep disturbance is primary and the headache is a symptom; (2) the headache syndrome is primary and leads to the sleep disturbance; (3) both complaints are symptoms of a different pathological entity, unrelated to sleep or headache; and (4) the individual has both a sleep disturbance syndrome and a headache syndrome (with or without interaction between the 2). The line of reasoning selected by the practitioner will influence the diagnostic evaluation and lead to different treatment strategies. We have previously suggested that a thorough clinical interview that includes determination of the time of onset of the cephalalgia related to the sleepwake cycle could be a helpful clinical tool. [5] We describe the application of these simple recommendations in subjects, seen successively at a headache clinic, who reported a frequent association between onset of headache and sleep timing.

To test the hypothesis that a sleep disturbance might be at the root of some headache complaints, experimental subjects were obtained from a headache clinic and not from a sleep disorders center. For ease of interpretation, subjects had to be diurnal and the sleep period had to occur between 10 pm and 8 am. Only cephalalgia complaints that had onset during the night or the early morning, at least 75% of the time, were considered. Subjects meeting these criteria were included in the study, independently of age, gender, or associated symptoms. All subjects underwent the same protocol, which included clinical evaluations of the headache complaint, nocturnal sleep and possible sleep disturbances, and a polygraphic recording during nocturnal sleep.

All first-time patients aged 20 years and older, seen successively during a 6-month period at a specialized headache clinic, and who met the entry criteria entered the protocol. There were no dropouts during the short investigation and all the subjects are included in the study report. This group represents 17% of all the headache complainers seen at the clinic during the same period.

Table 47.1. Demographic Characteristics of the Studied Population(*)

Characteristics	Total Population (N=49)	Men (n=18)
Age, y	45.9[+ or -]10.9	48.2[+ or -]9.1
Weight, kg	72.1[+ or -]13.66	76.9[+ or -]8.9
BMI, kg/[m.sup.2][dagger]	27.1[+ or -]4.5	25.8[+ or -]2.6
Years of headache complaint	18.6[+ or -]13.7	18.5[+ or -]15.0

Characteristics	Women (n=31)
Age, y	44.6[+ or -]11.8
Weight, kg	69.5[+ or -]15.16
BMI, kg/[m.sup.2)[dagger]	27.9[+ or -]5.3
Years of headache complaint	18.6[+ or -]13.2

(*) Values are mean ([+ or -1 SD). [dagger] Body mass index (BMI) is a measure of weight in kilograms divided by the square of the height in meters.

Results

Forty-nine subjects participated in the study. Demographics are presented in Table 47.1. A first analysis was made to compare the results of in-laboratory polysomnography with those of home monitoring. There were no statistical differences in total sleep time and number of arousals between the 2 groups. For this reason, the results presented are for the total patient group. Twenty six subjects (14 women) were identified as presenting a primary, sleep disorder; this group represents 53% of the studied population and 9% of all headache complainers (n=288).

Table 47.2 presents the different sleep-related pathological features noted in the population.

Table 47.2. Different Sleep-Rated Pathological Features Noted in the Population(*)

Pathological Features	n	Mean ([+ or -]SD) Age, y
OSAS	7	49.0[+ or -]8.3
PLM	8	44.3[+ or -]13.7
Psychophysologic insomnia	1	45.0
Fibromyalgia	10	50.4[+ or -]8.6
Headache without sleep disorders	23	43.7[+ or -]11.5

(*) OSAS indicates obstructive sleep apnea syndrome; PLM, periodic limb movement syndrome.

As seen in Table 47.2, all subjects identified with a sleep disorder reported fragmented sleep. The 1-night polysomnographic recordings did not show significant sleep differences between the 2 groups studied. Mean ([+ or -]SD) total sleep time was 372[+ or -]61 minutes and rapid eve movement sleep was 11.9%[+ or -]6.7% in the headache with sleep disorder group, while in the headache with other disorder group the mean ([+ or -]SD) total sleep time was 367[+ or -]65 minutes and rapid eye movement sleep was 16.2%[+ or -112%. Polysomnography identified, however, the presence of specific sleep disorders in the population. The subgroup of subjects with sleep-disordered breathing had a mean ([+ or -]SD) respiratory disturbance index (respiratory disturbance index equals apneas and hypopneas per hour of Sleep) of 18.7[+ or -]6, compared with a mean ([+ or -]SD) respiratory disturbance index of 2.2[+ or -] 1. 0 in the other subjects. More than 85% of the breathing events seen were obstructive in nature. The recording also identified a subgroup of subjects with periodic limb movements (PLMS) with a mean ([+ or -]SD) PLM-arousal index of 12.7[+ or -]7 events per hour of sleep.

Analysis of the sleep-wake questionnaire[7] (Table 47.3) showed that patients with sleep disorders, when queried, reported many more sleep-related complaints than other subjects with headache. This questionnaire investigated the presence or absence of sleep complaints over a period and, as such, differs from the 1-night polysomnography, a test that focuses on the presence or absence of an organic sleep disorder.

Seventy percent of the sleep disorders group had been prescribed hypnotics during the 3 years preceding the study because of prior report of poor sleep compared with 39% of the pure cephalalgia group (P=.03).

The subjects' descriptions of the cephalalgias were analyzed. Investigations of the predominant location of the pain, frequency of the reported event, and reported time of appearance of pain during the nocturnal period did not dissociate the different types of cephalalgia; more particularly, these investigations did not allow us to dissociate between the cephalalgias related to sleep disorders and those that were not. Also, it must be emphasized that the frequency of the complaints was daily in 67% of the total population and in 69% of the sleep disorders population.

All the subjects with sleep disorders were treated etiologically: patients with obstructive sleep apnea syndrome were treated with nasal continuous positive airway pressure; PLM syndrome was treated with clonazepam (0.5-1.5 mg at bedtime); fibromyalgia was treated with physical exercise and/or trazodone hydrochloride at bedtime

(100-mg tablet); patients with psychophysiological insomnia followed a sleep hygiene treatment program.

All the patients with obstructive sleep apnea syndrome had a complete disappearance of headache complaint (100%), as did 7 subjects with fibromyalgia (70%) and 3 subjects with PLM syndrome (37.5%). Degree of improvement was based on comparisons of reports before and after treatment of the sleep disorder—specifically, the change in frequency of reported cephalalgia, the severity score of the reported headache, the subjective quality of nocturnal sleep, subjective total sleep time, and overall well-being. A minimum change of 50% relative to baseline on the selected indexes was required (ie, a 50% decrease in number of days of cephalalgia per week, 50% reduction in the severity score, 50% improvement in quality of sleep score, and also an increase in subjective total sleep time of 30 minutes). Improvement of the headache complaint was noted in the remaining subjects; however, despite these changes in the selected subjective indexes, this group still presented complaints of cephalalgia and expressed a desire for further treatment for headache pain. They represented 3 (30%)

Table 47.3. Percentage of Sleep Complaints in the 2 Subgroups of Headache Complainers

Sleep-Related Complaint	Headache With Sleep Disorders Group, %	Other Headache Group, %	p
Work-related problems caused by daytime sleepiness	82	30	.02
Sleepiness while talking	20	0	.05
Midday excessive sleepiness	80	17	.04
Nocturnal sleep disturbance	90	53	.05
Feeling of waking up short of breath or not breathing during sleep	35	0	.007
Sleep walking	28	0	.03
Sleep paralysis at onset of sleep	70	46.0	.04

of the initial fibromyalgic and 5 (62.5%) of the subjects with initial PLM. The complaint led to the introduction of headache medications, given at a low dosage, in the sleep-related treatment regimen.

Comment

Our investigation demonstrates that about 26 subjects (10%) with identifiable sleep disorders present with a primary complaint of headache and are referred to a headache clinic. The neurological interview defined well the headache problems that were non-lesion related and were classified under several headache nosological labels. The headache classification of subjects was rational; for example, subjects classified with a certain headache diagnosis were not outliers as far as age, complaint, or location from what would be expected, epidemiologically, from patients with such a diagnosis. [7] We must stress, however, the high incidence of men in the studied population, which was 12 (50%) in the subgroup presenting with a sleep disorder. This is unusual in chronic headache sufferers, where women are usually represented in greater numbers.

Analysis of the frequency and anatomical locations of the pain, part of the standard headache., evaluation, was much less useful than questions about sleep disorders for identifying patients who responded well to nonheadache medication. The suspicion of the sleep disorder may need to lead to a more systematic investigation of sleep-related complaints, including the use of sleep questionnaires and possibly polysomnography. This nocturnal testing does not need to be performed in a sleep laboratory, as indicated by our own results, but the equipment used to perform a nonattended home study must allow appropriate recording of EEG, leg and body movements, and respiration. If the technical quality of the home recording does not allow appropriate determination of the possible sleep disorder, the test will have to be redone at home or in a sleep laboratory.

The sleep disorder identified in this headache population always led to significant sleep fragmentation and, interestingly, the use of a sleep disorders questionnaire identified a much higher frequency of excessive and disturbing daytime sleepiness that may have been responsible for the cephalalgia. Also in 2 cases of obstructive sleep apnea syndrome, subjects had been inappropriately treated by practitioners to the point where the amount of medication(s) prescribed—perhaps related to an absence of treatment response—had led to the development of long-term analgesic abuse, appropriately recognized by the headache clinic specialist.

Sleep walking has been previously reported in patients with migraine and nonmigraine headaches. [10-14] Our survey confirms the prior reports that considered the frequency of headaches in long-term sleepwalkers[10,11] and the frequency of sleepwalking in headache sufferers.[12-14] The association between sleepwalking and headaches, first described in children[10] and confirmed in adults, [11-14] is known to sleep disorders specialists but may be unfamiliar to general practitioners. It is a point worth emphasizing, as questions concerning presence or absence of sleepwalking in headache sufferers may reveal other possible associations between sleep problems and headaches.

The frequency of reported sleep paralysis at onset of sleep (ie, 11 [46%]) in the "other headache" group is similar to that reported in general population studies. The unusually low report (2 [7%]) of sleep paralysis at onset of sleep in the headache with sleep disorders group may be related to the short sleep latencies typical of patients with excessive daytime sleepiness. [15] In normal, middle-aged subjects the mean sleep latency is 15 to 20 minutes.[16] This onset of sleep period in normal subjects is characterized by intermittent brief arousals during which there is the recognition of sleep paralysis.[17-20] The demonstrated reduction of sleep latency in subjects with excessive daytime sleepiness eliminates many of the arousals typically associated with falling asleep. The only exception to this rule is observed in patients with narcolepsy.

In these patients, despite short sleep latencies, the abnormal occurrence of rapid eye movement sleep (and its associated complete muscle atonia) at onset of sleep leads to a much higher than expected report of sleep paralysis.[18] In the context of this report, the lower than usual frequency of reported sleep paralysis emphasizes the excessive daytime sleepiness component of the overall clinical picture for this subgroup, but the presence or absence of this symptom has little diagnostic value in a single-case medical history.

The follow-up results are of interest as they show that complete cure of the headache complaint may be obtained in 17 subjects (65.4%) with sleep disorders who selected headache as their most troublesome symptom. However, the rest of the subjects had persistence of some headache complaint, albeit much decreased in frequency and intensity. The largest group of subjects with such complaints was the PLM syndrome group (5 subjects [62.5%]). The presence of this group raises some theoretical questions. We know that control of the PLM syndrome led to improvement of the headache complaint. The interaction between the sleep disorder and the frequency of the cephalalgia is, thus, clear. Whether the nocturnal headache had an impact on PLM is less clear. The question left unresolved is whether there is a problem leading to the onset of both syndromes or 2 completely different syndromes interacting in the same individual.

References

1. Hopkins A, Menken M, DeFriese G, A record of patient encounters in neurological practice in the United Kingdom. *J Neurol Neurosurg Psychiatry*. 1989-52: 436-438.

2. Papapetropoulos T, Tsibre E, Pelekoudas V. The neurological content of general practice. *J Neurol Neurosurg Psychiatry*. 1989;52:434-43 5.

3. Menken M. Neurologic education for primary care: relevance of secondary diagnosis. *Arch Neurol* 1986-43:947-950.

4. Miller J. The neurologic content of family practice: implications for neurologists. *Arch Neurol* 1986;43:286-288.

5. Paiva T, Batista A, Martins P, Martins A. The relationship between headaches and sleep disturbances. *Headache*. 1995;35:590-596.

6. Headache Classification Committee of the International Headache Society. *Classification and diagnostic criteria for headache disorders, cranial neuraigias and facial pain.* Cephalalgia. 1988;8(suppl 7):10-73.

7. Miles L. Sleep questionnaires. In: Guilleminault C, ed. *Sleep and Waking Disorders, Indications and Techniques*. Reading, Mass: Addison-Wesley Publishing Co; 1982:383-413.

8. International Classification of Sleep Disorders of the American Sleep Disorders Association. *Diagnostic and Coding Manual* Rochester, Minn: American Sleep Disorders Association; 1990.

9. Rechtschaffen A, Kales A. *A Manual of Standardized Terminology: Techniques and Scoring System for Sleep Stages of Human Subjects*. Washington, DC: US Government Printing Office; 1968.

10. Barabas G, Ferrari M, Matthews WS. Childhood migraine and somnambulism. *Neurology*. 1983;33:948-949.

11. Dexter JD. The relationship between disorders of arousal from sleep and migraine. *Headache*. 1986;26-322.

12. Giraud M. D'Aghis P. Guard 0, Dumas R. Migraine et somnambulisme: une enquete portant sur 122 migraineux. *Revneurol* (Paris). 1986;142:42-46.

13. Pradalier A, Guroud M, Dry J. Somnambulism, migraine and propanolol. *Headache.* 1987;27:143-145.

14. Paiva T, Martins P, Batistaa, Esperanca P, Martins I. Sleep disturbances in chronic headache patients: a comparison with healthy controls. *Headache Q.* 1994;5: 135-141.

15. Roth T, Roehrs TA, Carskadon MA, Dement WC. Daytime sleepiness and alertness. In: Kryger M, Roth T, Dement WC, eds. *Principles and Practice of Sleep Medicine.* 2nd ed. Philadelphia, Pa: V~B Saunders Co; 1994:40-49.

16. Carskadon MA, Dement WC, Mitler MM, Guilleminault C, Zarcone VP, Speigel R. Self-reports versus sleep laboratory findings in 122 drug-free subjects with complaints of chronic insomnia. *Am J Psychiatry.* 1976;133:1382-1388.

17. Pivik RT. The several qualities of sleepiness: psychophysiological considerations. In: Monk TH, ed. *Sleep, Sleepiness and Performance.* New York, NY: John Wiley & Sons Inc; 1991:3-37.

18. Hishikawa Y. Sleep paralysis. In: Guilleminault C, Passouant P, Dement WC, eds. *Narcolepsy.* New York, NY: Spectrum Publishers; 1976:95-124.

19. Penn NE, Kripke DF, Scharff J. Sleep paralysis among medical students. *J Psychol* 1981;107:247-252.

20. Bell CC, Shakoor B, Thompson B, et al. Prevalence to isolated sleep paralysis in black subjects. *JAMA.* 1984;76:500-508.

—by Teresa Paiva;
Ana Farinha;
Antonio Martins;
Andre Batista;
Christian Guilleminault.

Chapter 48

Sleep Disorders and Multiple Sclerosis

Individuals with multiple sclerosis (MS) who believe they are fatigued may actually have a sleeping condition.

It is estimated that one-third of a person's life is spent sleeping. For those with MS who may also take naps during the day, that figure rises. Thus, quantity and quality of sleep are especially important to individuals with MS.

"MS is definitely a reason to have a sleep problem," says Lauren Caruso, PhD, a neuropsychologist at St. Agnes Hospital's Medical Rehabilitation Research and Training Center for MS in White Plains, N.Y., "because there is a possibility of brain lesions [plaques] in the areas that regulate sleep."

What Goes Wrong?

Normal sleep can be disrupted by psychological, behavioral, and physiological factors. It is the latter of these that should most often concern doctors when MS patients complain of sleep abnormalities.

Studies conducted by Campbell M. Clark, MD, associate professor of psychiatry at the University of British Columbia in Vancouver, Canada, found that three lesion sites serving the supplementary motor areas of the brain were significantly correlated to the presence

Reprinted with permission from V. Hinson-Smith, *Real Living with Multiple Sclerosis*, September 1997 Volume 4 Number 9. © 1997 Springhouse Corporation.

of sleep complaints in persons with MS: the right and left frontal white matter in the supraventricular section and the deep white matter of the right insula. He concluded that the presence of sleep disturbances and depression in MS "may be a function of the lesion sites."

According to Dr. Clark, sleep complaints in the normal population registered "about 6%," although "it was about 25%" in the MS population. "Therefore," he says, "we hypothesized that these lesion sites, because they serve motor areas, may be causing periodic leg movement syndrome [PLMS] and that the usual pattern of neuronal firings disturbs the person and he actually wakes himself up."

Art Walters, MD, is a neurologist and sleep disorders specialist at the Robert Wood Johnson Medical School in New Brunswick, N.J. Because of his work with MS patients, he has become quite familiar with studies reporting that, in patients with both MS and PLMS, "as the MS remits, the PLMS tends to disappear." When there is another MS exacerbation, however, he says PLMS reappears.

PLMS does not in itself cause drowsiness, says Dr. Walters, "but I don't think drowsiness is the only measure of the quality of life vis-a-vis sleep disruption." He says what is important is the high incidence of those sleep disruptions and how they can cause memory difficulties and depression in persons with PLMS.

Dr. Clark says his research team also found that MS patients with sleep disturbance had higher scores for depression. "There has always been the argument," he says, "that depression is associated with MS, but how do you clinically classify depression? Well, one of the symptoms [of depression] is sleep disturbance."

Studies indicate that a significant number of persons with MS also show evidence of sleep apnea above what Dr. Caruso calls the "expected range" for the MS age-group. She describes apnea, which is the cessation of airflow at the nostrils and mouth lasting at least 10 seconds, as either obstructive (blockage of the airway by bone structure or extra fleshy material), central (neural failure to initiate breathing, as is the case in MS), or mixed (components of both).

Apnea severely disrupts sleep continuity and leaves those who suffer from it feeling chronically tired and fatigued. It is often accompanied by gasping, choking, or pauses in breathing during sleep.

Nocturia, excessive urination at night, is another common cause of arousals from sleep and, consequently, a disruption of sleep continuity for MS patients. Additionally, persons with MS often take several medications and may have what Dr. Caruso calls "complex drug regimes" that may alter certain sleep stages.

What Does It All Add Up To?

The result of any or all of the sleep abnormalities described may, as Dr. Caruso explains, contribute to daytime fatigue, excessive daytime sleepiness, and narcoleptic-like occurrences in persons with MS. She reports that persons suffering from true narcolepsy (the inability to inhibit REM sleep) show certain immunologic changes similar to those found in MS.

Mark Mahawold, MD, professor of neurology at the University of Minnesota School of Medicine and director of the Minnesota Regional Sleep Disorders Center in Minneapolis, says that "the real 'take-home' message regarding excessive daytime sleepiness is that it is most likely due to some underlying primary sleep disorder that is diagnosable and treatable and not due to the fatigue of MS or depression."

When Sleep Is "Suspect"

If a person with MS has a sleep problem, Neil Kavey, MD, director of the Sleep Disorders Center at Columbia-Presbyterian Medical Center in New York, recommends being specific when talking with a physician. Tell the doctor whether or not you are having difficulty falling asleep, staying asleep, moving excessively or having restlessness in sleep, feeling uncomfortable during sleep, having muscle spasms or jerking during sleep, choking during sleep, mumbling or talking or 'calling out' during sleep, or waking often during the night." He emphasizes that "how a person feels during the day" is important too.

"Solid research needs to be done," says Dr. Kavey, "and clinicians should include 'sleep' in their patient histories and should understand that there exists a real expertise in determining and managing sleep disorders.

"If MS patients or their families think they are having a sleep problem, they are," said Dr. Kavey. And they're not "crazy" to think something is wrong, and their doctors should not make inquiry from the perspective of "anxiety or depression" as reaction to the disease. Now perhaps patients will open a door with their doctors, and from there it can only lead to something good.

Options

So what do doctors do about confirmed sleep problems in persons with MS? Depending on the diagnosis, experts suggest a number of things.

A doctor might take a fairly conservative approach and begin a behavioral remediation program for certain patients. Such a program might include education in sleep regimen (setting the proper times to rise and to go to bed) and sleep scheduling, along with the completion of "sleep logs," which average the amount of time spent sleeping against how the patient feels during the day—leading to a "magic number" of sleep hours needed. For patients complaining of daytime fatigue and tiredness, naps are sometimes scheduled at appropriate times.

Individuals will likely be told to eliminate stimulants (coffee and cola) before bedtime and be asked to evaluate their diets for "hidden" sources of caffeine. Alcohol, individuals will be told, may initially cause drowsiness and invite sleep, but that type of sleep is usually fragmented and of inferior quality. Patients also will learn that tobacco has been reported to disturb sleep.

Doctors treating sleep disturbances might adjust certain MS medications that could have an effect on sleep. Along those lines, a discussion about all other medications, including over-the-counter drugs, might warrant an increase, decrease, or withdrawal of some medicines.

Judicious use of medications to induce sleep might be considered, but many sleep specialists caution that "sleeping pills" can sometimes have an unintended effect and that different, more appropriate management of sleep disorders might make them unnecessary.

Persons who have been diagnosed with PLMS have options that may or may not include prescription drugs. Nutritional changes and additions might make a difference, but medical testing for nutritional deficiencies is critical before dietary supplements are added.

In mild apnea, an oral appliance (much like a dental retainer) might be fitted as treatment. The device fits in the mouth during sleep and pulls the jaw and tongue forward to open the airway. In more serious cases, the most common form of treatment for apnea is use of a continuous positive airway pressure mask resting over the nose during sleep. A small machine to which it is attached pumps air into the mask and through the nose. That airflow then holds open the walls of the throat.

Guard Your Sleep

"Sleep is so basic," concludes Dr. Caruso, "and persons with MS should be especially careful with their sleep. They should be jealous of it and not let anyone or anything hinder it. People with MS already have enough going wrong with their bodies, and they don't need another biological rhythm being thrown off....There's nobody more worthwhile to help by treating sleep disorders than these people, who are such a major part of our society."

Tell your doctor if:

- you have trouble falling or staying asleep
- you wake up often in the night
- you have twitching or jerking of the legs during sleep
- you snore, gasp, choke, or stop breathing at times during sleep
- you often mumble, talk, scream, or walk in your sleep
- you awaken too early in the morning
- you wake feeling tired and unrefreshed after a normal amount of sleep
- you are excessively sleepy during the day
- you have problems staying awake during the day
- you fall asleep at inappropriate times and places
- you have sleep attacks and fall asleep uncontrollably

—by Vicki Hinson-Smith

Vicki Hinson-Smith lives and works in Massachusetts and New York. She has MS.

Chapter 49

Sleep Disorders in Cancer Patients

Cancer patients are at great risk for developing insomnia and disorders of the sleep-wake cycle. Insomnia is the most common sleep disturbance in this population and is most often secondary to physical and/or psychological factors related to cancer and/or cancer treatment. Anxiety and depression, common psychological responses to the diagnosis of cancer, cancer treatment, and hospitalization, are highly correlated with insomnia.[1-3]

Sleep disturbances may be exacerbated by paraneoplastic syndromes associated with steroid production and by symptoms associated with tumor invasion, such as draining lesions, gastrointestinal (GI) and genitourinary (GU) alterations, pain, fever, cough, dyspnea, pruritus, and fatigue. Medications, including vitamins, administration of corticosteroids, neuroleptics for nausea and vomiting, and sympathomimetics for the treatment of dyspnea, as well as other treatment factors can impact negatively on sleep patterns.

Side effects of treatment that may affect the sleep-wake cycle include:[4]

- pain
- anxiety
- night sweats/hot flashes
- GI disturbances (i.e., incontinence, diarrhea, constipation, nausea)
- GU disturbances (i.e., incontinence, retention, GU irritation)
- respiratory disturbances

NIH Publication, National Cancer Institute, modified March 1998.

Hypnotic drugs can also cause insomnia in cancer patients. Sustained use of central nervous system stimulants (e.g., amphetamines, caffeine, diet pills), sedatives and hypnotics (e.g., glutethimide, benzodiazepines, pentobarbital, chloral hydrate, secobarbital sodium, amobarbital sodium), cancer chemotherapeutic agents (especially antimetabolites), anticonvulsants (e.g., phenytoin), adrenocorticotropin, oral contraceptives, monoamine oxidase inhibitors, methyldopa, propranolol, atenolol, alcohol, and thyroid preparations can cause insomnia. In addition, withdrawal from central nervous system depressants (barbiturates, opioids, glutethimide, chloral hydrate, methaqualone, ethchlorvynol, alcohol, and over-the-counter and prescription antihistamine sedatives), benzodiazepines, major tranquilizers, tricyclic and monamine oxidase inhibitor antidepressants, illicit drugs (e.g., marijuana, cocaine, phencyclidine, opioids) may cause insomnia. Agents containing aspirin may also cause insomnia. The most commonly prescribed hypnotics interfere with REM sleep resulting in increased irritability, apathy, and diminished mental alertness. Abrupt withdrawal of hypnotics and sedatives may lead to many symptoms including nervousness, jitteriness, seizures, and REM rebound. Berlin defined REM rebound as a "marked increase in REM sleep with increased frequency and intensity of dreaming, including nightmares."[5] The increased physiologic arousal that occurs during REM rebound may be dangerous for patients with peptic ulcers or a history of cardiovascular problems.

Hospitalized patients are likely to experience frequent interruptions of sleep due to treatment schedules, hospital routines, and roommates, which singularly or collectively alter the sleep-wake schedule. Other factors influencing sleep-wake schedules in the hospital setting include age, noise, temperature, comfort, pain, and anxiety.[6]

Consequences of sleep disturbances can influence outcomes of therapeutic and supportive care measures. The patient with mild to moderate sleep disturbances may experience irritability and inability to concentrate, which may in turn affect the patient's compliance with treatment protocols, ability to make decisions, and relationships with significant others. Depression and anxiety can also be end-results of sleep disturbances. Supportive care measures are directed toward promoting quality of life and adequate rest.

References

1. Coursey RD: Personality measures and evoked responses in chronic insomniacs. *Journal of Abnormal Psychology* 84(3): 239-249, 1975.

2. Freemon FR: *Sleep Research: A Critical Review*. Springfield, IL: Thomas Publishing, 1972.

3. Johns MW, Bruce DW, Masterton JP: Psychological correlates of sleep habits reported by healthy young adults. *British Journal of Medical Psychology* 47(2): 181-187, 1974.

4. Page M: Sleep pattern disturbance. In: McNally JC, Stair JC, Somerville ET, Eds.: *Guidelines for Cancer Nursing Practice*. Orlando, FL: Grune and Stratton, Inc., 1985, pp 89-95.

5. Berlin RM: Management of insomnia in hospitalized patients. *Annals of Internal Medicine* 100(3): 398-404, 1984.

6. Webster RA, Thompson DR: Sleep in hospital. *Journal of Advanced Nursing* 11(4): 447-457, 1986.

7. Clark J, Landis L, McGee R: Nursing management of outcomes of disease, psychological response, treatment, and complications. In: Ziegfeld CR, Ed.: *Core Curriculum for Oncology Nursing*. Philadelphia: W.B. Saunders, 1987, pp 271-319.

Assessment

Assessment is the initial step in management strategies. Assessment data should include documentation of predisposing factors, sleep patterns, emotional status, exercise and activity level, diet, symptoms, medications, and caregiver routines.[1] The sections below outline recommendations for a sleep history and physical examination. Data can be retrieved from multiple sources: the patient's subjective report of sleep difficulty, objective observations of behavioral and physiologic manifestations of sleep disturbances, and reports from the patient's significant others regarding the patient's quality of sleep.[2]

The diagnosis of insomnia is primarily based on a careful, detailed medical and psychiatric history. The American Sleep Disorders Association has produced guidelines for the use of polysomnography as an objective tool in evaluating insomnia. The routine polysomnogram includes the monitoring of EEG, electro-oculography, electromyography, effort of breathing and air flow, oxygen saturation, electrocardiography, and body position. Polysomnography is the major diagnostic tool in sleep disorders and is indicated in the evaluation of suspected sleep-related breathing disorders and periodic limb movement disorder, and when the cause of insomnia is uncertain or when behavioral or pharmacologic therapy is unsuccessful.[3]

Risk Factors for Sleep Disorders

- disease factors including paraneoplastic syndromes with increased steroid production; symptoms associated with tumor invasion (e.g., obstruction, pain, fever, shortness of breath, pruritus, fatigue)

- treatment factors including symptoms related to surgery (e.g., pain, frequent monitoring, narcotics); chemotherapy (e.g., exogenous corticosteroids); symptoms related to chemotherapy

- medications such as narcotics, sedatives/hypnotics, steroids, caffeine/nicotine, some antidepressants, vitamins

- environmental factors

- physical and/or psychological stressors

- depression (see the PDQ summary on depression)

- anxiety (see the PDQ summary on anxiety)

- delirium (see the PDQ summary on delirium)

- daytime seizures, snoring, headaches

Characterization of Sleep

- usual patterns of sleep, including usual bedtime, routine prior to retiring (e.g., food, bath, medications), length of time before onset of sleep, and duration of sleep (awaking episodes during night, ability to resume sleep, and usual time to awaken)

- characteristics of disturbed sleep (changes following diagnosis, treatment, and/or hospitalization)

- perception of significant others as to quantity and quality of patient's sleep

- family history of sleep disorders

References

1. Kaempfer SH: Insomnia. In: Baird SB, Ed.: *Decision Making in Oncology Nursing*. Philadelphia: B.C. Decker, Inc., 1988, pp 78-79.

2. Kaempfer SH: Comfort: Sleep. In: Johnson BL, Gross J, Eds.: *Handbook of Oncology Nursing*. New York: John Wiley & Sons, 1985, pp 167-184.

3. Standards of Practice Committee of the American Sleep Disorders Association: An *American Sleep Disorders Association Report*: practice parameters for the use of polysomnography in the evaluation of insomnia. Sleep 18(1): 55-57, 1995.

Management

Management of sleep disturbances should focus on treatment of symptoms related to the cancer and its treatment, and identification and management of environmental and psychological factors. Treatment of the malignancy may resolve the sleep disturbance. When sleep disturbances are caused by symptoms of cancer or treatment, measures that control or alleviate symptoms are often the key to resolving sleep disturbances. Management of sleep disturbances combines non-pharmacologic and pharmacologic approaches individualized for the patient.

Non-Pharmacologic Management of Sleep Disturbances

The environment can be modified to decrease sleep disruption. Minimizing noise, dimming or turning off lights, adjusting room temperature, and consolidating patient care tasks to decrease interruptions can increase the amount of uninterrupted sleep.

Other Actions or Interventions That May Promote Rest Include[1,2]

- keeping the patient's skin clean and dry

- giving backrubs and/or massaging areas of the body the patient might find comforting (e.g., bony prominences, head and scalp, shoulders, hands, feet)

- keeping bedding and/or surfaces of support devices (chairs, pillows) clean, dry, and wrinkle-free

- ensuring adequate bedcovers for warmth

- regulating fluid intake to avoid frequent awakening for elimination

- encouraging bowel and bladder elimination before sleep

- promoting optimal bowel function (increased fluids, fiber in diet, use of stool softeners and laxatives)

- using condom catheter for nocturnal incontinence

- providing high-protein snack 2 hours before bedtime, e.g., milk, turkey, foods high in tryptophan

- avoiding beverages with caffeine

- encouraging patient to dress in loose, soft clothing

- facilitating comfort through repositioning and support with pillows as needed

- encouraging exercise or activity no less than 2 hours before bedtime

- keeping regular bedtime and awakening hours

- minimizing and coordinating necessary bedside contacts for inpatients

Psychological interventions are directed toward facilitating the patient's coping processes through education, support, and reassurance. As the patient learns to cope with the stresses of illness, hospitalization, and treatment, sleep may improve.[3] Relaxation exercises and self-hypnosis performed at bedtime can be helpful in promoting calm and sleep. Cognitive behavioral interventions that diminish the distress associated with early insomnia and change the goal from "need to sleep" to "just relax" can diminish anxiety and promote sleep.[4] Communication and verbalization of concerns, and openness between the patient, family, and health care team should be encouraged.

Pharmacologic Management of Sleep Disturbances

When sleep disturbances are not resolved with other supportive care measures, the use of sleep medications on a short-term or intermittent basis may be helpful. However, prolonged use of sleep medications for persistent insomnia can impair natural sleep patterns (i.e., REM deprivation) and alter physiologic functions. Prolonged use (>1-2 weeks) of these medications may result in tolerance, psychological and physical dependence, drug intoxication, and drug hangover.[5]

A newer agent, zolpidem, has reportedly not been associated with tolerance, dependence, sleep cycle alterations, or rebound insomnia. Zolpidem tartrate (Ambien) is administered in doses of 5-10 mg, 30 minutes before bedtime. To date, it has not been widely used or studied in cancer patients.

Benzodiazepines have been widely used in the management of sleep disturbances. Used as an adjunct to other treatment for short periods of time, these agents are safe and effective in producing natural sleep because they are less disruptive of REM sleep than are other hypnotic agents. Benzodiazepines have an anti-anxiety effect in low doses and a hypnotic effect in high doses.

Benzodiazepines differ from each other in duration of action and pharmacokinetics. Liver disease has less effect on the metabolism of lorazepam, oxazepam, and temazepam than on the metabolism of other benzodiazepines. While long-acting agents may produce daytime hangover, short-acting agents are more often associated with dependence, rebound insomnia, early morning insomnia, daytime anxiety, and serious withdrawal effects, such as seizures.[3] The following general characterizations can be made:

Intermediate- and short-acting benzodiazepines are characterized by half-lives of from 4 to 24 hours.

Short-acting benzodiazepines are characterized by:

1. few active metabolites
2. rarely, accumulation with multiple doses
3. minimal affect on drug clearance by age and liver disease

Long-acting benzodiazepines are characterized by:

1. half-lives of longer than 24 hours
2. pharmacologically active metabolites
3. accumulation with multiple dosages, and
4. impaired clearance in the elderly and those with liver disease

In general, non-benzodiazepines are reserved for patients who cannot tolerate benzodiazepines. Antihistamines have become popular drugs for the management of sleep disturbances among cancer patients. The anticholinergic properties of antihistamines relieve nausea and vomiting as well as insomnia. These agents must be used with caution since daytime sedation and delirium can occur, especially in

Table 49.1a. Medications Commonly Used to Promote Sleep

drug category	medication	hypnotic dose (route)	onset (duration of action)
benzodiazepines	diazepam (Valium)	5-10 mg (capsule, tablet)	30-60 min (6-8 hours)
	temazepam (Restoril)	15-30 mg (capsule)	60 min, minimum (6-8 hrs)
	triazolam (Halcion)	0.125-0.5 mg (tablet)	30 min (peaks 1-1.5 hours)
	clonazepam (Klonopin)	0.5-2.0 mg (tablet)	30-60 min (8-12 hours)
tricyclic antidepressants	doxepin (Sinequan)	10-150 mg	30 min
	amitriptyline (Elavil)	10-15 mg	30 min
	nortriptyline (Pamelor)	10-50 mg	30 min
chloral derivatives	chloral hydrate	0.5-1.0 g (capsule, syrup, suppository)	30-60 min (4-8 hrs)

Table 49.1b. Medications Commonly Used to Promote Sleep

drug category	medication	hypnotic dose (route)	onset (duration of action)
second generation antidepressants	trazodone	25-150 mg	30 min
	nefazadone	50-100 mg	30 min
antihistamines 10-30 min	diphenhydramine		25-100 mg
	(Benadryl)	(tablet, capsule, syrup)	(4-6 hrs)
	hydroxyzine (Vistaril, Atarax)'	10-100 mg (tablet, capsule, syrup)	15-30 min (4-6 hrs)
neuroleptics	thioridazine (Mellaril)	10-50 mg	30-60 min
	chlorpromazine (Thorazine)	10-50 mg	30-60 min
other	zolpidem tartrate (Ambien)	5-20 mg	30 min (4-6 hours)

the elderly. Tricyclic antidepressants, such as amitriptyline or doxepin (Sinequan), may be effective in patients who are not depressed as well as those who are depressed. When given at bedtime, these sedating agents can eliminate the need for an additional hypnotic. Low doses of tricyclic antidepressants can be effective sleep agents and may be the treatment of choice for insomnia in patients who have neuropathic pain and appetite loss (e.g., doxepin 50-100 mg at bedtime; amitriptyline 25-100 mg at bedtime). In low doses, trazodone (50-150 mg) can promote sleep and is often combined with other antidepressants (e.g., fluoxetine 20 mg in the morning) in depressed patients with insomnia. The hypnotic effects of marijuana (tetrahydrocannabinol or THC) are similar to conventional hypnotics in reducing REM sleep; however, side effects prior to sleep induction and hangover make the use of THC less acceptable than benzodiazepines.[6]

Low potency neuroleptics (e.g., thioridazine 10-25 mg) are useful in promoting sleep in patients with insomnia associated with organic mental syndromes and delirium. A separate summary containing information on delirium is also available in PDQ.

Barbiturates are generally not recommended for the management of sleep disturbances in cancer patients. Barbiturates have a number of adverse effects, including the development of tolerance, and they also have a narrow margin of safety.

Most hypnotics are effective initially but lose efficacy when used regularly, and they can become a primary cause of sleep disturbances.[7]

Melatonin, a hormone produced by the pineal gland during the hours of darkness, plays a major role in the sleep/wake cycle. While further study is indicated, melatonin may play an important role in the treatment of certain types of chronic sleep disorders.[8,9] It is suggested that melatonin exerts a hypnotic effect through thermoregulatory mechanisms. By lowering the core body temperature, melatonin reduces arousal and increases sleep propensity. Melatonin is likely to be an effective hypnotic agent for sleep disruption associated with elevated temperature due to low circulating melatonin levels. The combined circadian and hypnotic effects of melatonin suggest a synergistic action in the treatment of sleep disorders related to the inappropriate timing of sleep and wakefulness. Adjuvant melatonin may also improve sleep disruption caused by drugs known to alter normal melatonin production (e.g., beta-blockers and benzodiazepines).[8]

Melatonin replacement has been shown to improve sleep in children with endocrine tumors that diminish the natural production of the hormone.[9] However, this efficacy has not been shown beyond this particular study. Melatonin may affect the way tumor cells respond to chemotherapy and radiation therapy. Some studies in colon and brain cancer suggest the effect of melatonin on chemotherapy and on radiation therapy may be beneficial.[10] However, not enough is known to assure patients on these therapies that melatonin treatment for insomnia is safe. The use of melatonin to treat insomnia in cancer patients is under evaluation. Because the effect of melatonin on chemotherapy can vary, it is important for patients taking chemotherapy to consult with their health care professionals before using melatonin.

Changes in sleep/wake patterns are among the hallmarks of biologic aging.[11] Evidence suggests that circulating melatonin levels may be significantly lower in physically healthy elderly people and in insomniacs than in age-matched control subjects. In view of these findings, melatonin replacement therapy may be beneficial in the initiation and maintenance of sleep in the elderly.[12] However, melatonin replacement has not been studied in elderly people with cancer as a treatment for insomnia.

References

1. Page M: Sleep pattern disturbance. In: McNally JC, Stair JC, Somerville ET, Eds.: *Guidelines for Cancer Nursing Practice.* Orlando, FL: Grune and Stratton, Inc., 1985, pp 89-95.

2. Kaempfer SH: Insomnia. In: Baird SB, Ed.: *Decision Making in Oncology Nursing.* Philadelphia: B.C. Decker, Inc., 1988, pp 78-79.

3. Berlin RM: Management of insomnia in hospitalized patients. *Annals of Internal Medicine* 100(3): 398-404, 1984.

4. Horowitz SA, Breitbart W: Relaxation and imagery for symptom control in cancer patients. In: Breitbart W, Holland JC, Eds.: *Psychiatric Aspects of Symptom Management in Cancer Patients.* Washington, DC: American Psychiatric Press, 1993, pp 147-171.

5. Kaempfer SH: Comfort: Sleep. In: Johnson BL, Gross J, Eds.: *Handbook of Oncology Nursing.* New York: John Wiley & Sons, 1985, pp 167-184.

6. Hollister LE: Health aspects of cannabis. *Pharmacological Reviews* 38(1): 1-20, 1986.

7. Hayter J: Advances in sleep research: implications for nursing practice. In: Tierney AJ, Ed.: *Recent Advances in Nursing: Clinical Nursing Practice*. Edinburgh, Scotland: Churchill Livingstone, 1986, pp 21-43.

8. Dawson D, Encel N: Melatonin and sleep in humans. *Journal of Pineal Research* 15(1): 1-12, 1993.

9. Jan JE, Espezel H, Appleton RE: The treatment of sleep disorders with melatonin. *Developmental Medicine and Child Neurology* 36(2): 97-107 1994.

10. Lissoni P, Meregalli S, Nosetto L, et al.: Increased survival time in brain glioblastomas by a radioneuroendocrine strategy with radiotherapy plus melatonin compared to radiotherapy alone. *Oncology* 53(1): 43-46, 1996.

11. Haimov I, Lavie L: Melatonin-a chronobiotic and soporific hormone. *Archives of Gerontology and Geriatrics* 24(2): 167-173, 1997.

12. Haimov I, Lavie P, Laudon M, et al.: Melatonin replacement therapy of elderly insomniacs. *Sleep* 18(7): 598-603, 1995.

Special Considerations

The Patient With Pain

Since enhanced pain control improves sleep, appropriate analgesics or non-pharmacologic pain management should be administered before introducing sleep medications. Tricyclic antidepressants can be particularly useful for the treatment of insomnia in patients with neuropathic pain and depression. Patients on high-dose opioids for pain may be at increased risk for the development of delirium and organic mental disorders. Such patients may benefit from the use of low-dose neuroleptics as sleep agents (e.g., thioridazine 25-50 mg or haloperidol 0.5-1.0 mg).

The Elderly

Elderly patients frequently have insomnia due to age-related changes in sleep. The sleep cycle in this population is characterized by lighter sleep, more frequent awakenings, and less total sleep time. Anxiety, depression, loss of social support, and a diagnosis of cancer are contributory factors in sleep disturbances in the elderly.[1]

Sleep problems in older adults are so common that nearly half of all hypnotic prescriptions written are for persons over 65 years of age. Although normal aging affects sleep, the clinician should evaluate the many factors that cause insomnia, such as medical illness, psychiatric illness, dementia, alcohol and/or polypharmacy, restless legs syndrome, periodic leg movements, and sleep apnea syndrome. Nonpharmacologic treatment of sleep disorders is the preferred initial management, with the use of medication when indicated, and referral to a sleep disorder center when specialized care is necessary.[2]

Providing a regular schedule of meals, discouraging daytime naps, and encouraging physical activity may improve sleep. Hypnotic prescriptions for elderly patients must be adjusted for variations in metabolism, increased fat stores, and increased sensitivity. Dosages should be reduced by 30%-50%. Problems associated with drug accumulation (especially flurazepam) must be weighed against the risks of more severe withdrawal or rebound effects associated with short-acting benzodiazepines. An alternate drug for elderly patients is chloral hydrate.[1]

Somnolence Syndrome in Children

Cranial irradiation and intrathecal methotrexate are used to prevent the development of central nervous system (CNS) leukemia in children with acute lymphocytic leukemia (ALL). Somnolence syndrome (SS) is a complication of cranial irradiation occurring in 30%-50% of patients who receive over 1,800 cGy at daily dose fractions of 150-200 cGy. The syndrome may appear 4-6 weeks following completion of therapy. SS is characterized by mild drowsiness to moderate lethargy and, occasionally, low-grade fever. The pathophysiology is unknown, but electroencephalogram and cerebral spinal fluid abnormalities are detectable in affected children. While supportive care measures cannot prevent the occurrence of SS, acknowledgment of the existence of this problem may prevent or minimize anxieties for children and parents when symptoms of SS appear.

Sleep Apnea Following Mandibulectomy

Anterior mandibulectomy can result in the development of sleep apnea. All patients with head and neck tumors who have had extensive anterior oral cavity resection should be evaluated prior to decannulation of the tracheostomy tube. Subsequent flap and/or reconstruction of the lower jaw seems to prevent the development of sleep apnea. In contrast, facial sling suspension of the lower lip does not prevent the development of sleep apnea.[3] Assessment for symptoms and preparation for the appearance of symptoms in this population provide indications for interventions related to sleep apnea.

References

1. Berlin RM: Management of insomnia in hospitalized patients. *Annals of Internal Medicine* 100(3): 398-404, 1984.

2. Johnston JE: Sleep problems in the elderly. *Journal of the American Academy of Nurse Practitioners* 6(4): 161-166, 1994.

3. Panje WR, Holmes DK: Mandibulectomy without reconstruction can cause sleep apnea. *Laryngoscope* 94(12, Part 1): 1591-1594, 1984.

Part Six

Additional Help and Information

Chapter 50

Glossary of Sleep-Related Terminology

adenoids: Gland-like tissue growths in the nose above the throat which obstruct breathing when swollen.

airway obstruction: Narrowing, clogging or blocking of the air passages to or in the lung.

apnea: Cessation of breathing.

arousal: An abrupt change from deep sleep to a lighter stage of sleep which may or may not lead to awakening.

cardiac arrest: Sudden cessation of cardiac function.

cardiac arrhythmia: Variation in the normal rhythm of the heartbeat.

cataplexy: Sudden episodes of loss of muscle function, ranging from slight weakness (such as limpness at the neck or knees, sagging facial muscles, or inability to speak clearly) to complete body collapse.

This chapter includes definitions excerpted from NIH Publication Numbers 96-3645, 96-3649, and 97-407; NICHD Public Information and Communications Branch, *Sudden Infant Death Syndrome,* April 1997; National Heart, Lung, and Blood Institute, *Sleep Apnea: Breathing Disorders During Sleep,* August 1994; and *Wake Up America: A National Sleep Alert,* Volume 1, Executive Summary and Executive Report, Report of the National Commission on Sleep Disorders Research, Submitted to the United States Congress and to the Secretary U.S. Department of Health and Human Services, January 1993.

circadian rhythm: Natural daily fluctuation of physiological and behavioral functions.

circadian rhythm sleep disorders: This cluster of disorders is characterized by a disruption in the biological clock in which there is a "misalignment between the patient's sleep pattern and that which is desired or regarded as the societal norm."

corpulmonale: Heart disease secondary to lung disease.

CPAP: A mechanical device used to deliver continuous positive airway pressure.

dyspnea: Difficult or labored breathing.

diaphragm: The major respiratory muscle that participates in the act of breathing. The diaphragm separates the chest and abdominal areas.

edema: Abnormal amount of fluid in body tissues.

extrinsic sleep disorder: Sleep upsets that "originate or develop from causes outside of the body.

hemorrhage: Escape of blood from blood-carrying tissue.

hypnagogic hallucinations: Vivid, often frightening, dream-like experiences that occur while dozing or falling asleep.

hypoxia: A state in which there is oxygen deficiency.

hyperventilation: A state in which abnormally fast and deep respiration results in the intake of excessive amount of oxygen into the lung and reduced carbon dioxide levels in the blood.

hypoventilation: A state in which there is an insufficient amount of air entering and leaving the lung to bring oxygen to the tissues and eliminate carbon dioxide.

insomnia: The perception or complaint of inadequate or poor-quality sleep because of one or more of the following:

- difficulty falling asleep.
- waking up frequently during the night with difficulty returning to sleep.

- waking up too early in the morning.
- unrefreshing sleep.

intrinsic sleep disorders: Those that "either originate or develop within the body, or arise from causes within the body," and include, among others, narcolepsy, sleep apnea, restless legs syndrome, and certain forms of insomnia.

ischemic heart disease: Heart disease from restricted blood supply due to obstruction in blood vessels.

narcolepsy: A neurological disorder whose main symptom is uncontrollable, excessive sleep, regardless of the time of day or whether the person has had enough sleep during the previous night.

nares: Openings in the nasal cavities—nostrils.

NONREM sleep: A nonuniform series of four stages of sleep which occur early in the night and are characterized by the absence of movement and slow wave brain activity.

parasomnias: "Clinical disorders that are not abnormalities of the processes responsible for sleep...but rather are undesirable physical phenomena that occur predominantly during sleep," such as SIDS and infant sleep apnea, REM behavior disorder, sleepwalking, and sleep terrors.

polysomnography: The continuous recording of a number of physiological functions and events during sleep.

problem sleepiness: Sleepiness that interferes with daily routines and activities, or reduces the ability to function.

prostaglandins: A group of fat-delivered chemicals involved in the regulation of a number of body functions.

pulmonary function tests: Tests to measure the degree of damage to the lung; the most common tests measure, using a device called the spirometer, the ability of the lung to move air into and out of the lung.

rapid eye movement: A stage of sleep in which dreaming is associated with mild involuntary muscle movements. Adults cycle in and out of REM at about 90 minute intervals. REM occupies about 20 percent of total sleep.

restless legs syndrome: A sleep disorder in which a person experiences unpleasant sensations in the legs described as creeping, crawling, tingling, pulling, or painful.

sleep fragmentation: Interruption of a sleep stage by awakening, arousal or appearance of another sleep stage.

sleep hygiene: Conditions and practices that promote effective and continuous sleep, e.g., regular bedtime and arise time; restriction of alcohol, coffee etc.

sleep latency: Time measured from "lights out" or bedtime to actually falling asleep.

sleep paralysis: Temporary inability to talk or move when falling asleep or waking up.

sudden infant death syndrome (SIDS): The diagnosis given for the sudden death of an infant under one year of age that remains unexplained after a complete investigation, which includes an autopsy, examination of the death scene, and review of the symptoms or illnesses the infant had prior to dying and any other pertinent medical history.

tracheostomy: Surgical insertion of a tube into the airway through the neck to maintain an opening for the outside air to enter the lungs.

uvulopalatopharyngoplasty: UPPP is a procedure used to remove excess tissue at the back of the throat (tonsils, adenoids, uvula, and part of the soft palate)

ventilation: The process of exchange of air between the lungs and the atmospheric air leading to exchange of gases with blood.

Chapter 51

How to Find Sleep Information on the Internet

The Internet can be a great source of information about nearly every topic under the sun, including sleep apnea. At the same time, it can be a source of misinformation, too. If you want to explore the Internet, the following tips may be of interest to you.

First of all, if you don't have your own access to the Internet, call your local public library: you may be able to get on-line there. If the library does not have this service, look into businesses that sell office services such as copying and shipping. Many also provide computer privileges for a fee.

There are three basic types of sites: web pages, chat rooms, and newsgroups. There are numerous web pages now devoted to sleep, sponsored by both not-for-profit organizations and for-profit entities, including authors and manufacturers of medical equipment. In addition, there are several other web pages on health in general that devote a significant portion of the space to sleep and sleep disorders. Some of these web pages are run by companies in the health information field, and some by companies with a broader interest, such as newspapers or television broadcast companies. In the former case, the sites typically provide information free to the public and cover their expenses by selling products on-line and/or by accepting advertising or sponsorship from for-profit entities. Some sites allow interaction and may also allow you to submit questions of a health care professional, but do note the health care professionals' credentials in sleep medicine.

To find sites on sleep apnea, enter "sleep" or "sleep apnea" in your search engine. (There are too many to list here, and addresses do change.) Most pages have links to others; these can bring you easily to many more sites. Of course, some pages are intended solely for health care professionals, some solely for people with sleep apnea, some for both. In cases where the page is for both, you are often asked to "click here" for the information you are seeking.

How the information posted is screened varies from one web page to another. The federal government, for example, has a stringent review process for all of its material published by the National Institutes of Health. Some pages run by companies or non-profits that specialize in the field of sleep also have a strong review process, while those run by other entities without a strong background in sleep may have less knowledge on what is valid and what is not. (The ASAA has all material reviewed by appropriate board members and members of our Medical and Research Advisory Committee.)

In addition, some pages and chatrooms are run by lay individuals with a personal interest in sleep disorders: they do not presume to take the place of a doctor but instead offer their experiences. Keep in mind that any information on web pages is typically of a general nature only; in fact, a disclaimer to that effect is often included in the site.

If you have a sleep disorder, the information provided may give you an idea of how to proceed with your diagnosis and treatment options or how to comply with your prescribed treatment. However, what works for one person may not work for you: everyone has a unique medical history. *Do talk to your doctor or other health care professionals involved with treating your sleep disorder about the suggestions— gleaned from the Internet* (your home care company representative or a sleep technician, for example, can be helpful). Take what you see with a grain of salt—consider the source and the goal of the site.

If you are researching more detailed medical articles, you can get on PubMed (part of Medline, a research tool) sponsored by the National Library of Medicine: www.ncbi.nlm.nih.gov/pubmed. Once on it, you can put in search terms such as "sleep apnea" and "Down's syndrome." The relevant scientific papers found can then be printed for your personal use. The National Library of Medicine also now has Medline and other resources available on-line at no charge: the address is www.nim.nih.gov. (You can get to PubMed on that page as well.)

Chat rooms can also be very helpful to people affected by sleep apnea, as well as to people who think they may have sleep apnea. Chat rooms enable people to learn about others' experiences and to learn more about options; they also help to remove the sense of isolation that may come with a sleep apnea diagnosis.

Newsgroups are similar to chat rooms although they are not "live." Instead, statements are posted for responses. To participate, your Internet software must be able to support joining a newsgroup (look under "mail preferences"). You can get to a newsgroup via some webpages as well. One popular newsgroup for sleep apnea is alt.support.sleep-disorder, but with both chat rooms and newsgroups, as it is with anything, what works for one person may or may not work for you.

If you ever have any questions about material found on the Internet or about sleep apnea in general or for more information on finding a chatroom, feel free to call or to write the ASAA or to send an e-mail to us at asaa@sleepapnea.com.

Chapter 52

Additional Reading on Sleep Disorders

Anch, M., Browman, C.P., Mitler, M.M., Walsh, J. *Sleep: A Scientific Perspective.* Prentice Hall, Englewood, New Jersey: 1988.

Bohr, Robert, Whybrow, Peter, *The Hibernation Response.* William Morrow, New York: 1988.

Borbely, Alexander, *Secrets of Sleep.* Basic Books, New York, NY: 1986.

Carskadon, M.A. (Ed.)., *Encyclopedia of Sleep and Dreaming.* Macmillan Publishing Company New York, NY: 1992.

Chopra, Deepak, MD., *Restful Sleep: The Complete Mind/Body Program for Overcoming Insomnia.* Harmony Books, New York: 1994.

Coleman, R.M., *Wide Awake at 3:00 A.M.: By Choice or by Chance?* W.H. Freeman & Company, New York, NY: 1986.

Courtensy, Anthea, *Natural Sleep: Beating Insomnia Without Drugs.* Thorsons, San Francisco: 1991.

Cuthbertson, Joanne, Schevill, Susie, *Helping Your Child Sleep Through the Night.* Doubleday, New York : 1985.

Dement, W., *Some Must Watch While Some Must Sleep.* Norton & Company, New York, NY: 1972.

Dement, W., *The Sleepwatchers.* Stanford Alumni Association, Stanford, CA: 1992.

Dinges, D.F., & Broughton, R.J. (Eds.), *Sleep and Alertness: Chronobiological, Behavioral, and Medical Aspects of Napping.* Raven Press, New York, NY: 1989.

Dotto, Lydia, *Losing Sleep, How Your Sleeping Habits Affect Your Life.* William Morrow and Company, Inc., New York, NY: 1990.

Dryer, Bernard, MD, Kaplan, Ellen S., *Inside Insomnia.* Villard Books, NY, 1986.

Ferber, Richard, M.D., Kryger, Meir, M.D., *Principles and Practice of Sleep Medicine in the Child.* Saunders, New York: 1995.

Ford, Norman, *The Sleep Rx, 75 Proven Ways to Get a good Night's Sleep.* Renard Books, 1994.

Gardner, David C., Beatty, Grace Joely, *Never Be Tired Again!* MacMillan, New York: 1988.

Garfield, Patricia, *Your Child's Dreams.* Ballantine, New York: 1984.

Goldberg, Philip, *Everybody's Guide to Natural Sleep.* St. Martin's Press, New York: 1990.

Goswami, Meeta, MPH., Ph.D., Thorpy, Michael J., M.D., *Narcolepsy Primer.* Bronx, New York: Montefiore Medical Center, 1991.

Halberstadt, Jerry, Johnson, T. Scott, M.D., *Phantom of the Night: Overcome Sleep Apnea Syndrome-Win Your Hidden Struggle to Breathe, Sleep, and Live.* New Technology Publishing Inc., 1994.

Hales, Dianne, *The Complete Book of Sleep.* Addison-Wesley, Reading, MA: 1981.

Hartmann, Ernest, M.D., *The Sleep Book: Understanding and Preventing Sleep Problems in People Over 50.* American Association of Retired Persons, Washington, DC: 1987.

Horne, James, *Why We Sleep: The Functions of Sleep in Humans and Other Mammals.* Oxford University Press, New York, NY: 1988.

Kavey, Neil B., *50 Ways to Sleep Better.* Publications International, Ltd: Illinois, In association with The Sleep Disorders Center, Columbia-Presbyterian Medical Center,1996.

Kryger, M.H., Roth, T., and Dement, W (Eds.), *Principles and Practice of Sleep Medicine.* Saunders, Philadelphia, PA: 1994.

Lamberg, Lynne, *The American Medical Association Guide to Better Sleep*. Random House, New York: 1984.

Lambley, Peter, *Insomnia and Other Sleeping Problems*. Pinnacle Books, New York: 1982.

Mendelson, Wallace, *Human Sleep: Research and Clinical Care*, Plenum Publishing Corp., New York: 1987.

Mitler, Elizabeth A., Mitler, Merrill M., *101 Questions About Sleep And Dreams*. Wakefulness-Sleep Education and Research Foundation, Del Mar, CA: 1993.

Morgan, Kevin, Sleep and Aging: *A Research-Based Guide to Sleep in Later Life*. Johns Hopkins University Press, Baltimore, M.D.: 1987.

Moorcroft, William H., *Sleep, Dreaming and Sleep Disorders*. University Press of America, Landham, MD: 1989.

Moore-Ede, M, Sulzman, F.M., and Fuller, C.A., *The Clocks That Time Us: Physiology of the Circadian Timing System*. Harvard University Press, Cambridge, MA: 1982.

Nagle, Kim, M.D., Reite, Martin L., M.D., *The Concise Guide to the Evaluation and Management of Sleep Disorders*. American Psychiatric Press, Washington, DC: 1990.

Narcolepsy Network. Narcolepsy: A Guide to Understanding. Order from the Narcolepsy Network, P.O. Box 42460, Cincinnati, OH 45242. Phone (513) 891-3522.

Philips, Elliot Richard, *A Good Night's Sleep*. Prentice-Hall, Englewood Cliffs, NJ: 1983.

Regestein, Quentin, *Sound Sleep*. Simon & Schuster, New York, NY: 1980.

Regestein, Quentin R., Ritchie, David and the editors of Consumers Union Reports Books, *Sleep: Problems and Solutions*. Mount Vernon, NY: 1990.

Rosenthal, Lois, *How to Stop Snoring*. Writer's Digest Books, Cincinnati, OH: 1986.

Rosenthal, Norman E., MD., *Winter Blues, Seasonal Affective Disorder: What It is and How to Overcome It*. Guilford Press, New York, NY: 1993.

Shapiro, Colin M., Ph.D., M.B., F.R.C.P., *Conquering Insomnia: An Illustrated Guide to Understanding Sleep and a Manual for Overcoming Sleep Disruption.* Empowering Press, Hamilton, Canada: 1994.

Shapiro, Colin M., Ph.D., *ABC of Sleep Disorders.* BMJ Publishing Group, London: 1993.

Simpson, Carolyn, *Coping with Sleep Disorders.* Rosen Publishing Group, Inc., New York, NY: 1996.

Suess, Dr., *The Sleep Book.* Harper & Row, New York, NY: 1974.

Sweeney, Donald R., MD, Ph.D., G.P., *Overcoming Insomnia.* Putnam's Sons, New York: 1989.

U.S. Congress, Office of Technology Assessment. *Biological Rhythms: Implications for the Worker.* U.S. Government Printing Office, Washington, DC: 1991. OTA-BA-463.

Webb, Wilse B., *Sleep, the Gentle Tyrant.* Prentice-Hall, New York: 1975

Wilson, Virginia N., Walters, Arthur, M.D., *Sleep Thief, Restless Legs Syndrome.* Galaxy Books, Inc.: December 1996.

Chapter 53

Resources for Patients with Sleep Disorders

American Academy of Otolaryngology–Head and Neck Surgery, Inc.
One Prince Street
Alexandria, VA. 22314-3357
(703) 836-4444 voice
(703) 683-5100 fax
e-mail: entnet@aol.com
website: http://www.entnet.org

American Association for Respiratory Care
11030 Ables Lane
Dallas, Texas 75229
(972) 243-2272 voice
(972) 484-2720 fax
e-mail: info@aarc.org
website: http://www.aarc.org

American Foundation for Urologic Disease
300 West Pratt Street, Suite 401
Baltimore, MD 21201
(410) 468-1800 voice
 (800) 242-2383 toll-free
 (410) 468-1808 fax
e-mail: admin@afud.org
website: http://www.access.digex.net/~afud

American Sleep Apnea Association
1424 K Street, NW, Suite 302
Washington, DC 20005
(202) 293-3650 voice
(202) 293-3656 fax
e-mail: asaa@nicom.com
website: http://www.sleepapnea.org

The American Sleep Disorders Association
6301 Bandel Rd, Suite 101
Rochester, MN 55901
(507) 287-6000
(507) 287-6008
e-mail: asaa@nicom.com
website: www.asda.org

American SIDS Institute
6065 Roswell Road, Suite 876
Atlanta, GA 30328
(404) 843-1030 voice
(800) 232-7437 toll-free
(404) 843-0577 (fax)
e-mail: prevent@sids.org
website: http://www.sids.org

Association of SIDS and Infant Mortality Programs
630 West Fayette Street
Room 5-684
Baltimore, MD 21201
(410) 706-5062 voice
(800) 808-7437 tollfree (in MD)
(410) 706-0146 fax
e-mail: jshaefer@peds.04.ab.umd.edu
website: http://www.asip1.org

Association of SIDS Program Professionals (ASPP)
c/o Maryland SIDS Program
630 West Fayette St
Room 5-684
Baltimore, MA 21201
(410) 706-5062 voice
(410) 706-0146 (fax)

Narcolepsy Network
277 Fairfield Road
Suite 310B
Fairfield, NJ 07004
(973) 276-0115 voice
(973) 227-8224 fax
e-mail: narnet@aol.com
website: http://www.websciences.org/narnet/

National Association For Continence
P.O. Box 8310
Spartanburg, SC 29305
(864) 579-7900 voice
(800) BLADDER tollfree
(864) 579-7902 fax
website: http://www.nafc.org

National Center on Sleep Disorders Research
Two Rockledge Centre, Suite 10038
6701 Rockledge Drive
Bethesda, MD 20892-7920
(301) 435-0199 voice
(301) 480-3451 fax
e-mail: NHLBIIC@dgsys.com
website: http://www.nhlbi.nih.gov/nhlbi/sleep/sleep.htm

National Heart, Lung, and Blood Institute (NBLBI)
Communications and Public Information Branch
31 Center Drive, MSC 2486
Bethesda, NM 20892-2470
(301) 496-5166 voice
(301) 402-0818 fax
e-mail: NHLBIIC@dgsys.com
website: http://www.nhlbi.nih.gov/nhlbi/nhlbi.htm

NICHD/Back to Sleep
31 Center Drive
Room 2A32
Bethesda, MD 20892-2425
(800) 505-CRIB tollfree
(301) 496-7101 fax
website: http://www.nih.gov/nichd/html/publications.html

National Institute for Occupational Safety and Health
Humbert H. Humphrey Bldg.
200 Independence Ave., SW
Room 715H
Washington, DC 20201
(202) 401-6997 voice
(800) 356-4674 tollfree
(513) 533-8573 fax
e-mail: pubstaft@cdc.gov
website http://www.cdc.gov/niosh

National Kidney Foundation
30 East 33rd Street
New York, NY 10016
(212) 889-2210 voice
(800) 622-9010 tollfree
(212) 689-9261 fax
website: http://www.kidney.org

National Sleep Foundation
729 15th Street NW
Fourth Floor
Washington, DC 20005
(202) 347-3471 voice
(202) 347-3472 fax
e-mail: natsleep@erols.com
website: http://www.sleepfoundation.org

National SIDS Resource Center
2070 Chain Bridge Road
Suite 450
Vienna, VA 22181
(703) 821-8955 voice
(703) 821-2098 fax
e-mail: info@circsol.com
website: http://www.circsol.com/sids/index.HTM

Restless Legs Syndrome Foundation, Inc.
4410 19th Street, NW
Rochester, MN 55901-6624
e-mail: rlsf@millcomm.com
http://www.rls.org

The Simon Foundation for Continence
P.O. Box 835
Wilmette, IL 60091
(847) 864-3913 voice
(800) 23-SIMON tollfree
(847) 864-9758 fax
e-mail: simoninfo@simonfoundation.org
website: http://www.simonfoundation.org/html/

Society for Urologic Nurses and Associates
P.O. Box 56 East Holly Avenue
Pitman, NJ 08071
(609) 256-2335 voice
(609) 589-7463 fax
e-mail: webmaster@inurse.com
website: http://www.inurse.com

SIDS Alliance (a national network of SIDS support groups)
1314 Bedford Avenue
Suite 210
Baltimore, MD 21208
(410) 653-8226 voice
(800)221-7437 tollfree
(410) 653-8709 fax
website http://chamd.org/sids.html

Southwest SIDS Research Institute, Inc.
Brazosport Memorial Hospital
100 Medical Drive
Lake Jackson, TX 77566
(409) 299-2814 voice
(800) 245-7437 tollfree
(409) 297-6682 fax

Index

Index

Page numbers followed by 'n' indicate a footnote. Page numbers in *italics* indicate a table or illustration

A

425

Diabetes Sourcebook, 2nd Edition

Basic Information about Insulin-Dependent Diabetes, Noninsulin-Dependent Diabetes, Gestational Diabetes, and Related Disorders, Including Diabetes Prevalence Data, Management Issues, the Role of Diet and Exercise in Controlling Diabetes, Insulin and Other Diabetes Medicines, and Complications of Diabetes Such as Eye Diseases, Digestive Disorders, Periodontal Disease, Amputation, and End-Stage Renal Disease; Along with Reports on Current Research Initiatives, a Glossary, and Resource Listings for Further Help and Information

Edited by Karen Bellenir. 800 pages. 1998. 0-7808-0224-1. $78.

Diet & Nutrition Sourcebook, 1st Edition

Basic Information about Nutrition, Including the Dietary Guidelines for Americans, the Food Guide Pyramid, and Their Applications in Daily Diet, Nutritional Advice for Specific Age Groups, Current Nutritional Issues and Controversies, the New Food Label and How to Use It to Promote Healthy Eating, and Recent Developments in Nutritional Research

Edited by Dan R. Harris. 662 pages. 1996. 0-7808-0084-2. $78.

"Useful reference as a food and nutrition sourcebook for the general consumer."
— *Booklist Health Sciences Supplement, Oct '97*

"Recommended for public libraries and medical libraries that receive general information requests on nutrition. It is readable and will appeal to those interested in learning more about healthy dietary practices."
— *Medical Reference Services Quarterly, Fall '97*

"An abundance of medical and social statistics is translated into readable information geared toward the general reader." — *Bookwatch, Mar '97*

"With dozens of questionable diet books on the market, it is so refreshing to find a reliable and factual reference book. Recommended to aspiring professionals, librarians, and others seeking and giving reliable dietary advice. An excellent compilation." — *Choice, Feb '97*

Diet & Nutrition Sourcebook, 2nd Edition

Basic Information about Nutrition, Including General Nutritional Recommendations, Recommendations for People with Specific Medical Concerns, Dieting for Weight Control, Nutritional Supplements, Food Safety Issues, the Relationship between Nutrition and Disease Development, and Other Nutritional Research Reports; Along with Statistical and Demographic Data, Lifestyle Modification Recommendations, and Sources of Additional Help and Information

Edited by Karen Bellenir. 600 pages. 1998. 0-7808-0228-4. $78.

Ear, Nose & Throat Disorders Sourcebook

Basic Information about Disorders of the Ears, Nose, Sinus Cavities, Pharynx, and Larynx, Including Ear Infections, Tinnitus, Vestibular Disorders, Allergic and Non-Allergic Rhinitis, Sore Throats, Tonsillitis, and Cancers That Affect the Ears, Nose, Sinuses, and Throat, Along with Reports on Current Research Initiatives, a Glossary of Related Medical Terms, and a Directory of Sources for Further Help and Information

Edited by Karen Bellenir and Linda M. Shin. 592 pages. 1998. 0-7808-0206-3. $78.

Endocrine & Metabolic Disorders Sourcebook

Basic Information for the Layperson about Pancreatic and Insulin-Related Disorders Such as Pancreatitis, Diabetes, and Hypoglycemia; Adrenal Gland Disorders Such as Cushing's Syndrome, Addison's Disease, and Congenital Adrenal Hyperplasia; Pituitary Gland Disorders Such as Growth Hormone Deficiency, Acromegaly, and Pituitary Tumors; Thyroid Disorders Such as Hypothyroidism, Graves' Disease, Hashimoto's Disease, and Goiter; Hyperparathyroidism; and Other Diseases and Syndromes of Hormone Imbalance or Metabolic Dysfunction, Along with Reports on Current Research Initiatives

Edited by Linda M. Shin. 632 pages. 1998. 0-7808-0207-1. $78.

Environmentally Induced Disorders Sourcebook

Basic Information about Diseases and Syndromes Linked to Exposure to Pollutants and Other Substances in Outdoor and Indoor Environments Such as Lead, Asbestos, Formaldehyde, Mercury, Emissions, Noise, and More

Edited by Allan R. Cook. 620 pages. 1997. 0-7808-0083-4. $78.

". . . a good survey of numerous environmentally induced physical disorders . . . a useful addition to anyone's library ."
— *Doody's Health Science Book Reviews, Jan '98*

". . . provide[s] introductory information from the best authorities around. Since this volume covers topics that potentially affect everyone, it will surely be one of the most frequently consulted volumes in the *Health Reference Series*." — *Rettig on Reference, Nov '97*

"Recommended reference source."
— *Booklist, Oct '97*

Fitness & Exercise Sourcebook

Basic Information on Fitness and Exercise, Including Fitness Activities for Specific Age Groups, Exercise for People with Specific Medical Conditions, How to Begin a Fitness Program in Running, Walking, Swimming, Cycling, and Other Athletic Activities, and Recent Research in Fitness and Exercise

Edited by Dan R. Harris. 663 pages. 1996. 0-7808-0186-5. $78.

"A good resource for general readers."
— Choice, Nov '97

"The perennial popularity of the topic . . . make this an appealing selection for public libraries."
— Rettig on Reference, Jun/Jul '97

Food & Animal Borne Diseases Sourcebook

Basic Information about Diseases That Can Be Spread to Humans through the Ingestion of Contaminated Food or Water or by Contact with Infected Animals and Insects, Such as Botulism, E. Coli, Hepatitis A, Trichinosis, Lyme Disease, and Rabies, Along with Information Regarding Prevention and Treatment Methods, and a Special Section for International Travelers Describing Diseases Such as Cholera, Malaria, Travelers' Diarrhea, and Yellow Fever, and Offering Recommendations for Avoiding Illness

Edited by Karen Bellenir and Peter D. Dresser. 535 pages. 1995. 0-7808-0033-8. $78.

"Targeting general readers and providing them with a single, comprehensive source of information on selected topics, this book continues, with the excellent caliber of its predecessors, to catalog topical information on health matters of general interest. Readable and thorough, this valuable resource is highly recommended for all libraries."
— Academic Library Book Review, Summer '96

"A comprehensive collection of authoritative information."
— Emergency Medical Services, Oct '95

Gastrointestinal Diseases & Disorders Sourcebook

Basic Information about Gastroesophageal Reflux Disease (Heartburn), Ulcers, Diverticulosis, Irritable Bowel Syndrome, Crohn's Disease, Ulcerative Colitis, Diarrhea, Constipation, Lactose Intolerance, Hemorrhoids, Hepatitis, Cirrhosis, and Other Digestive Problems, Featuring Statistics, Descriptions of Symptoms, and Current Treatment Methods of Interest for Persons Living with Upper and Lower Gastrointestinal Maladies

Edited by Linda M. Ross. 413 pages. 1996. 0-7808-0078-8. $78.

". . . very readable form. The successful editorial work that brought this material together into a useful and understandable reference makes accessible to all readers information that can help them more effectively understand and obtain help for digestive tract problems."
— Choice, Feb '97

Genetic Disorders Sourcebook

Basic Information about Heritable Diseases and Disorders Such as Down Syndrome, PKU, Hemophilia, Von Willebrand Disease, Gaucher Disease, Tay-Sachs Disease, and Sickle-Cell Disease, Along with Information about Genetic Screening, Gene Therapy, Home Care, and Including Source Listings for Further Help and Information on More Than 300 Disorders

Edited by Karen Bellenir. 642 pages. 1996. 0-7808-0034-6. $78.

"Provides essential medical information to both the general public and those diagnosed with a serious or fatal genetic disease or disorder." *— Choice, Jan '97*

". . . geared toward the lay public. It would be well placed in all public libraries and in those hospital and medical libraries in which access to genetic references is limited."
— Doody's Health Sciences Book Review, Oct '96

Head Trauma Sourcebook

Basic Information for the Layperson about Open-Head and Closed-Head Injuries, Treatment Advances, Recovery, and Rehabilitation, Along with Reports on Current Research Initiatives

Edited by Karen Bellenir. 414 pages. 1997. 0-7808-0208-X. $78.

Health Insurance Sourcebook

Basic Information about Managed Care Organizations, Traditional Fee-for-Service Insurance, Insurance Portability and Pre-Existing Conditions Clauses, Medicare, Medicaid, Social Security, and Military Health Care, Along with Information about Insurance Fraud

Edited by Wendy Wilcox. 530 pages. 1997. 0-7808-0222-5. $78.

"The layout of the book is particularly helpful as it provides easy access to reference material. A most useful addition to the vast amount of information about health insurance. The use of data from U.S. government agencies is most commendable. Useful in a library or learning center for healthcare professional students."
— Doody's Health Sciences Book Reviews, Nov '97

Immune System Disorders Sourcebook

Basic Information about Lupus, Multiple Sclerosis, Guillain-Barré Syndrome, Chronic Granulomatous Disease, and More, Along with Statistical and Demographic Data and Reports on Current Research Initiatives

Edited by Allan R. Cook. 608 pages. 1997. 0-7808-0209-8. $78.

Kidney & Urinary Tract Diseases & Disorders Sourcebook

Basic Information about Kidney Stones, Urinary Incontinence, Bladder Disease, End Stage Renal Disease, Dialysis, and More, Along with Statistical and Demographic Data and Reports on Current Research Initiatives

Edited by Linda M. Ross. 602 pages. 1997. 0-7808-0079-6. $78.

Learning Disabilities Sourcebook

Basic Information about Disorders Such as Dyslexia, Visual and Auditory Processing Deficits, Attention Deficit/Hyperactivity Disorder, and Autism, Along with Statistical and Demographic Data, Reports on Current Research Initiatives, an Explanation of the Assessment Process, and a Special Section for Adults with Learning Disabilities

Edited by Linda M. Shin. 579 pages. 1998. 0-7808-0210-1. $78.

Men's Health Concerns Sourcebook

Basic Information about Health Issues That Affect Men, Featuring Facts about the Top Causes of Death in Men, Including Heart Disease, Stroke, Cancers, Prostate Disorders, Chronic Obstructive Pulmonary Disease, Pneumonia and Influenza, Human Immunodeficiency Virus and Acquired Immune Deficiency Syndrome, Diabetes Mellitus, Stress, Suicide, Accidents and Homicides; and Facts about Common Concerns for Men, Including Impotence, Contraception, Circumcision, Sleep Disorders, Snoring, Hair Loss, Diet, Nutrition, Exercise, Kidney and Urological Disorders, and Backaches

Edited by Allan R. Cook. 760 pages. 1998. 0-7808-0212-8. $78.

Mental Health Disorders Sourcebook

Basic Information about Schizophrenia, Depression, Bipolar Disorder, Panic Disorder, Obsessive-Compulsive Disorder, Phobias and Other Anxiety Disorders, Paranoia and Other Personality Disorders, Eating Disorders, and Sleep Disorders, Along with Information about Treatment and Therapies

Edited by Karen Bellenir. 548 pages. 1995. 0-7808-0040-0. $78.

"This is an excellent new book . . . written in easy-to-understand language."
— *Booklist Health Science Supplement*, Oct '97

". . . useful for public and academic libraries and consumer health collections."
— *Medical Reference Services Quarterly*, Spring '97

"The great strengths of the book are its readability and its inclusion of places to find more information. Especially recommended." — *RQ, Winter '96*

". . . a good resource for a consumer health library."
— *Bulletin of the MLA*, Oct '96

"The information is data-based and couched in brief, concise language that avoids jargon. . . . a useful reference source." — *Readings*, Sept '96

"The text is well organized and adequately written for its target audience." — *Choice, Jun '96*

". . . provides information on a wide range of mental disorders, presented in nontechnical language."
— *Exceptional Child Education Resources*, Spring '96

"Recommended for public and academic libraries."
— *Reference Book Review*, '96

Ophthalmic Disorders Sourcebook

Basic Information about Glaucoma, Cataracts, Macular Degeneration, Strabismus, Refractive Disorders, and More, Along with Statistical and Demographic Data and Reports on Current Research Initiatives

Edited by Linda M. Ross. 631 pages. 1996. 0-7808-0081-8. $78.

Oral Health Sourcebook

Basic Information about Diseases and Conditions Affecting Oral Health, Including Cavities, Gum Disease, Dry Mouth, Oral Cancers, Fever Blisters, Canker Sores, Oral Thrush, Bad Breath, Temporomandibular Disorders, and other Craniofacial Syndromes, Along with Statistical Data on the Oral Health of Americans, Oral Hygiene, Emergency First Aid, Information on Treatment Procedures and Methods of Replacing Lost Teeth

Edited by Allan R. Cook. 558 pages. 1997. 0-7808-0082-6. $78.

"Recommended reference source." — *Booklist, Dec '97*

Pain Sourcebook

Basic Information about Specific Forms of Acute and Chronic Pain, Including Headaches, Back Pain, Muscular Pain, Neuralgia, Surgical Pain, and Cancer Pain, Along with Pain Relief Options Such as Analgesics, Narcotics, Nerve Blocks, Transcutaneous Nerve Stimulation, and Alternative Forms of Pain Control, Including Biofeedback, Imaging, Behavior Modification, and Relaxation Techniques

Edited by Allan R. Cook. 667 pages. 1997. 0-7808-0213-6. $78.

"The information is basic in terms of scholarship and is appropriate for general readers. Written in journalistic style . . . intended for non-professionals. Quite thorough in its coverage of different pain conditions and summarizes the latest clinical information regarding pain treatment." — *Choice, Jun '98*

"Recommended reference source."

— *Booklist, Mar '98*

Pregnancy & Birth Sourcebook

Basic Information about Planning for Pregnancy, Maternal Health, Fetal Growth and Development, Labor and Delivery, Postpartum and Perinatal Care, Pregnancy in Mothers with Special Concerns, and Disorders of Pregnancy, Including Genetic Counseling, Nutrition and Exercise, Obstetrical Tests, Pregnancy Discomfort, Multiple Births, Cesarean Sections, Medical Testing of Newborns, Breastfeeding, Gestational Diabetes, and Ectopic Pregnancy

Edited by Heather E. Aldred. 737 pages. 1997. 0-7808-0216-0. $78.

". . . for the layperson. A well-organized handbook. Recommended for college libraries . . . general readers." — *Choice, Apr '98*

"Recommended reference source."

— *Booklist, Mar '98*

"This resource is recommended for public libraries to have on hand."

— *American Reference Books Annual, '98*

Public Health Sourcebook

Basic Information about Government Health Agencies, Including National Health Statistics and Trends, Healthy People 2000 Program Goals and Objectives, the Centers for Disease Control and Prevention, the Food and Drug Administration, and the National Institutes of Health, Along with Full Contact Information for Each Agency

Edited by Wendy Wilcox. 698 pages. 1998. 0-7808-0220-9. $78.

Rehabilitation Sourcebook

Basic Information for the Layperson about Physical Medicine (Physiatry) and Rehabilitative Therapies, Including Physical, Occupational, Recreational, Speech, and Vocational Therapy; Along with Descriptions of Devices and Equipment Such as Orthotics, Gait Aids, Prostheses, and Adaptive Systems Used during Rehabilitation and for Activities of Daily Living, and Featuring a Glossary and Source Listings for Further Help and Information

Edited by Theresa K. Murray. 600 pages. 1998. 0-7808-0236-5. $78.

Respiratory Diseases & Disorders Sourcebook

Basic Information about Respiratory Diseases and Disorders, Including Asthma, Cystic Fibrosis, Pneumonia, the Common Cold, Influenza, and Others, Featuring Facts about the Respiratory System, Statistical and Demographic Data, Treatments, Self-Help Management Suggestions, and Current Research Initiatives

Edited by Allan R. Cook and Peter D. Dresser. 771 pages. 1995. 0-7808-0037-0. $78.

"Designed for the layperson and for patients and their families coping with respiratory illness. . . . an extensive array of information on diagnosis, treatment, management, and prevention of respiratory illnesses for the general reader."

— *Choice, Jun '96*

"A highly recommended text for all collections. It is a comforting reminder of the power of knowledge that good books carry between their covers."

— *Academic Library Book Review, Spring '96*

"This sourcebook offers a comprehensive collection of authoritative information presented in a nontechnical, humanitarian style for patients, families, and caregivers."

— *Association of Operating Room Nurses, Sept/Oct '95*

Sexually Transmitted Diseases Sourcebook

Basic Information about Herpes, Chlamydia, Gonorrhea, Hepatitis, Nongonoccocal Urethritis, Pelvic Inflammatory Disease, Syphilis, AIDS, and More, Along with Current Data on Treatments and Preventions

Edited by Linda M. Ross. 550 pages. 1997. 0-7808-0217-9. $78.